Principles of Epidemiology
in Public Health Practice

Third Edition

An Introduction
to Applied Epidemiology and Biostatistics

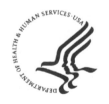

U.S. DEPARTMENT OF HEALTH AND HUMAN SERVICES
Centers for Disease Control and Prevention (CDC)
Office of Workforce and Career Development
Atlanta, GA 30333

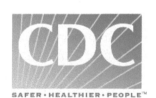

CONTENTS

Lesson Three: Measures of Risk

Lesson Four: Displaying Public Health Data

Lesson Five: Public Health Surveillance

Lesson Six: Investigating an Outbreak

Glossary

ACKNOWLEDGMENTS

Developed by

U.S. Department of Health and Human Services
Centers for Disease Control and Prevention (CDC)
Office of Workforce and Career Development (OWCD)
Career Development Division (CDD)
Atlanta, Georgia 30333

Technical Content

Richard C. Dicker, MD, MSc, Lead Author, CDC/OWCD/CDD (retired)
Fátima Coronado, MD, MPH, CDC/OWCD/CDD
Denise Koo, MD, MPH, CDC/OWCD/CDD
Roy Gibson Parrish, II, MD

Development Team

Sonya D. Arundar, MS, CDC (contractor)
Ron Teske, MS, CDC (contractor)
Susan Baker Toal, MPH, Public Health Consultant
Nancy M. Hunt, MPH, CDC (ORISE Fellow)
Susan D. Welch, MEd, Georgia Poison Center
Cassie Edwards, CDC (contractor)

Planning Committee

Christopher K. Allen, RPh, MPH, CDC
W. Randolph Daley, DVM, MPH, CDC
Patricia Drehobl, RN, MPH
Sharon Hall, RN, PhD, CDC
Dennis Jarvis, MPH, CHES, CDC
Denise Koo, MD, MPH, CDC

Graphics/Illustrations

Sonya D. Arundar, MS, CDC (contractor)
Lee Oakley, CDC (retired)
Jim Walters, CDC

Technical Reviewers

Tomas Aragon, MD, DrPH, San Francisco Department of Public Health
Diane Bennett, MD, MPH, CDC
Danae Bixler, MD, MPH, West Virginia Bureau for Public Health
R. Elliot Churchill, MS, MA, CDC (retired)
Roxanne Ereth, MPH, Arizona Department of Health Services
Stephen Everett, MPH, Yavapai County Community Health Services, Arizona
Michael Fraser, PhD, National Association of County and City Health Officials

Nancy C. Gathany, MEd, CDC
Marjorie A.Getz, MPHIL, Bradley University, Illinois
John Mosely Hayes, DrPH, MBA, MSPH, Tribal Epidemiology Center United South and
    Eastern Tribes, Inc., Tennessee
Richard Hopkins, MD, MSPH, Florida Department of Health
John M. Horan, MD, MPH, Georgia Division of Public Health
Christina M. Bruton Kwon, MSPH, Science Applications International Corporation,
    Atlanta
Edmond F. Maes, PhD, CDC
Sharon McDonnell, MD, MPH, Darmouth Medical School
William S. Paul, MD, MPH, Chicago Department of Public Health
James Ransom, MPH, National Association of County and City Health Officials
Lynn Steele, MS, CDC
Donna Stroup, PhD, MSc, American Cancer Society
Douglas A. Thoroughman, PhD, MS CDC
Kirsten T. Weiser, MD, Darmouth Hitchcock Medical School
Celia Woodfill, PhD, California Department of Health Services

Field Test Participants

Sean Altekruse, DVM, MPH, PhD, U.S. Public Health Service
Gwen A. Barnett, MPH, CHES, CDC
Jason Bell, MD, MPH
Lisa Benaise, MD, Med Immune, Inc., Maryland
Amy Binggeli, DrPH, RD, CHES, CLE, Imperial County Public Health Department,
    California
Kim M. Blindauer, DVM, MPH, Agency for Toxic Substances and Disease Registry
R. Bong, RN, BSN, Federal Bureau of Prisons
Johnna L. Burton, BS, CHES, Tennessee Department of Health
Catherine C. Chow, MD, MPH, Hawaii Department of Health
Janet Cliatt, MT, CLS(NCA), National Institutes of Health
Catherine Dentinger, FNP, MS, New York City Department of Health and Mental
    Hygiene
Veronica Gordon, BSN, MS, Indian Health Service, New Mexico
Susan E. Gorman, PharmD, DABAT, CDC
Deborah Gould, PhD, CDC
Juliana Grant, MD, MPH, CDC
Lori Evans Hall, PharmD, CDC
Nazmul Hassan, MS, Food and Drug Administration
Daniel L. Holcomb, BS, Agency for Toxic Substances and Disease Registry
Asim A. Jani, MD, MPH FACP, CDC
Charletta L. Lewis, BSN, Wellpinit Indian Health Service, Washington
Sheila F. Mahoney, CNM, MPH, National Institutes of Health
Cassandra Martin, MPH, CHES, Georgia Department of Human Resources
Joan Marie McFarland, AS, BSN, MS, Winslow Indian Health Care Center, Arizona
Rosemarie McIntyre, RN, MS, CHES, CDC

Gayle L. Miller, DVM, Jefferson County Department of Health and Environment, Colorado

Long S. Nguyen, MPH, CHES, NIH

Paras M. Patel, RPh, Food and Drug Administration

Rossanne M. Philen, MD, MS, CDC

Alyson Richmond, MPH, CHES, CDC (contractor)

Glenna A. Schindler, MPH, RN, CHES, Healthcare Services Group, Missouri

Sandra K. Schumacher, MD, MPH, CDC

Julie R. Sinclair, MA, DVM, MPH, CDC

Nita Sood, RPh, PharmD, U.S. Public Health Service

P. Lynne Stockton, VMD, MS, ELS(D), CDC

Jill B. Surrency, MPH, CHES, CDC (contractor)

Joyce K. Witt, RN, CDC

INTRODUCTION

This course was developed by the Centers for Disease Control and Prevention (CDC) as a self-study course. Continuing education credits are offered for certified public health educators, nurses, physicians, pharmacists, veterinarians, and public health professionals. CE credit is available only through the CDC/ATSDR Training and Continuing Education Online system at **http://www.cdc.gov/phtnonline**.

To receive CE credit, you must register for the course (SS1000) and complete the evaluation and examination online. You must achieve a score of 70% or higher to pass the examination. If you do not pass the first time, you can take the exam a second time.

For more information about continuing education, call **1-800-41-TRAIN** (1-800-418-7246) or by e-mail at **ce@cdc.gov**.

Course Design

This course covers basic epidemiology principles, concepts, and procedures useful in the surveillance and investigation of health-related states or events. It is designed for federal, state, and local government health professionals and private sector health professionals who are responsible for disease surveillance or investigation. A basic understanding of the practices of public health and biostatistics is recommended.

Course Materials

The course materials consist of six lessons. Each lesson presents instructional text interspersed with relevant exercises that apply and test knowledge and skills gained.

Lesson One: Introduction to Epidemiology

Key features and applications of descriptive and analytic epidemiology

Lesson Two: Summarizing Data

Calculation and interpretation of mean, median, mode, ranges, variance, standard deviation, and confidence interval

Lesson Three: Measures of Risk

Calculation and interpretation of ratios, proportions, incidence rates, mortality rates, prevalence, and years of potential life lost

Lesson Four: Displaying Public Health Data

Preparation and application of tables, graphs, and charts such as arithmetic-scale line, histograms, pie chart, and box plot

Lesson Five: Public Health Surveillance

Processes, uses, and evaluation of public health surveillance in the United States

Lesson Six: Investigating an Outbreak

Steps of an outbreak investigation

A Glossary that defines the major terms used in the course is also provided at the end of Lesson Six.

Supplementary Materials

In addition to the course materials, students may want to use the following:
- A calculator with square root and logarithmic functions for some of the exercises.
- A copy of Heymann, DL, ed. Control of Communicable Diseases Manual, 18th edition, 2004, for reference. Available from the American Public Health Association (202) 777-2742.

Objectives

Students who successfully complete this course should be able to correctly:
- Describe key features and applications of descriptive and analytic epidemiology.
- Calculate and interpret ratios, proportions, incidence rates, mortality rates, prevalence, and years of potential life lost.
- Calculate and interpret mean, median, mode, ranges, variance, standard deviation, and confidence interval.
- Prepare and apply tables, graphs, and charts such as arithmetic-scale line, scatter diagram, pie chart, and box plot.
- Describe the processes, uses, and evaluation of public health surveillance.
- Describe the steps of an outbreak investigation.

General Instructions

Self-study courses are "self-paced." We recommend that a lesson be completed within two weeks. To get the most out of this course, establish a regular time and method of study. Research has shown that these factors greatly influence learning ability.
Each lesson in the course consists of reading, exercises, and a self-assessment quiz.

Reading Assignments

Complete the assigned reading before attempting to answer the self-assessment questions. Read thoroughly and re-read for understanding as necessary. A casual reading may result in missing useful information which supports main themes. Assignments are designed to cover one or two major subject areas. However, as you progress, it is often necessary to combine previous learning to accomplish new skills. A review of previous lessons may be necessary. Frequent visits to the Glossary may also be useful.

Exercises

Exercises are included within each lesson to help you apply the lesson content. Some exercises may be more applicable to your workplace and background than others. You should review the answers to all exercises since the answers are very detailed. Answers to the exercises can be found at the end of each lesson. Your answers to these exercises are valuable study guides for the final examination.

Self-Assessment Quizzes

After completing the reading assignment, answer the self-assessment quizzes before continuing to the next lesson. Answers to the quizzes can be found at the end of the lesson. After passing all six lesson quizzes, you should be prepared for the final examination.

- Self-assessment quizzes are open book.
- Unless otherwise noted, choose ALL CORRECT answers.
- Do not guess at the answer.
- You should score at least 70% correct before continuing to the next lesson.

Tips for Answering Questions

- Carefully read the question.
  Note that it may ask, "Which is CORRECT?" as well as "Which is NOT CORRECT?" or "Which is the EXCEPTION?"
- Read all the choices given.
  One choice may be a correct statement, but another choice may be more nearly correct or complete for the question that is asked.

Final Examination and Course Evaluation

The final examination and course evaluation are available only on-line. The final requirement for the course is an open-book examination. We recommend that you thoroughly review the questions included with each lesson before completing the exam.

It is our sincere hope that you will find this undertaking to be a profitable and satisfying experience. We solicit your constructive criticism at all times and ask that you let us know whenever you have problems or need assistance.

Continuing Education Credit

To receive continuing education credit for completing the self-study course, go to the CDC/ATSDR Training and Continuing Education Online at http://www.cdc.gov/phtnonline and register as a participant. For individuals interested in obtaining RACE credit please contact the CDC Continuing Education office for details, 1-800-41 TRAIN or ce@cdc.gov. You will then need to register for the course (SS1000) and complete the course evaluation and exam online. You will have to answer at least 70% of the exam questions correctly to receive credit and to be awarded CDC's certificate of successful completion. For more information about continuing education credits, please call 1-800-41 TRAIN (1-800-418-7246).

Continuing Education Accreditation Statements

CDC is accredited by the Accreditation Council for Continuing Medical Education (ACCME) to provide continuing medical education for physicians.

CDC designates this educational activity for a maximum of 17 category 1 credits toward the AMA Physician's Recognition Award. Each physician should claim only those credits that he/she actually spent in the activity.

• • •

This activity for 17 contact hours is provided by CDC, which is accredited as a provider of continuing education in nursing by the American Nurses Credentialing Center's Commission on Accreditations.

• • •

CDC is a designated provider of continuing education contact hours (CECH) in health education by the National Commission for Health Education Credentialing, Inc. This program is a designated event for the CHES to receive 17 Category I contact hours in health education, CDC provider number GA0082.

• • •

CDC is accredited by the Accreditation Council for Pharmacy Education as a provider of continuing pharmacy education. This program is a designated event for pharmacists to receive 17 Contact Hours (1.7 CEUs) in pharmacy education. The Universal Program Number is 387-000-06-035-H04.

• • •

CDC has been approved as an Authorized Provider of continuing education and training programs by the International Association for Continuing Education and Training and awards 1.7 Continuing Education Units (CEUs).

• • •

This program was reviewed and approved by the AAVSB RACE program for continuing education. Please contact the AAVSB RACE program at race@aavsb.org with comments/concerns regarding this program's validity or relevancy to the veterinary profession.

Course Evaluation

Even if you are not interested in continuing education credits, we still encourage you to complete the course evaluation. To do this, go to http://www.cdc.gov/phtonline and register as a participant. You will then need to register for the course (SS1000) and complete the course evaluation online. Your comments are valuable to us and will help to revise the self-study course in the future.

Ordering Information

A hard-copy of the text can be obtained from the Public Health Foundation. Specify **Item No. SS1000** when ordering.

- Online at: http://bookstore.phf.org

- By phone:
  Toll-free within the US: 877-252-1200
  International: (301) 645-7773.

INTRODUCTION TO EPIDEMIOLOGY

Recently, a news story described an inner-city neighborhood's concern about the rise in the number of children with asthma. Another story reported the revised recommendations for who should receive influenza vaccine this year. A third story discussed the extensive disease-monitoring strategies being implemented in a city recently affected by a massive hurricane. A fourth story described a finding published in a leading medical journal of an association in workers exposed to a particular chemical and an increased risk of cancer. Each of these news stories included interviews with public health officials or researchers who called themselves epidemiologists. Well, who are these epidemiologists, and what do they do? What is epidemiology? This lesson is intended to answer those questions by describing what epidemiology is, how it has evolved and how it is used today, and what some of the key methods and concepts are. The focus is on epidemiology in public health practice, that is, the kind of epidemiology that is done at health departments.

Objectives

After studying this lesson and answering the questions in the exercises, you will be able to:
- *Define epidemiology*
- *Summarize the historical evolution of epidemiology*
- *Name some of the key uses of epidemiology*
- *Identify the core epidemiology functions*
- *Describe primary applications of epidemiology in public health practice*
- *Specify the elements of a case definition and state the effect of changing the value of any of the elements*
- *List the key features and uses of descriptive epidemiology*
- *List the key features and uses of analytic epidemiology*
- *List the three components of the epidemiologic triad*
- *Describe the different modes of transmission of communicable disease in a population*

Major Sections

Students of journalism are taught that a good news story, whether it be about a bank robbery, dramatic rescue, or presidential candidate's speech, must include the 5 W's: what, who, where, when and why (sometimes cited as why/how). The 5 W's are the essential components of a news story because if any of the five are missing, the story is incomplete.

The same is true in characterizing epidemiologic events, whether it be an outbreak of norovirus among cruise ship passengers or the use of mammograms to detect early breast cancer. The difference is that epidemiologists tend to use synonyms for the 5 W's: diagnosis or health event (what), person (who), place (where), time (when), and causes, risk factors, and modes of transmission (why/how).

Definition of Epidemiology

The word epidemiology comes from the Greek words *epi*, meaning on or upon, *demos*, meaning people, and *logos*, meaning the study of. In other words, the word epidemiology has its roots in the study of what befalls a population. Many definitions have been proposed, but the following definition captures the underlying principles and public health spirit of epidemiology:

> *Epidemiology is the **study** of the **distribution** and **determinants** of **health-related states or events** in **specified populations**, and the **application** of this study to the control of health problems.*[1]

Key terms in this definition reflect some of the important principles of epidemiology.

Study

Epidemiology is a scientific discipline with sound methods of scientific inquiry at its foundation. Epidemiology is data-driven and relies on a systematic and unbiased approach to the collection, analysis, and interpretation of data. Basic epidemiologic methods tend to rely on careful observation and use of valid comparison groups to assess whether what was observed, such as the number of cases of disease in a particular area during a particular time period or the frequency of an exposure among persons with disease, differs from what might be expected. However, epidemiology also draws on methods from other scientific fields, including biostatistics and informatics, with biologic, economic, social, and behavioral sciences.

In fact, epidemiology is often described as the basic science of public health, and for good reason. First, epidemiology is a quantitative discipline that relies on a working knowledge of probability, statistics, and sound research methods. Second, epidemiology is a method of causal reasoning based on developing and testing hypotheses grounded in such scientific fields as biology, behavioral sciences, physics, and ergonomics to explain health-related behaviors, states, and events. However, epidemiology is not just a research activity but an integral component of public health, providing the foundation for directing practical and appropriate public health action based on this science and causal reasoning.[2]

Distribution

Epidemiology is concerned with the **frequency** and **pattern** of health events in a population:

> **Frequency** refers not only to the number of health events such as the number of cases of meningitis or diabetes in a population, but also to the relationship of that number to the size of the population. The resulting rate allows epidemiologists to compare disease occurrence across different populations.

> **Pattern** refers to the occurrence of health-related events by time, place, and person. Time patterns may be annual, seasonal, weekly, daily, hourly, weekday versus weekend, or any other breakdown of time that may influence disease or injury occurrence. Place patterns include geographic variation, urban/rural differences, and location of work sites or schools. Personal characteristics include demographic factors which may be related to risk of illness, injury, or disability such as age, sex, marital status, and socioeconomic status, as well as behaviors and environmental exposures.

Characterizing health events by time, place, and person are activities of **descriptive epidemiology**, discussed in more detail later in this lesson.

Determinants

Determinant: any factor, whether event, characteristic, or other definable entity, that brings about a change in a health condition or other defined characteristic.[1]

Epidemiology is also used to search for **determinants**, which are the causes and other factors that influence the occurrence of disease and other health-related events. Epidemiologists assume that illness does not occur randomly in a population, but happens only when the right accumulation of risk factors or determinants exists in an individual. To search for these determinants, epidemiologists use analytic epidemiology or epidemiologic studies to provide the "Why" and "How" of such events. They assess whether groups with different rates of disease differ in their demographic characteristics, genetic or immunologic make-up, behaviors, environmental exposures, or other so-called potential risk factors. Ideally, the findings provide sufficient evidence to direct prompt and effective public health control and prevention measures.

Health-related states or events

Epidemiology was originally focused exclusively on epidemics of communicable diseases[3] but was subsequently expanded to address endemic communicable diseases and non-communicable infectious diseases. By the middle of the 20th Century, additional epidemiologic methods had been developed and applied to chronic diseases, injuries, birth defects, maternal-child health, occupational health, and environmental health. Then epidemiologists began to look at behaviors related to health and well-being, such as amount of exercise and seat belt use. Now, with the recent explosion in molecular methods, epidemiologists can make important strides in examining genetic markers of disease risk. Indeed, the term health-related states or events may be seen as anything that affects the well-being of a population. Nonetheless, many epidemiologists still use the term "disease" as shorthand for the wide range of health-related states and events that are studied.

Specified populations

Although epidemiologists and direct health-care providers (clinicians) are both concerned with occurrence and control of disease, they differ greatly in how they view "the patient." The clinician is concerned about the health of an individual; the epidemiologist is concerned about the collective health of the people in a community or population. In other words, the clinician's "patient" is the individual; the epidemiologist's "patient" is the community. Therefore, the clinician and the epidemiologist have different responsibilities when faced with a person with illness. For example, when a patient with diarrheal disease presents, both are interested in establishing the correct diagnosis. However, while the clinician usually focuses on treating and caring for the individual, the epidemiologist focuses on identifying the exposure or source that caused the illness; the number of other persons who may have been similarly exposed; the potential for further spread in the community; and interventions to prevent additional cases or recurrences.

Application

Epidemiology is not just "the study of" health in a population; it also involves applying the knowledge gained by the studies to community-based practice. Like the practice of medicine, the practice of epidemiology is both a science and an art. To make the proper diagnosis and prescribe appropriate treatment for a patient, the clinician combines medical (scientific) knowledge with experience, clinical judgment, and understanding of the patient.

Similarly, the epidemiologist uses the scientific methods of descriptive and analytic epidemiology as well as experience, epidemiologic judgment, and understanding of local conditions in "diagnosing" the health of a community and proposing appropriate, practical, and acceptable public health interventions to control and prevent disease in the community.

Summary

Epidemiology is the study (scientific, systematic, data-driven) of the distribution (frequency, pattern) and determinants (causes, risk factors) of health-related states and events (not just diseases) in specified populations (patient is community, individuals viewed collectively), and the application of (since epidemiology is a discipline within public health) this study to the control of health problems.

Exercise 1.1

Below are four key terms taken from the definition of epidemiology, followed by a list of activities that an epidemiologist might perform. Match the term to the activity that best describes it. You should match only one term per activity.

A. *Distribution*
B. *Determinants*
C. *Application*

_____ 1. Compare food histories between persons with *Staphylococcus* food poisoning and those without

_____ 2. Compare frequency of brain cancer among anatomists with frequency in general population

_____ 3. Mark on a map the residences of all children born with birth defects within 2 miles of a hazardous waste site

_____ 4. Graph the number of cases of congenital syphilis by year for the country

_____ 5. Recommend that close contacts of a child recently reported with meningococcal meningitis receive Rifampin

_____ 6. Tabulate the frequency of clinical signs, symptoms, and laboratory findings among children with chickenpox in Cincinnati, Ohio

 Check your answers on page 1-81

Historical Evolution of Epidemiology

Although epidemiology as a discipline has blossomed since World War II, epidemiologic thinking has been traced from Hippocrates through John Graunt, William Farr, John Snow, and others. The contributions of some of these early and more recent thinkers are described below.[5]

Circa 400 B.C.

Epidemiology's roots are nearly 2500 years old.

Hippocrates attempted to explain disease occurrence from a rational rather than a supernatural viewpoint. In his essay entitled "On Airs, Waters, and Places," Hippocrates suggested that environmental and host factors such as behaviors might influence the development of disease.

1662

Another early contributor to epidemiology was John Graunt, a London haberdasher and councilman who published a landmark analysis of mortality data in 1662. This publication was the first to quantify patterns of birth, death, and disease occurrence, noting disparities between males and females, high infant mortality, urban/rural differences, and seasonal variations.[5]

1800

William Farr built upon Graunt's work by systematically collecting and analyzing Britain's mortality statistics. Farr, considered the father of modern vital statistics and surveillance, developed many of the basic practices used today in vital statistics and disease classification. He concentrated his efforts on collecting vital statistics, assembling and evaluating those data, and reporting to responsible health authorities and the general public.[4]

1854

In the mid-1800s, an anesthesiologist named John Snow was conducting a series of investigations in London that warrant his being considered the "father of field epidemiology." Twenty years before the development of the microscope, Snow conducted studies of cholera outbreaks both to discover the cause of disease and to prevent its recurrence. Because his work illustrates the classic sequence from descriptive epidemiology to hypothesis generation to hypothesis testing (analytic epidemiology) to application, two of his investigations will be described in detail.

Snow conducted one of his now famous studies in 1854 when an epidemic of cholera erupted in the Golden Square of London.[5] He began his investigation by determining where in this area persons with cholera lived and worked. He marked each residence on a map of the area, as shown in Figure 1.1. Today, this type of map, showing the geographic distribution of cases, is called a spot map.

Figure 1.1 Spot map of deaths from cholera in Golden Square area, London, 1854 (redrawn from original)

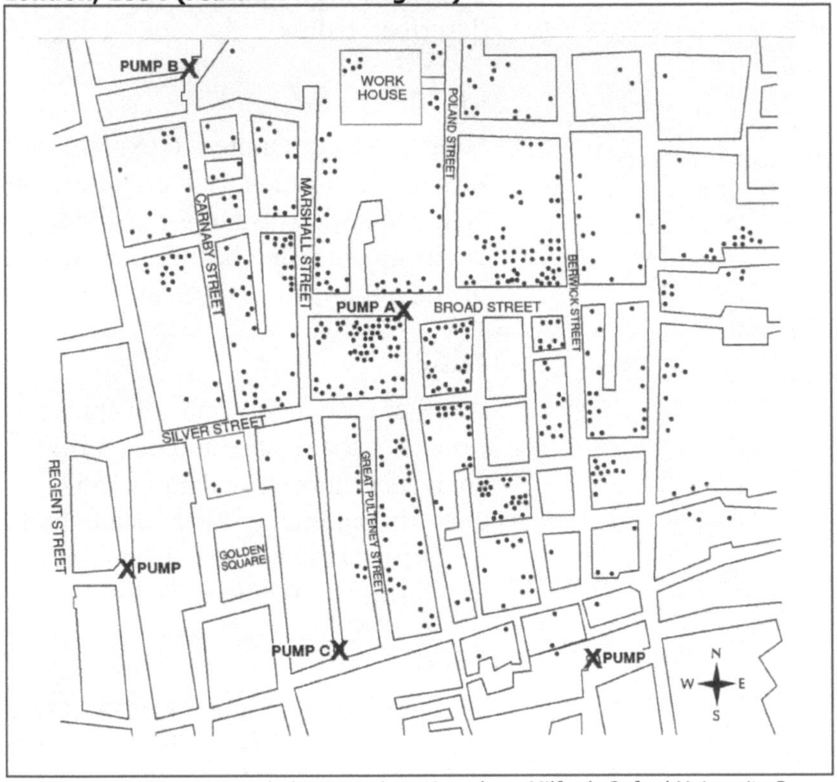

Source: Snow J. Snow on cholera. London: Humphrey Milford: Oxford University Press; 1936.

Because Snow believed that water was a source of infection for cholera, he marked the location of water pumps on his spot map, then looked for a relationship between the distribution of households with cases of cholera and the location of pumps. He noticed that more case households clustered around Pump A, the Broad Street pump, than around Pump B or C. When he questioned residents who lived in the Golden Square area, he was told that they avoided Pump B because it was grossly contaminated, and that Pump C was located too inconveniently for most of them. From this information, Snow concluded that the Broad Street pump (Pump A) was the primary source of water and the most likely source of infection for most persons with cholera in the Golden Square area. He noted with curiosity, however, that no cases of cholera had occurred in a two-block area just to the east of the Broad Street pump. Upon investigating, Snow found a brewery located there with a deep well on the premises. Brewery workers got their water from this well, and also received a daily portion of malt liquor. Access to these uncontaminated rations could explain why none of the brewery's employees contracted cholera.

To confirm that the Broad Street pump was the source of the epidemic, Snow gathered information on where persons with cholera had obtained their water. Consumption of water from the Broad Street pump was the one common factor among the cholera patients. After Snow presented his findings to municipal officials, the handle of the pump was removed and the outbreak ended. The site of the pump is now marked by a plaque mounted on the wall outside of the appropriately named John Snow Pub.

Figure 1.2 John Snow Pub, London

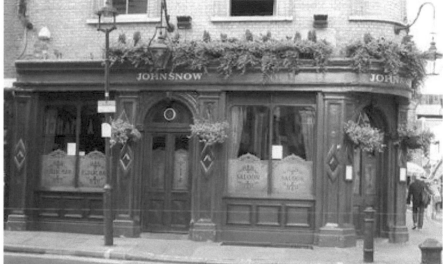

Source: The John Snow Society [Internet]. London: [updated 2005 Oct 14; cited 2006 Feb 6]. Available from: http://johnsnowsociety.org.

Snow's second investigation reexamined data from the 1854 cholera outbreak in London. During a cholera epidemic a few years earlier, Snow had noted that districts with the highest death rates were serviced by two water companies: the Lambeth Company and the Southwark and Vauxhall Company. At that time, both companies obtained water from the Thames River at intake points that were downstream from London and thus susceptible to contamination from London sewage, which was discharged directly into the Thames. To avoid contamination by London sewage, in 1852 the Lambeth Company moved its intake water works to a site on the Thames well upstream from London. Over a 7-week period during the summer of 1854, Snow compared cholera mortality among districts that received water from one or the other or both water companies. The results are shown in Table 1.1.

Table 1.1 Mortality from Cholera in the Districts of London Supplied by the Southwark and Vauxhall and the Lambeth Companies, July 9–August 26, 1854

Districts with Water Supplied By:	Population (1851 Census)	Number of Deaths from Cholera	Cholera Death Rate per 1,000 Population
Southwark and Vauxhall Only	167,654	844	5.0
Lambeth Only	19,133	18	0.9
Both Companies	300,149	652	2.2

Source: Snow J. Snow on cholera. London: Humphrey Milford: Oxford University Press; 1936.

The data in Table 1.1 show that the cholera death rate was more than 5 times higher in districts served only by the Southwark and Vauxhall Company (intake downstream from London) than in those served only by the Lambeth Company (intake upstream from London). Interestingly, the mortality rate in districts supplied by both companies fell between the rates for districts served exclusively by either company. These data were consistent with the hypothesis that water obtained from the Thames below London was a source of cholera. Alternatively, the populations supplied by the two companies may have differed on other factors that affected their risk of cholera.

To test his water supply hypothesis, Snow focused on the districts served by both companies, because the households within a district were generally comparable except for the water supply company. In these districts, Snow identified the water supply company for every house in which a death from cholera had occurred during the 7-week period. Table 1.2 shows his findings.

Table 1.2 Mortality from Cholera in London Related to the Water Supply of Individual Houses in Districts Served by Both the Southwark and Vauxhall Company and the Lambeth Company, July 9–August 26, 1854

Water Supply of Individual House	Population (1851 Census)	Number of Deaths from Cholera	Cholera Death Rate per 1,000 Population
Southwark and Vauxhall Only	98,862	419	4.2
Lambeth Only	154,615	80	0.5

Source: Snow J. Snow on cholera. London: Humphrey Milford: Oxford University Press; 1936.

This study, demonstrating a higher death rate from cholera among households served by the Southwark and Vauxhall Company in the mixed districts, added support to Snow's hypothesis. It also established the sequence of steps used by current-day epidemiologists to investigate outbreaks of disease. Based on a characterization of the cases and population at risk by time, place, and person, Snow developed a testable hypothesis. He then tested his hypothesis with a more rigorously designed study, ensuring that the groups to be compared were comparable. After this study, efforts to control the epidemic were directed at changing the location of the water intake of the Southwark and Vauxhall Company to avoid sources of contamination. Thus, with no knowledge of the existence of microorganisms, Snow demonstrated through epidemiologic studies that water could serve as a vehicle for transmitting cholera and that epidemiologic information could be used to direct prompt and appropriate public health action.

19th and 20th centuries

In the mid- and late-1800s, epidemiological methods began to be applied in the investigation of disease occurrence. At that time, most investigators focused on acute infectious diseases. In the 1930s and 1940s, epidemiologists extended their methods to noninfectious diseases. The period since World War II has seen an explosion in the development of research methods and the theoretical underpinnings of epidemiology. Epidemiology has been applied to the entire range of health-related outcomes, behaviors, and even knowledge and attitudes. The studies by Doll and Hill linking lung cancer to smoking[6] and the study of cardiovascular disease among residents of Framingham, Massachusetts[7] are two examples of how pioneering researchers have applied epidemiologic methods to chronic disease since World War II. During the 1960s and early 1970s health workers applied epidemiologic methods to eradicate naturally occurring smallpox worldwide.[8] This was an achievement in applied epidemiology of unprecedented proportions.

In the 1980s, epidemiology was extended to the studies of injuries and violence. In the 1990s, the related fields of molecular and genetic epidemiology (expansion of epidemiology to look at specific pathways, molecules and genes that influence risk of developing disease) took root. Meanwhile, infectious diseases continued to challenge epidemiologists as new infectious agents emerged (Ebola virus, Human Immunodeficiency virus (HIV)/ Acquired Immunodeficiency Syndrome (AIDS)), were identified (Legionella, Severe Acute Respiratory Syndrome (SARS)), or changed (drug-resistant Mycobacterium tuberculosis, Avian influenza). Beginning in the 1990s and accelerating after the terrorist attacks of September 11, 2001, epidemiologists have had to consider not only natural transmission of infectious organisms but also deliberate spread through biologic warfare and bioterrorism.

Today, public health workers throughout the world accept and use epidemiology regularly to characterize the health of their communities and to solve day-to-day problems, large and small.

Uses

Epidemiology and the information generated by epidemiologic methods have been used in many ways.[9] Some common uses are described below.

Assessing the community's health

Public health officials responsible for policy development, implementation, and evaluation use epidemiologic information as a factual framework for decision making. To assess the health of a population or community, relevant sources of data must be identified and analyzed by person, place, and time (descriptive epidemiology).

- What are the actual and potential health problems in the community?
- Where are they occurring?
- Which populations are at increased risk?
- Which problems have declined over time?
- Which ones are increasing or have the potential to increase?
- How do these patterns relate to the level and distribution of public health services available?

More detailed data may need to be collected and analyzed to determine whether health services are available, accessible, effective, and efficient. For example, public health officials used epidemiologic data and methods to identify baselines, to set health goals for the nation in 2000 and 2010, and to monitor progress toward these goals.[10-12]

Making individual decisions

Many individuals may not realize that they use epidemiologic information to make daily decisions affecting their health. When persons decide to quit smoking, climb the stairs rather than wait for an elevator, eat a salad rather than a cheeseburger with fries for lunch, or use a condom, they may be influenced, consciously or unconsciously, by epidemiologists' assessment of risk. Since World War II, epidemiologists have provided information related to all those decisions. In the 1950s, epidemiologists reported the increased risk of lung cancer among smokers. In the 1970s, epidemiologists documented the role of exercise and proper diet in reducing the risk of heart disease. In the mid-1980s, epidemiologists identified the increased risk of HIV infection associated with certain sexual and drug-related behaviors. These and hundreds of other epidemiologic findings are directly relevant to the choices people make every day, choices that affect their health over a lifetime.

Completing the clinical picture

When investigating a disease outbreak, epidemiologists rely on health-care providers and laboratorians to establish the proper diagnosis of individual patients. But epidemiologists also contribute to physicians' understanding of the clinical picture and natural history of disease. For example, in late 1989, a physician saw three patients with unexplained eosinophilia (an increase in the number of a specific type of white blood cell called an eosinophil) and myalgias (severe muscle pains). Although the physician could not make a definitive diagnosis, he notified public health authorities. Within weeks, epidemiologists had identified enough other cases to characterize the spectrum and course of the illness that came to be known as eosinophilia-myalgia syndrome.[13] More recently, epidemiologists, clinicians, and researchers around the world have collaborated to characterize SARS, a disease caused by a new type of coronavirus that emerged in China in late 2002.[14] Epidemiology has also been instrumental in characterizing many non-acute diseases, such as the numerous conditions associated with cigarette smoking — from pulmonary and heart disease to lip, throat, and lung cancer.

Searching for causes

Much epidemiologic research is devoted to searching for causal factors that influence one's risk of disease. Ideally, the goal is to identify a cause so that appropriate public health action might be taken. One can argue that epidemiology can never prove a causal relationship between an exposure and a disease, since much of epidemiology is based on ecologic reasoning. Nevertheless, epidemiology often provides enough information to support effective action. Examples date from the removal of the handle from the Broad St. pump following John Snow's investigation of cholera in the Golden Square area of London in 1854,[5] to the withdrawal of a vaccine against rotavirus in 1999 after epidemiologists found that it increased the risk of intussusception, a potentially life-threatening condition.[15] Just as often, epidemiology and laboratory science converge to provide the evidence needed to establish causation. For example, epidemiologists were able to identify a variety of risk factors during an outbreak of pneumonia among persons attending the American Legion Convention in Philadelphia in 1976, even though the Legionnaires' bacillus was not identified in the laboratory from lung tissue of a person who had died from Legionnaires' disease until almost 6 months later.[16]

Exercise 1.2

In August 1999, epidemiologists learned of a cluster of cases of encephalitis caused by West Nile virus infection among residents of Queens, New York. West Nile virus infection, transmitted by mosquitoes, had never before been identified in North America.

Describe how this information might be used for each of the following:

1. Assessing the community's health

2. Making decisions about individual patients

3. Documenting the clinical picture of the illness

4. Searching for causes to prevent future outbreaks

 Check your answers on page 1-81

Core Epidemiologic Functions

In the mid-1980s, five major tasks of epidemiology in public health practice were identified: **public health surveillance, field investigation, analytic studies, evaluation, and linkages.**[17] A sixth task, **policy development**, was recently added. These tasks are described below.

Public health surveillance

Public health surveillance is the ongoing, systematic collection, analysis, interpretation, and dissemination of health data to help guide public health decision making and action. Surveillance is equivalent to monitoring the pulse of the community. The purpose of public health surveillance, which is sometimes called "information for action,"[18] is to portray the ongoing patterns of disease occurrence and disease potential so that investigation, control, and prevention measures can be applied efficiently and effectively. This is accomplished through the systematic collection and evaluation of morbidity and mortality reports and other relevant health information, and the dissemination of these data and their interpretation to those involved in disease control and public health decision making.

Figure 1.3. Surveillance Cycle

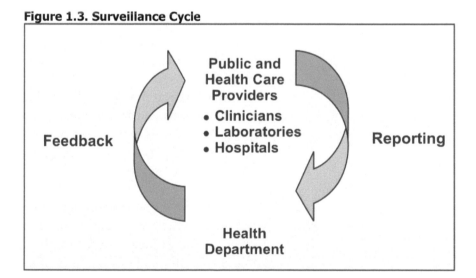

Morbidity and mortality reports are common sources of surveillance data for local and state health departments. These reports generally are submitted by health-care providers, infection control practitioners, or laboratories that are required to notify the health department of any patient with a reportable disease such as pertussis, meningococcal meningitis, or AIDS. Other sources of health-related data that are used for surveillance include reports from investigations of individual cases and disease clusters, public health program data such as immunization coverage in a community, disease registries, and health surveys.

Most often, surveillance relies on simple systems to collect a limited amount of information about each case. Although not every case of disease is reported, health officials regularly review the case reports they do receive and look for patterns among them. These practices have proven invaluable in detecting problems, evaluating programs, and guiding public health action.

While public health surveillance traditionally has focused on communicable diseases, surveillance systems now exist that target injuries, chronic diseases, genetic and birth defects, occupational and potentially environmentally-related diseases, and health behaviors. Since September 11, 2001, a variety of systems that rely on electronic reporting have been developed, including those that report daily emergency department visits, sales of over-the-counter medicines, and worker absenteeism.[19,20] Because epidemiologists are likely to be called upon to design and use these and other new surveillance systems, an epidemiologist's core competencies must include design of data collection instruments, data management, descriptive methods and graphing, interpretation of data, and scientific writing and presentation.

Field investigation

As noted above, surveillance provides information for action. One of the first actions that results from a surveillance case report or report of a cluster is investigation by the public health department. The investigation may be as limited as a phone call to the health-care provider to confirm or clarify the circumstances of the reported case, or it may involve a field investigation requiring the coordinated efforts of dozens of people to characterize the extent of an epidemic and to identify its cause.

The objectives of such investigations also vary. Investigations often lead to the identification of additional unreported or unrecognized ill persons who might otherwise continue to spread infection to others. For example, one of the hallmarks of investigations of persons with sexually transmitted disease is the identification of sexual partners or contacts of patients. When interviewed, many of these contacts are found to be infected without knowing it, and are given treatment they did not realize they needed. Identification and treatment of these contacts prevents further spread.

For some diseases, investigations may identify a source or vehicle of infection that can be controlled or eliminated. For example, the investigation of a case of *Escherichia coli* O157:H7 infection usually focuses on trying to identify the vehicle, often ground beef but sometimes something more unusual such as fruit juice. By identifying the vehicle, investigators may be able to determine how many other persons might have already been exposed and how many continue to be at risk. When a commercial product turns out to be the culprit, public announcements and recalling the product may prevent many additional cases.

Occasionally, the objective of an investigation may simply be to learn more about the natural history, clinical spectrum, descriptive epidemiology, and risk factors of the disease before determining what disease intervention methods might be appropriate. Early investigations of the epidemic of SARS in 2003 were needed to establish a case definition based on the clinical presentation, and to characterize the populations at risk by time, place, and person. As more was learned about the epidemiology of the disease and communicability of the virus, appropriate recommendations regarding isolation and quarantine were issued.[21]

Symbol of EIS

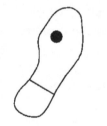

Field investigations of the type described above are sometimes referred to as "shoe leather epidemiology," conjuring up images of dedicated, if haggard, epidemiologists beating the pavement in search of additional cases and clues regarding source and mode of transmission. This approach is commemorated in the symbol of the Epidemic Intelligence Service (EIS), CDC's training program for disease detectives — a shoe with a hole in the sole.

Analytic studies

Surveillance and field investigations are usually sufficient to identify causes, modes of transmission, and appropriate control and prevention measures. But sometimes analytic studies employing more rigorous methods are needed. Often the methods are used in combination — with surveillance and field investigations providing clues or hypotheses about causes and modes of transmission, and analytic studies evaluating the credibility of those hypotheses.

Clusters or outbreaks of disease frequently are investigated initially with descriptive epidemiology. The descriptive approach involves the study of disease incidence and distribution by time, place, and person. It includes the calculation of rates and identification of parts of the population at higher risk than others. Occasionally, when the association between exposure and disease is quite strong, the investigation may stop when descriptive epidemiology is complete and control measures may be implemented immediately. John Snow's 1854 investigation of cholera is an example. More frequently, descriptive studies, like case investigations, generate hypotheses that can be tested with analytic studies. While some field investigations are conducted in response to acute health problems such as outbreaks, many others are planned studies.

The hallmark of an analytic epidemiologic study is the use of a valid comparison group. Epidemiologists must be skilled in all aspects of such studies, including design, conduct, analysis, interpretation, and communication of findings.

- **Design** includes determining the appropriate research strategy and study design, writing justifications and protocols, calculating sample sizes, deciding on criteria for subject selection (e.g., developing case definitions), choosing an appropriate comparison group, and designing questionnaires.
- **Conduct** involves securing appropriate clearances and approvals, adhering to appropriate ethical principles, abstracting records, tracking down and interviewing subjects, collecting and handling specimens, and managing the data.
- **Analysis** begins with describing the characteristics of the subjects. It progresses to calculation of rates, creation of comparative tables (e.g., two-by-two tables), and computation of measures of association (e.g., risk ratios or odds ratios), tests of significance (e.g., chi-square test), confidence intervals, and the like. Many epidemiologic studies require more advanced analytic techniques such as stratified analysis, regression, and modeling.
- Finally, **interpretation** involves putting the study findings into perspective, identifying the key take-home messages, and making sound recommendations. Doing so requires that the epidemiologist be knowledgeable about the subject matter and the strengths and weaknesses of the study.

Evaluation

Epidemiologists, who are accustomed to using systematic and quantitative approaches, have come to play an important role in evaluation of public health services and other activities. Evaluation is the process of determining, as systematically and objectively as possible, the relevance, effectiveness, efficiency, and impact of activities with respect to established goals.[22]

- **Effectiveness** refers to the ability of a program to produce the intended or expected results in the field; effectiveness differs from **efficacy**, which is the ability to produce results under ideal conditions.
- **Efficiency** refers to the ability of the program to produce

the intended results with a minimum expenditure of time and resources.

The evaluation itself may focus on plans (formative evaluation), operations (process evaluation), impact (summative evaluation), or outcomes — or any combination of these. Evaluation of an immunization program, for example, might assess the efficiency of the operations, the proportion of the target population immunized, and the apparent impact of the program on the incidence of vaccine-preventable diseases. Similarly, evaluation of a surveillance system might address operations and attributes of the system, its ability to detect cases or outbreaks, and its usefulness.[23]

Linkages

Epidemiologists working in public health settings rarely act in isolation. In fact, field epidemiology is often said to be a "team sport." During an investigation an epidemiologist usually participates as either a member or the leader of a multidisciplinary team. Other team members may be laboratorians, sanitarians, infection control personnel, nurses or other clinical staff, and, increasingly, computer information specialists. Many outbreaks cross geographical and jurisdictional lines, so co-investigators may be from local, state, or federal levels of government, academic institutions, clinical facilities, or the private sector. To promote current and future collaboration, the epidemiologists need to maintain relationships with staff of other agencies and institutions. Mechanisms for sustaining such linkages include official memoranda of understanding, sharing of published or on-line information for public health audiences and outside partners, and informal networking that takes place at professional meetings.

Policy development

The definition of epidemiology ends with the following phrase: "...and the application of this study to the control of health problems." While some academically minded epidemiologists have stated that epidemiologists should stick to research and not get involved in policy development or even make recommendations,[24] public health epidemiologists do not have this luxury. Indeed, epidemiologists who understand a problem and the population in which it occurs are often in a uniquely qualified position to recommend appropriate interventions. As a result, epidemiologists working in public health regularly provide input, testimony, and recommendations regarding disease control strategies, reportable disease regulations, and health-care policy.

Exercise 1.3

Match the appropriate core function to each of the statements below.

A. Public health surveillance
B. Field investigation
C. Analytic studies
D. Evaluation
E. Linkages
F. Policy development

_____ 1. Reviewing reports of test results for *Chlamydia trachomatis* from public health clinics

_____ 2. Meeting with directors of family planning clinics and college health clinics to discuss *Chlamydia* testing and reporting

_____ 3. Developing guidelines/criteria about which patients coming to the clinic should be screened (tested) for *Chlamydia* infection

_____ 4. Interviewing persons infected with *Chlamydia* to identify their sex partners

_____ 5. Conducting an analysis of patient flow at the public health clinic to determine waiting times for clinic patients

_____ 6. Comparing persons with symptomatic versus asymptomatic *Chlamydia* infection to identify predictors

 Check your answers on page 1-82

The Epidemiologic Approach

An epidemiologist:
- Counts
- Divides
- Compares

As with all scientific endeavors, the practice of epidemiology relies on a systematic approach. In very simple terms, the epidemiologist:

- **Counts** cases or health events, and describes them in terms of time, place, and person;
- **Divides** the number of cases by an appropriate denominator to calculate rates; and
- **Compares** these rates over time or for different groups of people.

Before counting cases, however, the epidemiologist must decide what a case is. This is done by developing a case definition. Then, using this case definition, the epidemiologist finds and collects information about the case-patients. The epidemiologist then performs descriptive epidemiology by characterizing the cases collectively according to time, place, and person. To calculate the disease rate, the epidemiologist divides the number of cases by the size of the population. Finally, to determine whether this rate is greater than what one would normally expect, and if so to identify factors contributing to this increase, the epidemiologist compares the rate from this population to the rate in an appropriate comparison group, using analytic epidemiology techniques. These epidemiologic actions are described in more detail below. Subsequent tasks, such as reporting the results and recommending how they can be used for public health action, are just as important, but are beyond the scope of this lesson.

Defining a case

Before counting cases, the epidemiologist must decide what to count, that is, what to call a case. For that, the epidemiologist uses a **case definition**. A case definition is a set of standard criteria for classifying whether a person has a particular disease, syndrome, or other health condition. Some case definitions, particularly those used for national surveillance, have been developed and adopted as national standards that ensure comparability. Use of an agreed-upon standard case definition ensures that every case is equivalent, regardless of when or where it occurred, or who identified it. Furthermore, the number of cases or rate of disease identified in one time or place can be compared with the number or rate from another time or place. For example, with a standard case definition, health officials could compare the number of cases of listeriosis that occurred in Forsyth County, North Carolina in 2000 with the number that occurred there in 1999. Or they could compare the rate of listeriosis in Forsyth County in 2000 with the national rate in that same year. When everyone uses the same standard case definition and a difference is observed, the difference is likely to be real rather than the result of variation in how cases are classified.

To ensure that all health departments in the United States use the same case definitions for surveillance, the Council of State and Territorial Epidemiologists (CSTE), CDC, and other interested parties have adopted standard case definitions for the notifiable infectious diseases[25]. These definitions are revised as needed. In 1999, to address the need for common definitions and methods for state-level chronic disease surveillance, CSTE, the Association of State and Territorial Chronic Disease Program Directors, and CDC adopted standard definitions for 73 chronic disease indicators[29].

Other case definitions, particularly those used in local outbreak investigations, are often tailored to the local situation. For example, a case definition developed for an outbreak of viral illness might require laboratory confirmation where such laboratory services are available, but likely would not if such services were not readily available.

Components of a case definition for outbreak investigations

A case definition consists of clinical criteria and, sometimes, limitations on time, place, and person. The clinical criteria usually include confirmatory laboratory tests, if available, or combinations of symptoms (subjective complaints), signs (objective physical findings), and other findings. Case definitions used during outbreak investigations are more likely to specify limits on time, place, and/or person than those used for surveillance. Contrast the case definition used for surveillance of listeriosis (see box below) with the case definition used during an investigation of a listeriosis outbreak in North Carolina in 2000.[25,26]

Both the national surveillance case definition and the outbreak case definition require a clinically compatible illness and laboratory confirmation of *Listeria monocytogenes* from a normally sterile site, but the outbreak case definition adds restrictions on time and place, reflecting the scope of the outbreak.

> **Listeriosis — Surveillance Case Definition**
>
> **Clinical description**
> Infection caused by *Listeria monocytogenes*, which may produce any of several clinical syndromes, including stillbirth, listeriosis of the newborn, meningitis, bacteriemia, or localized infections
>
> **Laboratory criteria for diagnosis**
> Isolation of *L. monocytogenes* from a normally sterile site (e.g., blood or cerebrospinal fluid or, less commonly, joint, pleural, or pericardial fluid)
>
> **Case classification**
> *Confirmed*: a clinically compatible case that is laboratory confirmed
>
> *Source: Centers for Disease Control and Prevention. Case definitions for infectious conditions under public health surveillance. MMWR Recommendations and Reports 1997:46(RR-10):49-50.*
>
> **Listeriosis — Outbreak Investigation**
>
> **Case definition**
> Clinically compatible illness with *L. monocytogenes* isolated
> - From a normally sterile site
> - In a resident of Winston-Salem, North Carolina
> - With onset between October 24, 2000 and January 4, 2001
>
> *Source: MacDonald P, Boggs J, Whitwam R, Beatty M, Hunter S, MacCormack N, et al. Listeria-associated birth complications linked with homemade Mexican-style cheese, North Carolina, October 2000 [abstract]. 50th Annual Epidemic Intelligence Service Conference; 2001 Apr 23-27; Atlanta, GA.*

Many case definitions, such as that shown for listeriosis, require laboratory confirmation. This is not always necessary, however; in fact, some diseases have no distinctive laboratory findings. Kawasaki syndrome, for example, is a childhood illness with fever and rash that has no known cause and no specifically distinctive laboratory findings. Notice that its case definition (see box below) is based on the presence of fever, at least four of five specified clinical findings, and the lack of a more reasonable explanation.

Criteria in case definitions

A case definition may have several sets of criteria, depending on how certain the diagnosis is. For example, during an investigation of a possible case or outbreak of measles, a person with a fever and rash might be classified as having a suspected, probable, or confirmed case of measles, depending on what evidence of measles is present (see box below).

Measles (Rubeola) — 1996 Case Definition

Clinical description

An illness characterized by all the following:

- A generalized rash lasting greater than or equal to 3 days
- A temperature greater than or equal to 101.0°F (greater than or equal to 38.3°C)
- Cough, coryza, or conjunctivitis

Laboratory criteria for diagnosis

- Positive serologic test for measles immunoglobulin M antibody, or
- Significant rise in measles antibody level by any standard serologic assay, or
- Isolation of measles virus from a clinical specimen

Case classification

Suspected: Any febrile illness accompanied by rash

Probable: A case that meets the clinical case definition, has noncontributory or no serologic or virologic testing, and is not epidemiologically linked to a confirmed case

Confirmed: A case that is laboratory confirmed or that meets the clinical case definition and is epidemiologically linked to a confirmed case. (A laboratory-confirmed case does not need to meet the clinical case definition.)

Comment: Confirmed cases should be reported to National Notifiable Diseases Surveillance System. An imported case has its source outside the country or state. Rash onset occurs within 18 days after entering the jurisdiction, and illness cannot be linked to local transmission. Imported cases should be classified as:

- International. A case that is imported from another country
- Out-of-State. A case that is imported from another state in the United States. The possibility that a patient was exposed within his or her state of residence should be excluded; therefore, the patient either must have been out of state continuously for the entire period of possible exposure (at least 7-18 days before onset of rash) or have had one of the following types of exposure while out of state: a) face-to-face contact with a person who had either a probable or confirmed case or b) attendance in the same institution as a person who had a case of measles (e.g., in a school, classroom, or day care center).

An indigenous case is defined as a case of measles that is not imported. Cases that are linked to imported cases should be classified as indigenous if the exposure to the imported case occurred in the reporting state. Any case that cannot be proved to be imported should be classified as indigenous.

Source: Centers for Disease Control and Prevention. Case definitions for infectious conditions under public health surveillance. MMWR Recommendations and Reports 1997:46(RR-10):23–24.

A case might be classified as suspected or probable while waiting for the laboratory results to become available. Once the laboratory provides the report, the case can be reclassified as either confirmed or "not a case," depending on the laboratory results. In the midst of a large outbreak of a disease caused by a known agent, some cases may be permanently classified as suspected or probable because officials may feel that running laboratory tests on every patient with a consistent clinical picture and a history of exposure (e.g., chickenpox) is unnecessary and even wasteful. Case definitions should not rely on laboratory culture results alone, since organisms are sometimes present without causing disease.

Modifying case definitions

Case definitions can also change over time as more information is obtained. The first case definition for SARS, based on clinical symptoms and either contact with a case or travel to an area with SARS transmission, was published in CDC's Morbidity and Mortality Weekly Report (MMWR) on March 21, 2003 (see box below).[27] Two weeks later it was modified slightly. On March 29, after a novel coronavirus was determined to be the causative agent, an interim surveillance case definition was published that included laboratory criteria for evidence of infection with the SARS-associated coronavirus. By June, the case definition had changed several more times. In anticipation of a new wave of cases in 2004, a revised and much more complex case definition was published in December 2003.[28]

CDC Preliminary Case Definition for Severe Acute Respiratory Syndrome (SARS) — March 21, 2003

Suspected case
Respiratory illness of unknown etiology with onset since February 1, 2003, and the following criteria:

- Documented temperature > 100.4°F (>38.0°C)
- One or more symptoms with respiratory illness (e.g., cough, shortness of breath, difficulty breathing, or radiographic findings of pneumonia or acute respiratory distress syndrome)
- Close contact* within 10 days of onset of symptoms with a person under investigation for or suspected of having SARS or travel within 10 days of onset of symptoms to an area with documented transmission of SARS as defined by the World Health Organization (WHO)

* Defined as having cared for, having lived with, or having had direct contact with respiratory secretions and/or body fluids of a person suspected of having SARS.

Source: Centers for Disease Control and Prevention. Outbreak of severe acute respiratory syndrome–worldwide, 2003. MMWR 2003;52:226–8.

Variation in case definitions

Case definitions may also vary according to the purpose for classifying the occurrences of a disease. For example, health officials need to know as soon as possible if anyone has symptoms of plague or anthrax so that they can begin planning what actions to take. For such rare but potentially severe communicable diseases, for which it is important to identify every possible case, health officials use a sensitive case definition. A sensitive case definition is one that is broad or "loose," in the hope of capturing most or all of the true cases. For example, the case definition for a suspected case of rubella (German measles) is "any generalized rash illness of acute onset."[25] This definition is quite broad, and would include not only all cases of rubella, but also measles, chickenpox, and rashes due to other causes such as drug allergies. So while the advantage of a sensitive case definition is that it includes most or all of the true cases, the disadvantage is that it sometimes includes other illnesses as well.

On the other hand, an investigator studying the causes of a disease outbreak usually wants to be certain that any person included in a study really had the disease. That investigator will prefer a specific or "strict" case definition. For instance, in an outbreak of *Salmonella* Agona infection, the investigators would be more likely to identify the source of the infection if they included only persons who were confirmed to have been infected with that organism, rather than including anyone with acute diarrhea, because some persons may have had diarrhea from a different cause. In this setting, the only disadvantages of a strict case definition are the requirement that everyone with symptoms be tested and an underestimation of the total number of cases if some people with salmonellosis are not tested.

Exercise 1.4

Investigators of an outbreak of trichinosis used a case definition with the following categories:

Clinical Criteria

Confirmed case: Signs and symptoms plus laboratory confirmation

Probable case: Acute onset of at least three of the following four features: myalgia, fever, facial edema, or eosinophil count greater than 500/mm3

Possible case: Acute onset of two of the four features plus a physician diagnosis of trichinosis

Suspect case: Unexplained eosinophilia

Not a case: Failure to fulfill the criteria for a confirmed, probable, possible, or suspect case

Time: Onset after October 1, 2006
Place: Metropolitan Atlanta
Person: Any

Using this case definition, assign the appropriate classification to each of the persons included in the line listing below. Use the highest rate classification possible. (All were residents of Atlanta with acute onset of symptoms in November.)

ID #	Last Name	Myalgias	Fever	Facial Edema	Eosinophil Count	Physician Diagnosis	Laboratory Confirmation	Classification
1	Anderson	yes	yes	no	495	trichinosis	yes	_____
2	Buffington	yes	yes	yes	pending	possible trichinosis	pending	_____
3	Callahan	yes	yes	no	1,100	possible trichinosis	pending	_____
4	Doll	yes	yes	no	2,050	EMS*	pending	_____
5	Ehrlich	no	yes	no	600	trichinosis	not done	_____

*Eosinophilia-Myalgia Syndrome

 Check your answers on page 1-82

Exercise 1.5

Consider the initial case definition for SARS presented on page 1-26.
Explain how the case definition might address the purposes listed below.

1. Diagnosing and caring for individual patients

2. Tracking the occurrence of disease

3. Doing research to identify the cause of the disease

4. Deciding who should be quarantined (quarantine is the separation or restriction of movement of persons who are not ill but are believed to have been exposed to infection, to prevent further transmission)

 Check your answers on page 1-82

Using counts and rates

As noted, one of the basic tasks in public health is identifying and counting cases. These counts, usually derived from case reports submitted by health-care workers and laboratories to the health department, allow public health officials to determine the extent and patterns of disease occurrence by time, place, and person. They may also indicate clusters or outbreaks of disease in the community.

Counts are also valuable for health planning. For example, a health official might use counts (i.e., numbers) to plan how many infection control isolation units or doses of vaccine may be needed.

Rate:

the number of cases

divided by

the size of the population per unit of time

However, simple counts do not provide all the information a health department needs. For some purposes, the counts must be put into context, based on the population in which they arose. Rates are measures that relate the numbers of cases during a certain period of time (usually per year) to the size of the population in which they occurred. For example, 42,745 new cases of AIDS were reported in the United States in 2002.[30] This number, divided by the estimated 2002 population, results in a rate of 15.3 cases per 100,000 population. Rates are particularly useful for comparing the frequency of disease in different locations whose populations differ in size. For example, in 2003, Pennsylvania had over twelve times as many births (140,660) as its neighboring state, Delaware (11,264). However, Pennsylvania has nearly ten times the population of Delaware. So a more fair way to compare is to calculate rates. In fact, the birth rate was greater in Delaware (13.8 per 1,000 women aged 15–44 years) than in Pennsylvania (11.4 per 1,000 women aged 15–44 years).[31]

Rates are also useful for comparing disease occurrence during different periods of time. For example, 19.5 cases of chickenpox per 100,000 were reported in 2001 compared with 135.8 cases per 100,000 in 1991. In addition, rates of disease among different subgroups can be compared to identify those at increased risk of disease. These so-called high risk groups can be further assessed and targeted for special intervention. High risk groups can also be studied to identify risk factors that cause them to have increased risk of disease. While some risk factors such as age and family history of breast cancer may not be modifiable, others, such as smoking and unsafe sexual practices, are. Individuals can use knowledge of the modifiable risk factors to guide decisions about behaviors that influence their health.

Descriptive Epidemiology

The 5W's of descriptive epidemiology:
What = health issue of concern
Who = person
Where = place
When = time
Why/how = causes, risk factors, modes of transmission

As noted earlier, every novice newspaper reporter is taught that a story is incomplete if it does not describe the what, who, where, when, and why/how of a situation, whether it be a space shuttle launch or a house fire. Epidemiologists strive for similar comprehensiveness in characterizing an epidemiologic event, whether it be a pandemic of influenza or a local increase in all-terrain vehicle crashes. However, epidemiologists tend to use synonyms for the five W's listed above: case definition, person, place, time, and causes/risk factors/modes of transmission. Descriptive epidemiology covers **time**, **place**, and **person**.

Compiling and analyzing data by time, place, and person is desirable for several reasons.

- First, by looking at the data carefully, the epidemiologist becomes very familiar with the data. He or she can see what the data can or cannot reveal based on the variables available, its limitations (for example, the number of records with missing information for each important variable), and its eccentricities (for example, all cases range in age from 2 months to 6 years, plus one 17-year-old.).

- Second, the epidemiologist learns the extent and pattern of the public health problem being investigated — which months, which neighborhoods, and which groups of people have the most and least cases.

- Third, the epidemiologist creates a detailed description of the health of a population that can be easily communicated with tables, graphs, and maps.

- Fourth, the epidemiologist can identify areas or groups within the population that have high rates of disease. This information in turn provides important clues to the causes of the disease, and these clues can be turned into testable hypotheses.

Time

The occurrence of disease changes over time. Some of these changes occur regularly, while others are unpredictable. Two diseases that occur during the same season each year include influenza (winter) and West Nile virus infection (August–September). In contrast, diseases such as hepatitis B and salmonellosis can occur at any time. For diseases that occur seasonally, health officials can anticipate their occurrence and implement control and prevention measures, such as an influenza vaccination campaign or mosquito spraying. For diseases that occur sporadically, investigators can conduct studies to identify the causes and modes of spread, and then develop appropriately targeted actions to control or prevent further occurrence of the disease.

In either situation, displaying the patterns of disease occurrence by time is critical for monitoring disease occurrence in the community and for assessing whether the public health interventions made a difference.

Time data are usually displayed with a two-dimensional graph. The vertical or y-axis usually shows the number or rate of cases; the horizontal or x-axis shows the time periods such as years, months, or days. The number or rate of cases is plotted over time. Graphs of disease occurrence over time are usually plotted as line graphs (Figure 1.4) or histograms (Figure 1.5).

Figure 1.4 Reported Cases of Salmonellosis per 100,000 Population, by Year — United States, 1972–2002

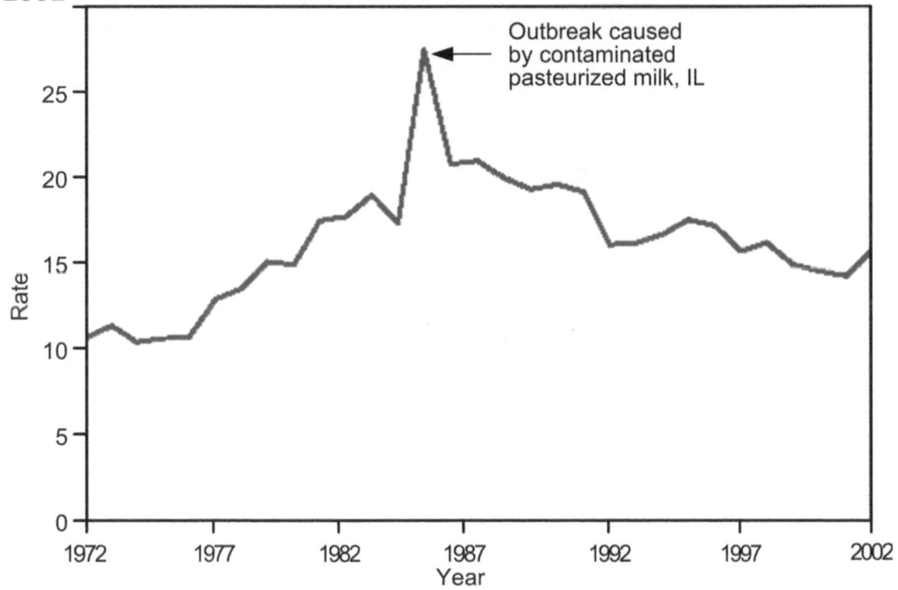

Source: Centers for Disease Control and Prevention. Summary of notifiable diseases–United States, 2002. Published April 30, 2004, for MMWR 2002;51(No. 53): p. 59.

Figure 1.5 Number of Intussusception Reports After the Rhesus Rotavirus Vaccine-tetravalent (RRV-TV) by Vaccination Date—United States, September 1998–December 1999

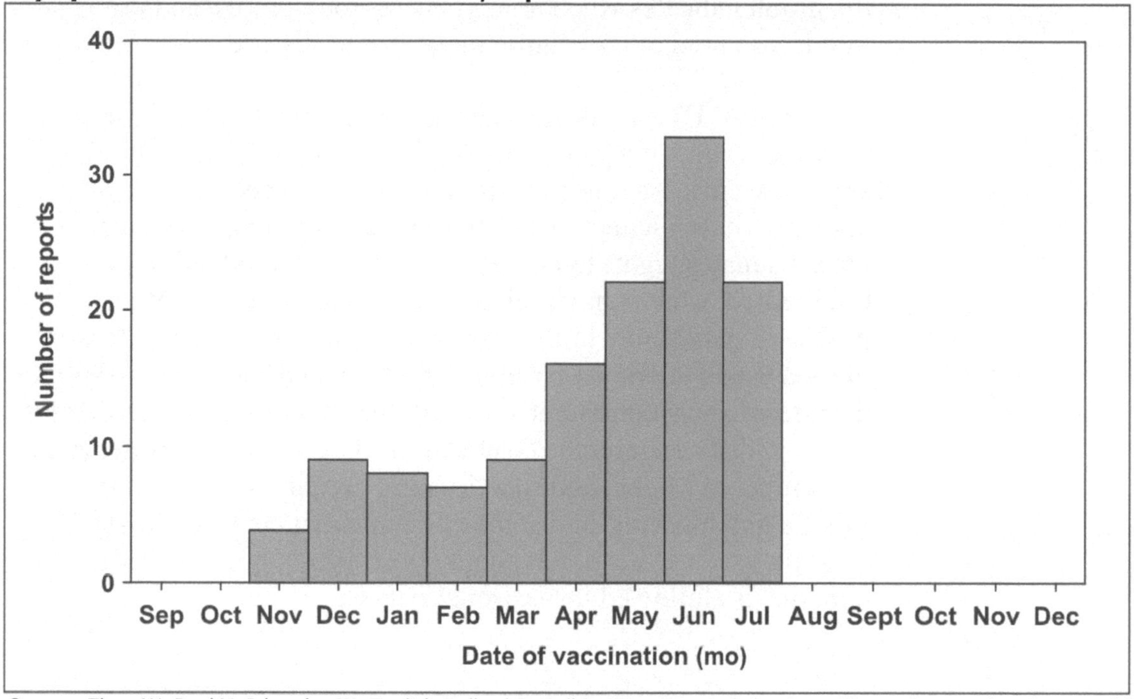

Source: Zhou W, Pool V, Iskander JK, English-Bullard R, Ball R, Wise RP, et al. In: Surveillance Summaries, January 24, 2003. MMWR 2003;52(No. SS-1):1–26.

Sometimes a graph shows the timing of events that are related to disease trends being displayed. For example, the graph may indicate the period of exposure or the date control measures were implemented. Studying a graph that notes the period of exposure may lead to insights into what may have caused illness. Studying a graph that notes the timing of control measures shows what impact, if any, the measures may have had on disease occurrence.

As noted above, time is plotted along the x-axis. Depending on the disease, the time scale may be as broad as years or decades, or as brief as days or even hours of the day. For some conditions — many chronic diseases, for example — epidemiologists tend to be interested in long-term trends or patterns in the number of cases or the rate. For other conditions, such as foodborne outbreaks, the relevant time scale is likely to be days or hours. Some of the common types of time-related graphs are further described below. These and other graphs are described in more detail in Lesson 4.

Secular (long-term) trends. Graphing the annual cases or rate of a disease over a period of years shows long-term or secular trends in the occurrence of the disease (Figure 1.4). Health officials use these graphs to assess the prevailing direction of disease occurrence (increasing, decreasing, or essentially flat), help them evaluate programs or make policy decisions, infer what caused an increase or decrease in the occurrence of a disease (particularly if the graph indicates when related events took place), and use past trends as a predictor of future incidence of disease.

Seasonality. Disease occurrence can be graphed by week or month over the course of a year or more to show its seasonal pattern, if any. Some diseases such as influenza and West Nile infection are known to have characteristic seasonal distributions. Seasonal patterns may suggest hypotheses about how the infection is transmitted, what behavioral factors increase risk, and other possible contributors to the disease or condition. Figure 1.6 shows the seasonal patterns of rubella, influenza, and rotavirus. All three diseases display consistent seasonal distributions, but each disease peaks in different months – rubella in March to June, influenza in November to March, and rotavirus in February to April. The rubella graph is striking for the epidemic that occurred in 1963 (rubella vaccine was not available until 1969), but this epidemic nonetheless followed the seasonal pattern.

Figure 1.6 Seasonal Pattern of Rubella, Influenza and Rotavirus

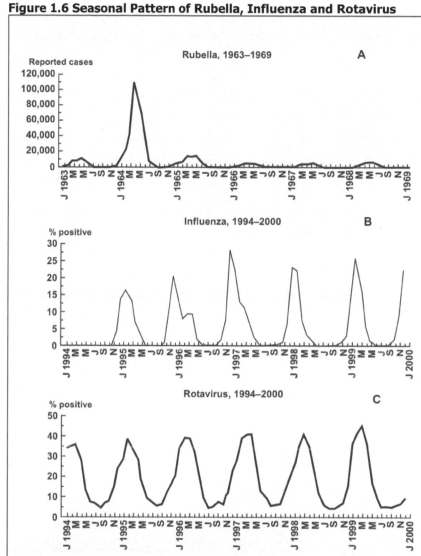

Source: Dowell SF. Seasonal Variation in Host Susceptibility and Cycles of Certain Infectious Diseases. Emerg Infect Dis. 2001;5:369–74.

Day of week and time of day. For some conditions, displaying data by day of the week or time of day may be informative. Analysis at these shorter time periods is particularly appropriate for conditions related to occupational or environmental exposures that tend to occur at regularly scheduled intervals. In Figure 1.7, farm tractor fatalities are displayed by days of the week.[32] Note that the number of farm tractor fatalities on Sundays was about half the number on the other days. The pattern of farm tractor injuries by hour, as displayed in Figure 1.8 peaked at 11:00 a.m., dipped at noon, and peaked again at 4:00 p.m. These patterns may suggest hypotheses and possible explanations that could be evaluated with further study. Figure 1.9 shows the hourly number of survivors and rescuers presenting to local hospitals in New York following the attack on the World Trade Center on September 11, 2001.

Figure 1.7 Farm Tractor Injuries by Day of Week

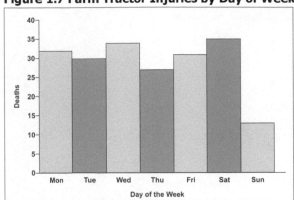

Figure 1.8 Farm Tractor Injuries by Hour of Day

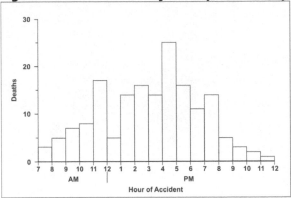

Source: Goodman RA, Smith JD, Sikes RK, Rogers DL, Mickey JL. Fatalities associated with farm tractor injuries: an epidemiologic study. Public Health Rep 1985;100:329–33.

Figure 1.9 World Trade Center Survivors and Rescuers

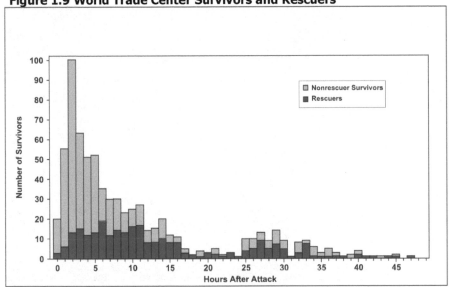

*N=723. Time of assessment data missing for 67 (8%) of the survivors with injuries.
Source: Centers for Disease Control and Prevention. Rapid Assessment of Injuries Among Survivors of the Terrorist Attack on the World Trade Center — New York City, September 2001. MMWR 2002;51:1–5.

Epidemic period. To show the time course of a disease outbreak or epidemic, epidemiologists use a graph called an epidemic curve. As with the other graphs presented so far, an epidemic curve's y-axis shows the number of cases, while the x-axis shows time as either date of symptom onset or date of diagnosis. Depending on the incubation period (the length of time between exposure and onset of symptoms) and routes of transmission, the scale on the x-axis can be as broad as weeks (for a very prolonged epidemic) or as narrow as minutes (e.g., for food poisoning by chemicals that cause symptoms within minutes). Conventionally, the data are displayed as a histogram (which is similar to a bar chart but has no gaps between adjacent columns). Sometimes each case is displayed as a square, as in Figure 1.10. The shape and other features of an epidemic curve can suggest hypotheses about the time and source of exposure, the mode of transmission, and the causative agent. Epidemic curves are discussed in more detail in Lessons 4 and 6.

Figure 1.10 Cases of *Salmonella* Eneriditis — Chicago, February 13–21, by Date and Time of Symptom Onset

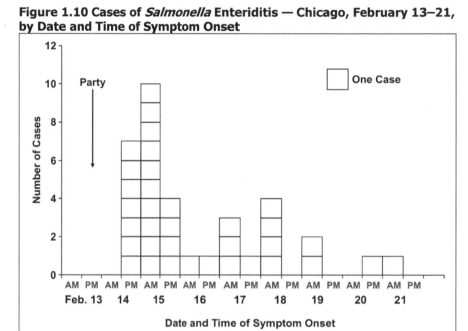

Source: Cortese M, Gerber S, Jones E, Fernandez J. A Salmonella Enteriditis outbreak in Chicago. Presented at the Eastern Regional Epidemic Intelligence Service Conference, March 23, 2000, Boston, Massachusetts.

Place

Describing the occurrence of disease by place provides insight into the geographic extent of the problem and its geographic variation. Characterization by place refers not only to place of residence but to any geographic location relevant to disease occurrence. Such locations include place of diagnosis or report, birthplace, site of employment, school district, hospital unit, or recent travel destinations. The unit may be as large as a continent or country or as small as a street address, hospital wing, or operating room. Sometimes place refers not to a specific location at all but to a place category such as urban or rural, domestic or foreign, and institutional or noninstitutional.

Consider the data in Tables 1.3 and 1.4. Table 1.3 displays SARS data by source of report, and reflects where a person with possible SARS is likely to be quarantined and treated.[33] In contrast, Table 1.4 displays the same data by where the possible SARS patients had traveled, and reflects where transmission may have occurred.

Table 1.3 Reported Cases of SARS through November 3, 2004 — United States, by Case Definition Category and State of Residence

Location	Total Cases Reported	Total Suspect Cases Reported	Total Probable Cases Reported	Total Confirmed Cases Reported
Alaska	1	1	0	0
California	29	22	5	2
Colorado	2	2	0	0
Florida	8	6	2	0
Georgia	3	3	0	0
Hawaii	1	1	0	0
Illinois	8	7	1	0
Kansas	1	1	0	0
Kentucky	6	4	2	0
Maryland	2	2	0	0
Massachusetts	8	8	0	0
Minnesota	1	1	0	0
Mississippi	1	0	1	0
Missouri	3	3	0	0
Nevada	3	3	0	0
New Jersey	2	1	0	1
New Mexico	1	0	0	1
New York	29	23	6	0
North Carolina	4	3	0	1
Ohio	2	2	0	0
Pennsylvania	6	5	0	1
Rhode Island	1	1	0	0
South Carolina	3	3	0	0
Tennessee	1	1	0	0
Texas	5	5	0	0
Utah	7	6	0	1
Vermont	1	1	0	0
Virginia	3	2	0	1
Washington	12	11	1	0
West Virginia	1	1	0	0
Wisconsin	2	1	1	0
Puerto Rico	1	1	0	0
Total	**158**	**131**	**19**	**8**

Adapted from: Centers for Disease Control and Prevention. Severe Acute Respiratory Syndrome (SARS) Report of Cases in the United States; Available from:
http://cdc.gov/od/oc/media/presskits/sars/cases.htm.

Table 1.4 Reported Cases of SARS through November 3, 2004 — United States, by High-Risk Area Visited

Area	Count*	Percent
Hong Kong City, China	45	28
Toronto, Canada	35	22
Guangdong Province, China	34	22
Beijing City, China	25	16
Shanghai City, China	23	15
Singapore	15	9
China, mainland	15	9
Taiwan	10	6
Anhui Province, China	4	3
Hanoi, Vietnam	4	3
Chongqing City, China	3	2
Guizhou Province, China	2	1
Macoa City, China	2	1
Tianjin City, China	2	1
Jilin Province, China	2	1
Xinjiang Province	1	1
Zhejiang Province, China	1	1
Guangxi Province, China	1	1
Shanxi Province, China	1	1
Liaoning Province, China	1	1
Hunan Province, China	1	1
Sichuan Province, China	1	1
Hubei Province, China	1	1
Jiangxi Province, China	1	1
Fujian Province, China	1	1
Jiangsu Province, China	1	1
Yunnan Province, China	0	0
Hebei Province, China	0	0
Qinghai Province, China	0	0
Tibet (Xizang) Province, China	0	0
Hainan Province	0	0
Henan Province, China	0	0
Gansu Province, China	0	0
Shandong Province, China	0	0

* 158 reported case-patients visited 232 areas

Data Source: Heymann DL, Rodier G. Global Surveillance, National Surveillance, and SARS. Emerg Infect Dis. 2004;10:173–175.

Although place data can be shown in a table such as Table 1.3 or Table 1.4, a map provides a more striking visual display of place data. On a map, different numbers or rates of disease can be depicted using different shadings, colors, or line patterns, as in Figure 1.11.

Figure 1.11 Mortality Rates for Asbestosis, by State — United States, 1968–1981 and 1982–2000

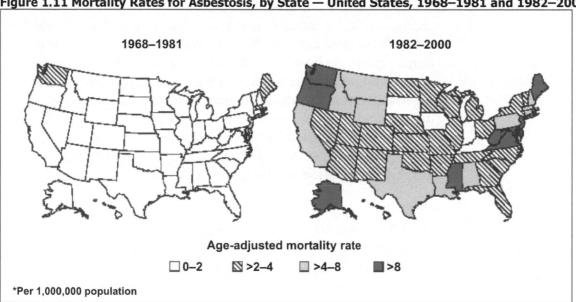

1968–1981   1982–2000

Age-adjusted mortality rate

☐ 0–2   ☒ >2–4   ☐ >4–8   ■ >8

*Per 1,000,000 population

Source: Centers for Disease Control and Prevention. Changing patterns of pneumoconiosis mortality–United States, 1968-2000. MMWR 2004;53:627–32.

Another type of map for place data is a spot map, such as Figure 1.12. Spot maps generally are used for clusters or outbreaks with a limited number of cases. A dot or X is placed on the location that is most relevant to the disease of interest, usually where each victim lived or worked, just as John Snow did in his spot map of the Golden Square area of London (Figure 1.1). If known, sites that are relevant, such as probable locations of exposure (water pumps in Figure 1.1), are usually noted on the map.

Figure 1.12 Spot Map of Giardia Cases

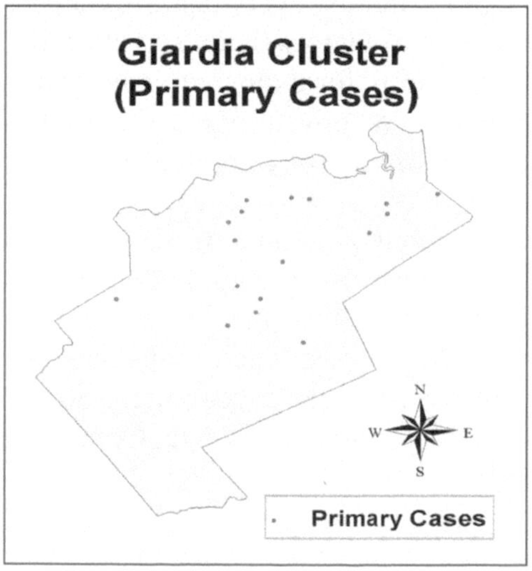

Giardia Cluster (Primary Cases)

N
W ✦ E
S

· Primary Cases

Analyzing data by place can identify communities at increased risk of disease. Even if the data cannot reveal why these people have an increased risk, it can help generate hypotheses to test with additional studies. For example, is a community at increased risk because of characteristics of the people in the community such as genetic susceptibility, lack of immunity, risky behaviors, or exposure to local toxins or contaminated food? Can the increased risk, particularly of a communicable disease, be attributed to characteristics of the causative agent such as a particularly virulent strain, hospitable breeding sites, or availability of the vector that transmits the organism to humans? Or can the increased risk be attributed to the environment that brings the agent and the host together, such as crowding in urban areas that increases the risk of disease transmission from person to person, or more homes being built in wooded areas close to deer that carry ticks infected with the organism that causes Lyme disease? (More techniques for graphic presentation are discussed in Lesson 4.)

Person

"Person" attributes include age, sex, ethnicity/race, and socioeconomic status.

Because personal characteristics may affect illness, organization and analysis of data by "person" may use inherent characteristics of people (for example, age, sex, race), biologic characteristics (immune status), acquired characteristics (marital status), activities (occupation, leisure activities, use of medications/tobacco/drugs), or the conditions under which they live (socioeconomic status, access to medical care). Age and sex are included in almost all data sets and are the two most commonly analyzed "person" characteristics. However, depending on the disease and the data available, analyses of other person variables are usually necessary. Usually epidemiologists begin the analysis of person data by looking at each variable separately. Sometimes, two variables such as age and sex can be examined simultaneously. Person data are usually displayed in tables or graphs.

Age. Age is probably the single most important "person" attribute, because almost every health-related event varies with age. A number of factors that also vary with age include: susceptibility, opportunity for exposure, latency or incubation period of the disease, and physiologic response (which affects, among other things, disease development).

When analyzing data by age, epidemiologists try to use age groups that are narrow enough to detect any age-related patterns that may be present in the data. For some diseases, particularly chronic diseases, 10-year age groups may be adequate. For other diseases, 10-year and even 5-year age groups conceal important variations in disease occurrence by age. Consider the graph of pertussis occurrence by standard 5-year age groups shown in Figure 1.13a. The highest rate is clearly among children 4 years old and younger. But is the rate equally high in all children within that age group, or do some children have higher rates than others?

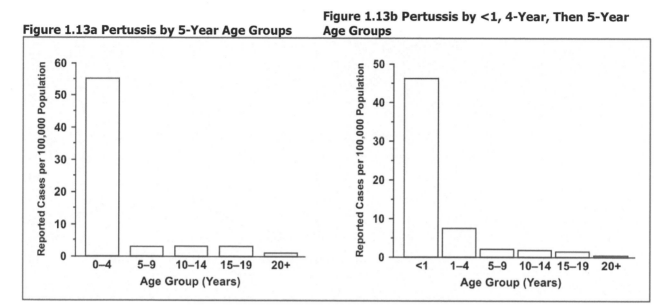

Figure 1.13a Pertussis by 5-Year Age Groups

Figure 1.13b Pertussis by <1, 4-Year, Then 5-Year Age Groups

To answer this question, different age groups are needed. Examine Figure 1.13b, which shows the same data but displays the rate of pertussis for children under 1 year of age separately. Clearly, infants account for most of the high rate among 0–4 year olds. Public health efforts should thus be focused on children less than 1 year of age, rather than on the entire 5-year age group.

Sex. Males have higher rates of illness and death than do females for many diseases. For some diseases, this sex-related difference is because of genetic, hormonal, anatomic, or other inherent differences between the sexes. These inherent differences affect susceptibility or physiologic responses. For example, premenopausal women have a lower risk of heart disease than men of the same age. This difference has been attributed to higher estrogen levels in women. On the other hand, the sex-related differences in the occurrence of many diseases reflect differences in opportunity or levels of exposure. For example, Figure 1.14 shows the differences in lung cancer rates over time among men and women.[34] The difference noted in earlier years has been attributed to the higher prevalence of smoking among men in the past. Unfortunately, prevalence of smoking among women now equals that among men, and lung cancer rates in women have been climbing as a result.[35]

Figure 1.14 Lung Cancer Rates — United States, 1930–1999

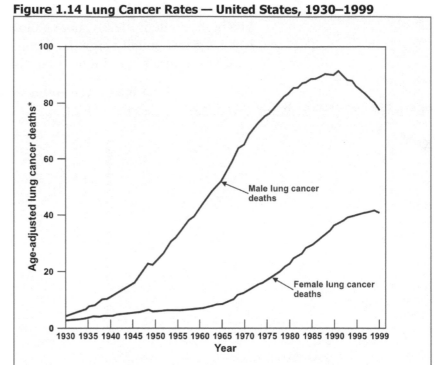

Data Source: American Cancer Society [Internet]. Atlanta: The American Cancer Society, Inc. Available from: http://cancer.org/docroot/PRO/content/PRO_1_1_ Cancer_ Statistics_2005_Presentation.asp.

Ethnic and racial groups. Sometimes epidemiologists are interested in analyzing person data by biologic, cultural or social groupings such as race, nationality, religion, or social groups such as tribes and other geographically or socially isolated groups. Differences in racial, ethnic, or other group variables may reflect differences in susceptibility or exposure, or differences in other factors that influence the risk of disease, such as socioeconomic status and access to health care. In Figure 1.15, infant mortality rates for 2002 are shown by race and Hispanic origin of the mother.

Figure 1.15 Infant Mortality Rates for 2002, by Race and Ethnicity of Mother

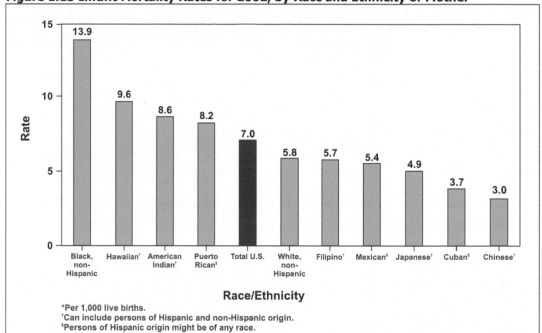

*Per 1,000 live births.
†Can include persons of Hispanic and non-Hispanic origin.
§Persons of Hispanic origin might be of any race.

Source: Centers for Disease Control and Prevention. QuickStats: Infant mortality rates, by selected racial/ethnic populations—United States, 2002, MMWR 2005;54(05):126.*

Socioeconomic status. Socioeconomic status is difficult to quantify. It is made up of many variables such as occupation, family income, educational achievement or census track, living conditions, and social standing. The variables that are easiest to measure may not accurately reflect the overall concept. Nevertheless, epidemiologists commonly use occupation, family income, and educational achievement, while recognizing that these variables do not measure socioeconomic status precisely.

The frequency of many adverse health conditions increases with decreasing socioeconomic status. For example, tuberculosis is more common among persons in lower socioeconomic strata. Infant mortality and time lost from work due to disability are both associated with lower income. These patterns may reflect more harmful exposures, lower resistance, and less access to health care. Or they may in part reflect an interdependent relationship that is impossible to untangle: Does low socioeconomic status contribute to disability, or does disability contribute to lower socioeconomic status, or both? What accounts for the disproportionate prevalence of diabetes and asthma in lower socioeconomic areas?[36,37]

A few adverse health conditions occur more frequently among persons of higher socioeconomic status. Gout was known as the "disease of kings" because of its association with consumption of rich foods. Other conditions associated with higher socioeconomic status include breast cancer, Kawasaki syndrome, chronic fatigue syndrome, and tennis elbow. Differences in exposure account for at least some if not most of the differences in the frequency of these conditions.

Exercise 1.6

Using the data in Tables 1.5 and 1.6, describe the death rate patterns for the "Unusual Event." For example, how do death rates vary between men and women overall, among the different socioeconomic classes, among men and women in different socioeconomic classes, and among adults and children in different socioeconomic classes? Can you guess what type of situation might result in such death rate patterns?

Table 1.5 Deaths and Death Rates for an Unusual Event, by Sex and Socioeconomic Status

| Sex | Measure | Socioeconomic Status | | | Total |
		High	Middle	Low	
Males	Persons at risk	179	173	499	851
	Deaths	120	148	441	709
	Death rate (%)	67.0%	85.5%	88.4%	83.3%
Females	Persons at risk	143	107	212	462
	Deaths	9	13	132	154
	Death rate (%)	6.3%	12.6%	62.3%	33.3%
Both sexes	Persons at risk	322	280	711	1313
	Deaths	129	161	573	863
	Death rate (%)	40.1%	57.5%	80.6%	65.7%

Table 1.6 Deaths and Death Rates for an Unusual Event, by Age and Socioeconomic Status

| Age Group | Measure | Socioeconomic Status | | Total |
		High/Middle	Low	
Adults	Persons at risk	566	664	1230
	Deaths	287	545	832
	Death rate (%)	50.7%	82.1%	67.6%
Children	Persons at risk	36	47	83
	Deaths	3	28	31
	Death rate (%)	8.3%	59.6%	37.3%
All Ages	Persons at risk	602	711	1313
	Deaths	290	573	863
	Death rate (%)	48.2%	80.6%	65.7%

✔ **Check your answers on page 1-82**

Analytic Epidemiology

As noted earlier, descriptive epidemiology can identify patterns among cases and in populations by time, place and person. From these observations, epidemiologists develop hypotheses about the causes of these patterns and about the factors that increase risk of disease. In other words, epidemiologists can use descriptive epidemiology to generate hypotheses, but only rarely to test those hypotheses. For that, epidemiologists must turn to analytic epidemiology.

Key feature of analytic epidemiology = Comparison group

The key feature of analytic epidemiology is a comparison group. Consider a large outbreak of hepatitis A that occurred in Pennsylvania in 2003.[38] Investigators found almost all of the case-patients had eaten at a particular restaurant during the 2–6 weeks (i.e., the typical incubation period for hepatitis A) before onset of illness. While the investigators were able to narrow down their hypotheses to the restaurant and were able to exclude the food preparers and servers as the source, they did not know which particular food may have been contaminated. The investigators asked the case-patients which restaurant foods they had eaten, but that only indicated which foods were popular. The investigators, therefore, also enrolled and interviewed a comparison or control group — a group of persons who had eaten at the restaurant during the same period but who did not get sick. Of 133 items on the restaurant's menu, the most striking difference between the case and control groups was in the proportion that ate salsa (94% of case-patients ate, compared with 39% of controls). Further investigation of the ingredients in the salsa implicated green onions as the source of infection. Shortly thereafter, the Food and Drug Administration issued an advisory to the public about green onions and risk of hepatitis A. This action was in direct response to the convincing results of the analytic epidemiology, which compared the exposure history of case-patients with that of an appropriate comparison group.

When investigators find that persons with a particular characteristic are more likely than those without the characteristic to contract a disease, the characteristic is said to be associated with the disease. The characteristic may be a:
- Demographic factor such as age, race, or sex;
- Constitutional factor such as blood group or immune status;
- Behavior or act such as smoking or having eaten salsa; or
- Circumstance such as living near a toxic waste site.

Identifying factors associated with disease help health officials appropriately target public health prevention and control activities. It also guides additional research into the causes of disease.

Thus, analytic epidemiology is concerned with the search for causes and effects, or the why and the how. Epidemiologists use analytic epidemiology to quantify the association between exposures and outcomes and to test hypotheses about causal relationships. It has been said that epidemiology by itself can never prove that a particular exposure caused a particular outcome. Often, however, epidemiology provides sufficient evidence to take appropriate control and prevention measures.

Epidemiologic studies fall into two categories: **experimental** and **observational**.

Experimental studies

In an experimental study, the investigator determines through a controlled process the exposure for each individual (clinical trial) or community (community trial), and then tracks the individuals or communities over time to detect the effects of the exposure. For example, in a clinical trial of a new vaccine, the investigator may randomly assign some of the participants to receive the new vaccine, while others receive a placebo shot. The investigator then tracks all participants, observes who gets the disease that the new vaccine is intended to prevent, and compares the two groups (new vaccine vs. placebo) to see whether the vaccine group has a lower rate of disease. Similarly, in a trial to prevent onset of diabetes among high-risk individuals, investigators randomly assigned enrollees to one of three groups — placebo, an anti-diabetes drug, or lifestyle intervention. At the end of the follow-up period, investigators found the lowest incidence of diabetes in the lifestyle intervention group, the next lowest in the anti-diabetic drug group, and the highest in the placebo group.[39]

Observational studies

In an observational study, the epidemiologist simply observes the exposure and disease status of each study participant. John Snow's studies of cholera in London were observational studies. The two most common types of observational studies are cohort studies and case-control studies; a third type is cross-sectional studies.

Cohort study. A cohort study is similar in concept to the experimental study. In a cohort study the epidemiologist records whether each study participant is exposed or not, and then tracks the participants to see if they develop the disease of interest. Note that this differs from an experimental study because, in a cohort study, the investigator observes rather than determines the participants' exposure status. After a period of time, the investigator compares the disease rate in the exposed group with the disease rate in the unexposed group. The unexposed group serves as the comparison group, providing an estimate of the baseline or expected amount of disease occurrence in the community. If the disease rate is substantively different in the exposed group compared to the unexposed group, the exposure is said to be associated with illness.

The length of follow-up varies considerably. In an attempt to respond quickly to a public health concern such as an outbreak, public health departments tend to conduct relatively brief studies. On the other hand, research and academic organizations are more likely to conduct studies of cancer, cardiovascular disease, and other chronic diseases which may last for years and even decades. The Framingham study is a well-known cohort study that has followed over 5,000 residents of Framingham, Massachusetts, since the early 1950s to establish the rates and risk factors for heart disease.[7] The Nurses Health Study and the Nurses Health Study II are cohort studies established in 1976 and 1989, respectively, that have followed over 100,000 nurses each and have provided useful information on oral contraceptives, diet, and lifestyle risk factors.[40] These studies are sometimes called **follow-up** or **prospective** cohort studies, because participants are enrolled as the study begins and are then followed prospectively over time to identify occurrence of the outcomes of interest.

An alternative type of cohort study is a **retrospective** cohort study. In this type of study both the exposure and the outcomes have already occurred. Just as in a prospective cohort study, the investigator calculates and compares rates of disease in the exposed and unexposed groups. Retrospective cohort studies are commonly used in investigations of disease in groups of easily identified people such as workers at a particular factory or attendees at a wedding. For example, a retrospective cohort study was used to determine the source of infection of cyclosporiasis, a parasitic disease that caused an outbreak among members of a residential facility in Pennsylvania in 2004.[41] The investigation indicated that consumption of snow peas was implicated as the vehicle of the cyclosporiasis outbreak.

Case-control study. In a case-control study, investigators start by enrolling a group of people with disease (at CDC such persons are called case-patients rather than cases, because case refers to occurrence of disease, not a person). As a comparison group, the investigator then enrolls a group of people without disease (controls). Investigators then compare previous exposures between the two groups. The control group provides an estimate of the baseline or expected amount of exposure in that population. If the amount of exposure among the case group is substantially higher than the amount you would expect based on the control group, then illness is said to be associated with that exposure. The study of hepatitis A traced to green onions, described above, is an example of a case-control study. The key in a case-control study is to identify an appropriate control group, comparable to the case group in most respects, in order to provide a reasonable estimate of the baseline or expected exposure.

Cross-sectional study. In this third type of observational study, a sample of persons from a population is enrolled and their exposures and health outcomes are measured simultaneously. The cross-sectional study tends to assess the presence (prevalence) of the health outcome at that point of time without regard to duration. For example, in a cross-sectional study of diabetes, some of the enrollees with diabetes may have lived with their diabetes for many years, while others may have been recently diagnosed.

From an analytic viewpoint the cross-sectional study is weaker than either a cohort or a case-control study because a cross-sectional study usually cannot disentangle risk factors for occurrence of disease (incidence) from risk factors for survival with the disease. (Incidence and prevalence are discussed in more detail in Lesson 3.) On the other hand, a cross-sectional study is a perfectly fine tool for descriptive epidemiology purposes. Cross-sectional studies are used routinely to document the prevalence in a community of health behaviors (prevalence of smoking), health states (prevalence of vaccination against measles), and health outcomes, particularly chronic conditions (hypertension, diabetes).

In summary, the purpose of an analytic study in epidemiology is to identify and quantify the relationship between an exposure and a health outcome. The hallmark of such a study is the presence of at least two groups, one of which serves as a comparison group. In an experimental study, the investigator determines the exposure for the study subjects; in an observational study, the subjects are exposed under more natural conditions. In an observational cohort study, subjects are enrolled or grouped on the basis of their exposure, then are followed to document occurrence of disease. Differences in disease rates between the exposed and unexposed groups lead investigators to conclude that exposure is associated with disease. In an observational case-control study, subjects are enrolled according to whether they have the disease or not, then are questioned or tested to determine their prior exposure. Differences in exposure prevalence between the case and control groups allow investigators to conclude that the exposure is associated with the disease. Cross-sectional studies measure exposure and disease status at the same time, and are better suited to descriptive epidemiology than causation.

Exercise 1.7

Classify each of the following studies as:

A. *Experimental*
B. *Observational cohort*
C. *Observational case-control*
D. *Observational cross-sectional*
E. *Not an analytical or epidemiologic study*

_____ 1. Representative sample of residents were telephoned and asked how much they exercise each week and whether they currently have (have ever been diagnosed with) heart disease.

_____ 2. Occurrence of cancer was identified between April 1991 and July 2002 for 50,000 troops who served in the first Gulf War (ended April 1991) and 50,000 troops who served elsewhere during the same period.

_____ 3. Persons diagnosed with new-onset Lyme disease were asked how often they walk through woods, use insect repellant, wear short sleeves and pants, etc. Twice as many patients without Lyme disease from the same physician's practice were asked the same questions, and the responses in the two groups were compared.

_____ 4. Subjects were children enrolled in a health maintenance organization. At 2 months, each child was randomly given one of two types of a new vaccine against rotavirus infection. Parents were called by a nurse two weeks later and asked whether the children had experienced any of a list of side-effects.

 Check your answers on page 1-83

Concepts of Disease Occurrence

A critical premise of epidemiology is that disease and other health events do not occur randomly in a population, but are more likely to occur in some members of the population than others because of risk factors that may not be distributed randomly in the population. As noted earlier, one important use of epidemiology is to identify the factors that place some members at greater risk than others.

Causation

A number of models of disease causation have been proposed. Among the simplest of these is the epidemiologic triad or triangle, the traditional model for infectious disease. The triad consists of an external **agent**, a susceptible **host**, and an **environment** that brings the host and agent together. In this model, disease results from the interaction between the agent and the susceptible host in an environment that supports transmission of the agent from a source to that host. Two ways of depicting this model are shown in Figure 1.16.

Agent, host, and environmental factors interrelate in a variety of complex ways to produce disease. Different diseases require different balances and interactions of these three components. Development of appropriate, practical, and effective public health measures to control or prevent disease usually requires assessment of all three components and their interactions.

Figure 1.16 Epidemiologic Triad

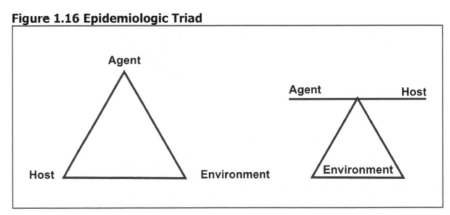

Agent originally referred to an infectious microorganism or pathogen: a virus, bacterium, parasite, or other microbe. Generally, the agent must be present for disease to occur; however, presence of that agent alone is not always sufficient to cause disease. A variety of factors influence whether exposure to an organism will result in disease, including the organism's pathogenicity (ability to cause disease) and dose.

Over time, the concept of agent has been broadened to include chemical and physical causes of disease or injury. These include chemical contaminants (such as the L-tryptophan contaminant responsible for eosinophilia-myalgia syndrome), as well as physical forces (such as repetitive mechanical forces associated with carpal tunnel syndrome). While the epidemiologic triad serves as a useful model for many diseases, it has proven inadequate for cardiovascular disease, cancer, and other diseases that appear to have multiple contributing causes without a single necessary one.

Host refers to the human who can get the disease. A variety of factors intrinsic to the host, sometimes called risk factors, can influence an individual's exposure, susceptibility, or response to a causative agent. Opportunities for exposure are often influenced by behaviors such as sexual practices, hygiene, and other personal choices as well as by age and sex. Susceptibility and response to an agent are influenced by factors such as genetic composition, nutritional and immunologic status, anatomic structure, presence of disease or medications, and psychological makeup.

Environment refers to extrinsic factors that affect the agent and the opportunity for exposure. Environmental factors include physical factors such as geology and climate, biologic factors such as insects that transmit the agent, and socioeconomic factors such as crowding, sanitation, and the availability of health services.

Component causes and causal pies

Because the agent-host-environment model did not work well for many non-infectious diseases, several other models that attempt to account for the multifactorial nature of causation have been proposed. One such model was proposed by Rothman in 1976, and has come to be known as the Causal Pies.[42] This model is illustrated in Figure 1.17. An individual factor that contributes to cause disease is shown as a piece of a pie. After all the pieces of a pie fall into place, the pie is complete — and disease occurs. The individual factors are called **component causes**. The complete pie, which might be considered a causal pathway, is called a **sufficient cause**. A disease may have more than one sufficient cause, with each sufficient cause being composed of several component causes that may or may not overlap. A component that appears in every pie or pathway is called a **necessary cause**, because without it, disease does not occur. Note in Figure 1.17 that component cause A is a necessary cause because it appears in every pie.

Figure 1.17 Rothman's Causal Pies

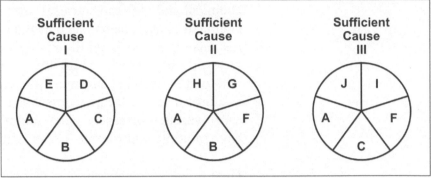

Source: Rothman KJ. Causes. Am J Epidemiol 1976;104:587–592.

The component causes may include intrinsic host factors as well as the agent and the environmental factors of the agent-host-environment triad. A single component cause is rarely a sufficient cause by itself. For example, even exposure to a highly infectious agent such as measles virus does not invariably result in measles disease. Host susceptibility and other host factors also may play a role.

At the other extreme, an agent that is usually harmless in healthy persons may cause devastating disease under different conditions. *Pneumocystis carinii* is an organism that harmlessly colonizes the respiratory tract of some healthy persons, but can cause potentially lethal pneumonia in persons whose immune systems have been weakened by human immunodeficiency virus (HIV). Presence of *Pneumocystis carinii* organisms is therefore a necessary but not sufficient cause of pneumocystis pneumonia. In Figure 1.17, it would be represented by component cause A.

As the model indicates, a particular disease may result from a variety of different sufficient causes or pathways. For example, lung cancer may result from a sufficient cause that includes smoking as a component cause. Smoking is not a sufficient cause by itself, however, because not all smokers develop lung cancer. Neither is smoking a necessary cause, because a small fraction of lung cancer victims have never smoked. Suppose Component Cause B is smoking and Component Cause C is asbestos. Sufficient Cause I includes both smoking (B) and asbestos (C). Sufficient Cause II includes asbestos without smoking, and Sufficient Cause C includes smoking without asbestos. But because lung cancer can develop in persons who have never been exposed to either smoking or asbestos, a proper model for lung cancer would have to show at least one more Sufficient Cause Pie that does not include either component B or component C.

Note that public health action does not depend on the identification of every component cause. Disease prevention can be accomplished by blocking any single component of a sufficient cause, at least through that pathway. For example, elimination of smoking (component B) would prevent lung cancer from sufficient causes I and II, although some lung cancer would still occur through sufficient cause III.

Exercise 1.8

Read the Anthrax Fact Sheet on the following 2 pages, then answer the questions below.

1. Describe its causation in terms of agent, host, and environment.

   a. Agent:

   b. Host:

   c. Environment:

2. For each of the following risk factors and health outcomes, identify whether they are necessary causes, sufficient causes, or component causes.

	Risk Factor	Health Outcome
_____	a. Hypertension	Stroke
_____	b. *Treponema pallidum*	Syphilis
_____	c. Type A personality	Heart disease
_____	d. Skin contact with a strong acid	Burn

 Check your answers on page 1-83

Anthrax Fact Sheet

What is anthrax?

Anthrax is an acute infectious disease that usually occurs in animals such as livestock, but can also affect humans. Human anthrax comes in three forms, depending on the route of infection: cutaneous (skin) anthrax, inhalation anthrax, and intestinal anthrax. Symptoms usually occur within 7 days after exposure.

Cutaneous: Most (about 95%) anthrax infections occur when the bacterium enters a cut or abrasion on the skin after handling infected livestock or contaminated animal products. Skin infection begins as a raised itchy bump that resembles an insect bite but within 1-2 days develops into a vesicle and then a painless ulcer, usually 1-3 cm in diameter, with a characteristic black necrotic (dying) area in the center. Lymph glands in the adjacent area may swell. About 20% of untreated cases of cutaneous anthrax will result in death. Deaths are rare with appropriate antimicrobial therapy.

Inhalation: Initial symptoms are like cold or flu symptoms and can include a sore throat, mild fever, and muscle aches. After several days, the symptoms may progress to cough, chest discomfort, severe breathing problems and shock. Inhalation anthrax is often fatal. Eleven of the mail-related cases were inhalation; 5 (45%) of the 11 patients died.

Intestinal: Initial signs of nausea, loss of appetite, vomiting, and fever are followed by abdominal pain, vomiting of blood, and severe diarrhea. Intestinal anthrax results in death in 25% to 60% of cases.

While most human cases of anthrax result from contact with infected animals or contaminated animal products, anthrax also can be used as a biologic weapon. In 1979, dozens of residents of Sverdlovsk in the former Soviet Union are thought to have died of inhalation anthrax after an unintentional release of an aerosol from a biologic weapons facility. In 2001, 22 cases of anthrax occurred in the United States from letters containing anthrax spores that were mailed to members of Congress, television networks, and newspaper companies.

What causes anthrax?

Anthrax is caused by the bacterium *Bacillus anthracis*. The anthrax bacterium forms a protective shell called a spore. B. anthracis spores are found naturally in soil, and can survive for many years.

How is anthrax diagnosed?

Anthrax is diagnosed by isolating *B. anthracis* from the blood, skin lesions, or respiratory secretions or by measuring specific antibodies in the blood of persons with suspected cases.

Is there a treatment for anthrax?

Antibiotics are used to treat all three types of anthrax. Treatment should be initiated early because the disease is more likely to be fatal if treatment is delayed or not given at all.

How common is anthrax and where is it found?

Anthrax is most common in agricultural regions of South and Central America, Southern and Eastern Europe, Asia, Africa, the Caribbean, and the Middle East, where it occurs in animals. When anthrax affects humans, it is usually the result of an occupational exposure to infected animals or their products. Naturally occurring anthrax is rare in the United States (28 reported cases between 1971 and 2000), but 22 mail-related cases were identified in 2001.

Infections occur most commonly in wild and domestic lower vertebrates (cattle, sheep, goats, camels, antelopes, and other herbivores), but it can also occur in humans when they are exposed to infected animals or tissue from infected animals.

How is anthrax transmitted?

Anthrax can infect a person in three ways: by anthrax spores entering through a break in the skin, by inhaling anthrax spores, or by eating contaminate, undercooked meat. Anthrax is not spread from person to person. The skin ("cutaneous") form of anthrax is usually the result of contact with infected livestock, wild animals, or contaminated animal products such as carcasses, hides, hair, wool, meat, or bone meal. The inhalation form is from breathing in spores from the same sources. Anthrax can also be spread as a bioterrorist agent.

Anthrax Fact Sheet (Continued)

Who has an increased risk of being exposed to anthrax?

Susceptibility to anthrax is universal. Most naturally occurring anthrax affects people whose work brings them into contact with livestock or products from livestock. Such occupations include veterinarians, animal handlers, abattoir workers, and laboratorians. Inhalation anthrax was once called Woolsorter's Disease because workers who inhaled spores from contaminated wool before it was cleaned developed the disease. Soldiers and other potential targets of bioterrorist anthrax attacks might also be considered at increased risk.

Is there a way to prevent infection?

In countries where anthrax is common and vaccination levels of animal herds are low, humans should avoid contact with livestock and animal products and avoid eating meat that has not been properly slaughtered and cooked. Also, an anthrax vaccine has been licensed for use in humans. It is reported to be 93% effective in protecting against anthrax. It is used by veterinarians, laboratorians, soldiers, and others who may be at increased risk of exposure, but is not available to the general public at this time.

For a person who has been exposed to anthrax but is not yet sick, antibiotics combined with anthrax vaccine are used to prevent illness.

Sources: Centers for Disease Control and Prevention [Internet]. Atlanta: Anthrax. Available from: http://www.cdc.gov/ncidod/dbmd/diseaseinfo/anthrax_t.htm and Anthrax Public Health Fact Sheet, Mass. Dept. of Public Health, August 2002.

Natural History and Spectrum of Disease

Natural history of disease refers to the progression of a disease process in an individual over time, in the absence of treatment. For example, untreated infection with HIV causes a spectrum of clinical problems beginning at the time of seroconversion (primary HIV) and terminating with AIDS and usually death. It is now recognized that it may take 10 years or more for AIDS to develop after seroconversion.[43] Many, if not most, diseases have a characteristic natural history, although the time frame and specific manifestations of disease may vary from individual to individual and are influenced by preventive and therapeutic measures.

Figure 1.18 Natural History of Disease Timeline

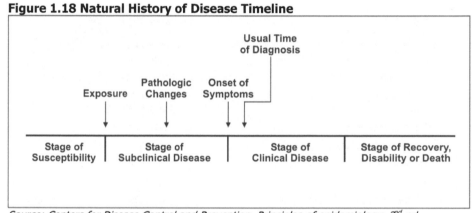

Source: Centers for Disease Control and Prevention. Principles of epidemiology, 2nd ed. Atlanta: U.S. Department of Health and Human Services;1992.

The process begins with the appropriate exposure to or accumulation of factors sufficient for the disease process to begin in a susceptible host. For an infectious disease, the exposure is a microorganism. For cancer, the exposure may be a factor that initiates the process, such as asbestos fibers or components in tobacco smoke (for lung cancer), or one that promotes the process, such as estrogen (for endometrial cancer).

After the disease process has been triggered, pathological changes then occur without the individual being aware of them. This stage of subclinical disease, extending from the time of exposure to onset of disease symptoms, is usually called the **incubation period** for infectious diseases, and the **latency period** for chronic diseases. During this stage, disease is said to be asymptomatic (no symptoms) or inapparent. This period may be as brief as seconds for hypersensitivity and toxic reactions to as long as decades for certain chronic diseases. Even for a single disease, the characteristic incubation period has a range. For example, the typical incubation period for hepatitis A is as long as 7 weeks. The latency period for leukemia to become evident among survivors of the atomic bomb blast in Hiroshima ranged from 2 to 12 years, peaking at 6-7 years.[44] Incubation periods of selected exposures and diseases varying from minutes to decades are displayed in Table 1.7.

Table 1.7 Incubation Periods of Selected Exposures and Diseases

Exposure	Clinical Effect	Incubation/Latency Period
Saxitoxin and similar toxins from shellfish	Paralytic shellfish poisoning (tingling, numbness around lips and fingertips, giddiness, incoherent speech, respiratory paralysis, sometimes death)	few minutes-30 minutes
Organophosphorus ingestion	Nausea, vomiting, cramps, headache, nervousness, blurred vision, chest pain, confusion, twitching, convulsions	few minutes-few hours
Salmonella	Diarrhea, often with fever and cramps	usually 6–48 hours
SARS-associated corona virus	Severe Acute Respiratory Syndrome (SARS)	3–10 days, usually 4–6 days
Varicella-zoster virus	Chickenpox	10–21 days, usually 14–16 days
Treponema pallidum	Syphilis	10–90 days, usually 3 weeks
Hepatitis A virus	Hepatitis	14–50 days, average 4 weeks
Hepatitis B virus	Hepatitis	50–180 days, usually 2–3 months
Human immunodeficiency virus	AIDS	<1 to 15+ years
Atomic bomb radiation (Japan)	Leukemia	2–12 years
Radiation (Japan, Chernobyl)	Thyroid cancer	3–20+ years
Radium (watch dial painters)	Bone cancer	8–40 years

Although disease is not apparent during the incubation period, some pathologic changes may be detectable with laboratory, radiographic, or other screening methods. Most screening programs attempt to identify the disease process during this phase of its natural history, since intervention at this early stage is likely to be more effective than treatment given after the disease has progressed and become symptomatic.

The onset of symptoms marks the transition from subclinical to clinical disease. Most diagnoses are made during the stage of clinical disease. In some people, however, the disease process may never progress to clinically apparent illness. In others, the disease process may result in illness that ranges from mild to severe or fatal. This range is called the **spectrum of disease**. Ultimately, the disease process ends either in recovery, disability or death.

For an infectious agent, **infectivity** refers to the proportion of exposed persons who become infected. **Pathogenicity** refers to the proportion of infected individuals who develop clinically apparent disease. **Virulence** refers to the proportion of clinically apparent cases that are severe or fatal.

Because the spectrum of disease can include asymptomatic and mild cases, the cases of illness diagnosed by clinicians in the community often represent only the tip of the iceberg. Many additional cases may be too early to diagnose or may never progress to the clinical stage. Unfortunately, persons with inapparent or undiagnosed infections may nonetheless be able to transmit infection to others. Such persons who are infectious but have subclinical disease are called **carriers**. Frequently, carriers are persons with incubating disease or inapparent infection. Persons with measles, hepatitis A, and several other diseases become infectious a few days before the onset of symptoms. However carriers may also be persons who appear to have recovered from their clinical illness but remain infectious, such as chronic carriers of hepatitis B virus, or persons who never exhibited symptoms. The challenge to public health workers is that these carriers, unaware that they are infected and infectious to others, are sometimes more likely to unwittingly spread infection than are people with obvious illness.

Chain of Infection

As described above, the traditional epidemiologic triad model holds that infectious diseases result from the interaction of agent, host, and environment. More specifically, transmission occurs when the agent leaves its **reservoir** or host through a **portal of exit**, is conveyed by some **mode of transmission**, and enters through an appropriate **portal of entry** to infect a **susceptible host**. This sequence is sometimes called the chain of infection.

Figure 1.19 Chain of Infection

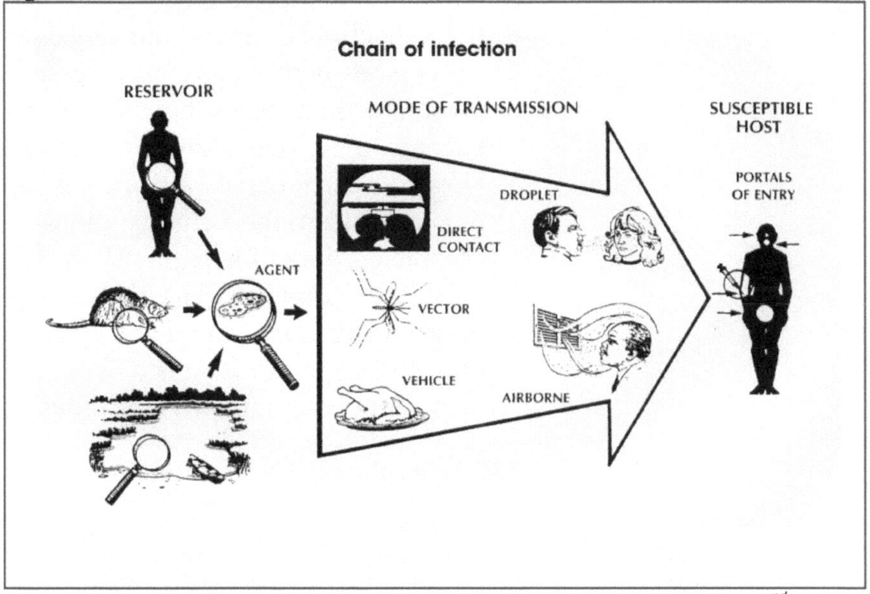

Source: Centers for Disease Control and Prevention. Principles of epidemiology, 2nd ed. Atlanta: U.S. Department of Health and Human Services;1992.

Reservoir

The reservoir of an infectious agent is the habitat in which the agent normally lives, grows, and multiplies. Reservoirs include humans, animals, and the environment. The reservoir may or may not be the source from which an agent is transferred to a host. For example, the reservoir of *Clostridium botulinum* is soil, but the source of most botulism infections is improperly canned food containing *C. botulinum* spores.

Human reservoirs. Many common infectious diseases have human reservoirs. Diseases that are transmitted from person to person without intermediaries include the sexually transmitted diseases, measles, mumps, streptococcal infection, and many respiratory pathogens. Because humans were the only reservoir for the smallpox virus, naturally occurring smallpox was eradicated after the last human case was identified and isolated.[8]

Human reservoirs may or may not show the effects of illness. As noted earlier, a carrier is a person with inapparent infection who is capable of transmitting the pathogen to others. Asymptomatic or passive or healthy carriers are those who never experience symptoms despite being infected. Incubatory carriers are those who can transmit the agent during the incubation period before clinical illness begins. Convalescent carriers are those who have recovered from their illness but remain capable of transmitting to others. Chronic carriers are those who continue to harbor a pathogen such as hepatitis B virus or *Salmonella* Typhi, the causative agent of typhoid fever, for months or even years after their initial infection. One notorious carrier is Mary Mallon, or Typhoid Mary, who was an asymptomatic chronic carrier of *Salmonella* Typhi. As a cook in New York City and New Jersey in the early 1900s, she unintentionally infected dozens of people until she was placed in isolation on an island in the East River, where she died 23 years later.[45]

Carriers commonly transmit disease because they do not realize they are infected, and consequently take no special precautions to prevent transmission. Symptomatic persons who are aware of their illness, on the other hand, may be less likely to transmit infection because they are either too sick to be out and about, take precautions to reduce transmission, or receive treatment that limits the disease.

Animal reservoirs. Humans are also subject to diseases that have animal reservoirs. Many of these diseases are transmitted from animal to animal, with humans as incidental hosts. The term **zoonosis** refers to an infectious disease that is transmissible under natural conditions from vertebrate animals to humans. Long recognized zoonotic diseases include brucellosis (cows and pigs), anthrax (sheep), plague (rodents), trichinellosis/trichinosis (swine), tularemia (rabbits), and rabies (bats, raccoons, dogs, and other mammals). Zoonoses newly emergent in North America include West Nile encephalitis (birds), and monkeypox (prairie dogs). Many newly recognized infectious diseases in humans, including HIV/AIDS, Ebola infection and SARS, are thought to have emerged from animal hosts, although those hosts have not yet been identified.

Environmental reservoirs. Plants, soil, and water in the environment are also reservoirs for some infectious agents. Many fungal agents, such as those that cause histoplasmosis, live and multiply in the soil. Outbreaks of Legionnaires disease are often traced to water supplies in cooling towers and evaporative condensers, reservoirs for the causative organism *Legionella pneumophila.*

Portal of exit

Portal of exit is the path by which a pathogen leaves its host. The portal of exit usually corresponds to the site where the pathogen is localized. For example, influenza viruses and *Mycobacterium tuberculosis* exit the respiratory tract, schistosomes through urine, cholera vibrios in feces, *Sarcoptes scabiei* in scabies skin lesions, and enterovirus 70, a cause of hemorrhagic conjunctivitis, in conjunctival secretions. Some bloodborne agents can exit by crossing the placenta from mother to fetus (rubella, syphilis, toxoplasmosis), while others exit through cuts or needles in the skin (hepatitis B) or blood-sucking arthropods (malaria).

Modes of transmission

An infectious agent may be transmitted from its natural reservoir to a susceptible host in different ways. There are different classifications for modes of transmission. Here is one classification:

- Direct
    - Direct contact
    - Droplet spread
- Indirect
    - Airborne
    - Vehicleborne
    - Vectorborne (mechanical or biologic)

In **direct transmission**, an infectious agent is transferred from a reservoir to a susceptible host by direct contact or droplet spread.

> **Direct contact** occurs through skin-to-skin contact, kissing, and sexual intercourse. Direct contact also refers to contact with soil or vegetation harboring infectious organisms. Thus, infectious mononucleosis ("kissing disease") and gonorrhea are spread from person to person by direct contact. Hookworm is spread by direct contact with contaminated soil.

> **Droplet spread** refers to spray with relatively large, short-range aerosols produced by sneezing, coughing, or even talking. Droplet spread is classified as direct because transmission is by direct spray over a few feet, before the droplets fall to the ground. Pertussis and meningococcal infection are examples of diseases transmitted from an infectious patient to a susceptible host by droplet spread.

Indirect transmission refers to the transfer of an infectious agent from a reservoir to a host by suspended air particles, inanimate objects (vehicles), or animate intermediaries (vectors).

Airborne transmission occurs when infectious agents are carried by dust or droplet nuclei suspended in air. Airborne dust includes material that has settled on surfaces and become resuspended by air currents as well as infectious particles blown from the soil by the wind. Droplet nuclei are dried residue of less than 5 microns in size. In contrast to droplets that fall to the ground within a few feet, droplet nuclei may remain suspended in the air for long periods of time and may be blown over great distances. Measles, for example, has occurred in children who came into a physician's office after a child with measles had left, because the measles virus remained suspended in the air.[46]

Vehicles that may indirectly transmit an infectious agent include food, water, biologic products (blood), and fomites (inanimate objects such as handkerchiefs, bedding, or surgical scalpels). A vehicle may passively carry a pathogen — as food or water may carry hepatitis A virus. Alternatively, the vehicle may provide an environment in which the agent grows, multiplies, or produces toxin — as improperly canned foods provide an environment that supports production of botulinum toxin by *Clostridium botulinum*.

Vectors such as mosquitoes, fleas, and ticks may carry an infectious agent through purely mechanical means or may support growth or changes in the agent. Examples of mechanical transmission are flies carrying *Shigella* on their appendages and fleas carrying *Yersinia pestis*, the causative agent of plague, in their gut. In contrast, in biologic transmission, the causative agent of malaria or guinea worm disease undergoes maturation in an intermediate host before it can be transmitted to humans (Figure 1.20).

Portal of entry

The portal of entry refers to the manner in which a pathogen enters a susceptible host. The portal of entry must provide access to tissues in which the pathogen can multiply or a toxin can act. Often, infectious agents use the same portal to enter a new host that they used to exit the source host. For example, influenza virus exits the respiratory tract of the source host and enters the respiratory tract of the new host. In contrast, many pathogens that cause gastroenteritis follow a so-called "fecal-oral" route because they exit the source host in feces, are carried on inadequately washed hands to a vehicle such as food, water, or utensil, and enter a new host through the mouth. Other portals of entry include the skin (hookworm), mucous membranes (syphilis), and blood (hepatitis B, human immunodeficiency virus).

Figure 1.20 Complex Life Cycle of *Dracunculus medinensis* (Guinea worm)

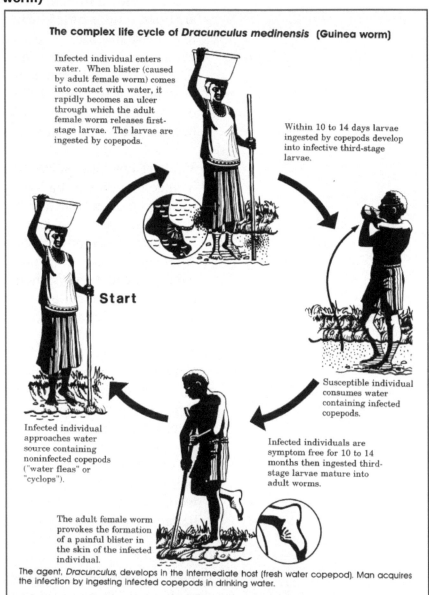

Source: Centers for Disease Control and Prevention. Principles of epidemiology, 2nd ed. Atlanta: U.S. Department of Health and Human Services;1992.

Host

The final link in the chain of infection is a susceptible host. Susceptibility of a host depends on genetic or constitutional factors, specific immunity, and nonspecific factors that affect an individual's ability to resist infection or to limit pathogenicity. An individual's genetic makeup may either increase or decrease susceptibility. For example, persons with sickle cell trait seem to be at least partially protected from a particular type of malaria. Specific immunity refers to protective antibodies that are directed against a specific agent. Such antibodies may develop in response to infection, vaccine, or toxoid (toxin that has been deactivated but retains its capacity to stimulate production of toxin antibodies) or may be acquired by transplacental transfer from mother to fetus or by injection of antitoxin or immune globulin. Nonspecific factors that defend against infection include the skin, mucous membranes, gastric acidity, cilia in the respiratory tract, the cough reflex, and nonspecific immune response. Factors that may increase susceptibility to infection by disrupting host defenses include malnutrition, alcoholism, and disease or therapy that impairs the nonspecific immune response.

Implications for public health

Knowledge of the portals of exit and entry and modes of transmission provides a basis for determining appropriate control measures. In general, control measures are usually directed against the segment in the infection chain that is most susceptible to intervention, unless practical issues dictate otherwise.

Interventions are directed at:
- Controlling or eliminating agent at source of transmission
- Protecting portals of entry
- Increasing host's defenses

For some diseases, the most appropriate intervention may be directed at controlling or eliminating the agent at its source. A patient sick with a communicable disease may be treated with antibiotics to eliminate the infection. An asymptomatic but infected person may be treated both to clear the infection and to reduce the risk of transmission to others. In the community, soil may be decontaminated or covered to prevent escape of the agent.

Some interventions are directed at the mode of transmission. Interruption of direct transmission may be accomplished by isolation of someone with infection, or counseling persons to avoid the specific type of contact associated with transmission. Vehicleborne transmission may be interrupted by elimination or decontamination of the vehicle. To prevent fecal-oral transmission, efforts often focus on rearranging the environment to reduce the risk of contamination in the future and on changing behaviors, such as promoting handwashing. For airborne diseases, strategies may be directed at modifying ventilation or air pressure, and filtering or treating the air. To interrupt vectorborne transmission, measures may be directed toward controlling the vector population, such as spraying to reduce the mosquito population.

Some strategies that protect portals of entry are simple and effective. For example, bed nets are used to protect sleeping persons from being bitten by mosquitoes that may transmit malaria. A dentist's mask and gloves are intended to protect the dentist from a patient's blood, secretions, and droplets, as well to protect the patient from the dentist. Wearing of long pants and sleeves and use of insect repellent are recommended to reduce the risk of Lyme disease and West Nile virus infection, which are transmitted by the bite of ticks and mosquitoes, respectively.

Some interventions aim to increase a host's defenses. Vaccinations promote development of specific antibodies that protect against infection. On the other hand, prophylactic use of antimalarial drugs, recommended for visitors to malaria-endemic areas, does not prevent exposure through mosquito bites, but does prevent infection from taking root.

Finally, some interventions attempt to prevent a pathogen from encountering a susceptible host. The concept of **herd immunity** suggests that if a high enough proportion of individuals in a population are resistant to an agent, then those few who are susceptible will be protected by the resistant majority, since the pathogen will be unlikely to "find" those few susceptible individuals. The degree of herd immunity necessary to prevent or interrupt an outbreak varies by disease. In theory, herd immunity means that not everyone in a community needs to be resistant (immune) to prevent disease spread and occurrence of an outbreak. In practice, herd immunity has not prevented outbreaks of measles and rubella in populations with immunization levels as high as 85% to 90%. One problem is that, in highly immunized populations, the relatively few susceptible persons are often clustered in subgroups defined by socioeconomic or cultural factors. If the pathogen is introduced into one of these subgroups, an outbreak may occur.

Exercise 1.9

Information about dengue fever is provided on the following pages. After studying this information, outline the chain of infection by identifying the reservoir(s), portal(s) of exit, mode(s) of transmission, portal(s) of entry, and factors in host susceptibility.

Reservoirs:

Portals of exit:

Modes of transmission:

Portals of entry:

Factors in host susceptibility:

 Check your answers on page 1-84

Dengue Fact Sheet

What is dengue?

Dengue is an acute infectious disease that comes in two forms: dengue and dengue hemorrhagic fever. The principal symptoms of dengue are high fever, severe headache, backache, joint pains, nausea and vomiting, eye pain, and rash. Generally, younger children have a milder illness than older children and adults.

Dengue hemorrhagic fever is a more severe form of dengue. It is characterized by a fever that lasts from 2 to 7 days, with general signs and symptoms that could occur with many other illnesses (e.g., nausea, vomiting, abdominal pain, and headache). This stage is followed by hemorrhagic manifestations, tendency to bruise easily or other types of skin hemorrhages, bleeding nose or gums, and possibly internal bleeding. The smallest blood vessels (capillaries) become excessively permeable ("leaky"), allowing the fluid component to escape from the blood vessels. This may lead to failure of the circulatory system and shock, followed by death, if circulatory failure is not corrected. Although the average case-fatality rate is about 5%, with good medical management, mortality can be less than 1%.

What causes dengue?

Dengue and dengue hemorrhagic fever are caused by any one of four closely related flaviviruses, designated DEN-1, DEN-2, DEN-3, or DEN-4.

How is dengue diagnosed?

Diagnosis of dengue infection requires laboratory confirmation, either by isolating the virus from serum within 5 days after onset of symptoms, or by detecting convalescent-phase specific antibodies obtained at least 6 days after onset of symptoms.

What is the treatment for dengue or dengue hemorrhagic fever?

There is no specific medication for treatment of a dengue infection. Persons who think they have dengue should use analgesics (pain relievers) with acetaminophen and avoid those containing aspirin. They should also rest, drink plenty of fluids, and consult a physician. Persons with dengue hemorrhagic fever can be effectively treated by fluid replacement therapy if an early clinical diagnosis is made, but hospitalization is often required.

How common is dengue and where is it found?

Dengue is endemic in many tropical countries in Asia and Latin America, most countries in Africa, and much of the Caribbean, including Puerto Rico. Cases have occurred sporadically in Texas. Epidemics occur periodically. Globally, an estimated 50 to 100 million cases of dengue and several hundred thousand cases of dengue hemorrhagic fever occur each year, depending on epidemic activity. Between 100 and 200 suspected cases are introduced into the United States each year by travelers.

How is dengue transmitted?

Dengue is transmitted to people by the bite of an Aedes mosquito that is infected with a dengue virus. The mosquito becomes infected with dengue virus when it bites a person who has dengue or DHF and after about a week can transmit the virus while biting a healthy person. Monkeys may serve as a reservoir in some parts of Asia and Africa. Dengue cannot be spread directly from person to person.

Who has an increased risk of being exposed to dengue?

Susceptibility to dengue is universal. Residents of or visitors to tropical urban areas and other areas where dengue is endemic are at highest risk of becoming infected. While a person who survives a bout of dengue caused by one serotype develops lifelong immunity to that serotype, there is no cross-protection against the three other serotypes.

Dengue Fact Sheet (Continued)

What can be done to reduce the risk of acquiring dengue?

There is no vaccine for preventing dengue. The best preventive measure for residents living in areas infested with Aedes aegypti is to eliminate the places where the mosquito lays her eggs, primarily artificial containers that hold water.

Items that collect rainwater or are used to store water (for example, plastic containers, 55-gallon drums, buckets, or used automobile tires) should be covered or properly discarded. Pet and animal watering containers and vases with fresh flowers should be emptied and scoured at least once a week. This will eliminate the mosquito eggs and larvae and reduce the number of mosquitoes present in these areas.

For travelers to areas with dengue, as well as people living in areas with dengue, the risk of being bitten by mosquitoes indoors is reduced by utilization of air conditioning or windows and doors that are screened. Proper application of mosquito repellents containing 20% to 30% DEET as the active ingredient on exposed skin and clothing decreases the risk of being bitten by mosquitoes. The risk of dengue infection for international travelers appears to be small, unless an epidemic is in progress.

Can epidemics of dengue hemorrhagic fever be prevented?

The emphasis for dengue prevention is on sustainable, community-based, integrated mosquito control, with limited reliance on insecticides (chemical larvicides and adulticides). Preventing epidemic disease requires a coordinated community effort to increase awareness about dengue/DHF, how to recognize it, and how to control the mosquito that transmits it. Residents are responsible for keeping their yards and patios free of sites where mosquitoes can be produced.

Source: Centers for Disease Control and Prevention [Internet]. Dengue Fever. [updated 2005 Aug 22]. Available from http://www.cdc.gov/ncidod/dvbid/dengue/index.htm.

Epidemic Disease Occurrence

Level of disease

The amount of a particular disease that is usually present in a community is referred to as the baseline or **endemic** level of the disease. This level is not necessarily the desired level, which may in fact be zero, but rather is the observed level. In the absence of intervention and assuming that the level is not high enough to deplete the pool of susceptible persons, the disease may continue to occur at this level indefinitely. Thus, the baseline level is often regarded as the expected level of the disease.

While some diseases are so rare in a given population that a single case warrants an epidemiologic investigation (e.g., rabies, plague, polio), other diseases occur more commonly so that only deviations from the norm warrant investigation. **Sporadic** refers to a disease that occurs infrequently and irregularly. **Endemic** refers to the constant presence and/or usual prevalence of a disease or infectious agent in a population within a geographic area. **Hyperendemic** refers to persistent, high levels of disease occurrence.

Occasionally, the amount of disease in a community rises above the expected level. **Epidemic** refers to an increase, often sudden, in the number of cases of a disease above what is normally expected in that population in that area. **Outbreak** carries the same definition of epidemic, but is often used for a more limited geographic area. **Cluster** refers to an aggregation of cases grouped in place and time that are suspected to be greater than the number expected, even though the expected number may not be known. **Pandemic** refers to an epidemic that has spread over several countries or continents, usually affecting a large number of people.

Epidemics occur when an agent and susceptible hosts are present in adequate numbers, and the agent can be effectively conveyed from a source to the susceptible hosts. More specifically, an epidemic may result from:
- A recent increase in amount or virulence of the agent,
- The recent introduction of the agent into a setting where it has not been before,
- An enhanced mode of transmission so that more susceptible persons are exposed,
- A change in the susceptibility of the host response to the agent, and/or
- Factors that increase host exposure or involve introduction

through new portals of entry.[47]

The previous description of epidemics presumes only infectious agents, but non-infectious diseases such as diabetes and obesity exist in epidemic proportion in the U.S.[51,52]

Exercise 1.10

For each of the following situations, identify whether it reflects:

A. *Sporadic disease*
B. *Endemic disease*
C. *Hyperendemic disease*
D. *Pandemic disease*
E. *Epidemic disease*

_____ 1. 22 cases of legionellosis occurred within 3 weeks among residents of a particular neighborhood (usually 0 or 1 per year)

_____ 2. Average annual incidence was 364 cases of pulmonary tuberculosis per 100,000 population in one area, compared with national average of 134 cases per 100,000 population

_____ 3. Over 20 million people worldwide died from influenza in 1918-1919

_____ 4. Single case of histoplasmosis was diagnosed in a community

_____ 5. About 60 cases of gonorrhea are usually reported in this region per week, slightly less than the national average

 Check your answers on page 1-84

Epidemic Patterns

Epidemics can be classified according to their manner of spread through a population:

- Common-source
  - Point
  - Continuous
  - Intermittent
- Propagated
- Mixed
- Other

A **common-source outbreak** is one in which a group of persons are all exposed to an infectious agent or a toxin from the same source.

If the group is exposed over a relatively brief period, so that everyone who becomes ill does so within one incubation period, then the common-source outbreak is further classified as a **point-source outbreak**. The epidemic of leukemia cases in Hiroshima following the atomic bomb blast and the epidemic of hepatitis A among patrons of the Pennsylvania restaurant who ate green onions each had a point source of exposure.[38, 44] If the number of cases during an epidemic were plotted over time, the resulting graph, called an epidemic curve, would typically have a steep upslope and a more gradual downslope (a so-called "log-normal distribution").

Figure 1.21 Hepatitis A Cases by Date of Onset, November–December, 1978

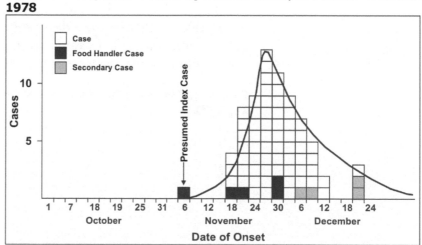

Source: Centers for Disease Control and Prevention. Unpublished data; 1979.

In some common-source outbreaks, case-patients may have been exposed over a period of days, weeks, or longer. In a **continuous common-source outbreak**, the range of exposures and range of incubation periods tend to flatten and widen the peaks of the epidemic curve (Figure 1.22) The epidemic curve of an **intermittent common-source outbreak** often has a pattern reflecting the intermittent nature of the exposure.

Figure 1.22 Diarrheal Illness in City Residents by Date of Onset and Character of Stool, December 1989–January 1990

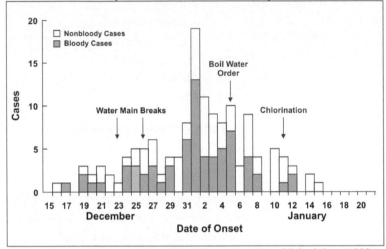

Source: Centers for Disease Control and Prevention. Unpublished data; 1990.

A **propagated outbreak** results from transmission from one person to another. Usually, transmission is by direct person-to-person contact, as with syphilis. Transmission may also be vehicleborne (e.g., transmission of hepatitis B or HIV by sharing needles) or vectorborne (e.g., transmission of yellow fever by mosquitoes). In propagated outbreaks, cases occur over more than one incubation period. In Figure 1.23, note the peaks occurring about 11 days apart, consistent with the incubation period for measles. The epidemic usually wanes after a few generations, either because the number of susceptible persons falls below some critical level required to sustain transmission, or because intervention measures become effective.

Figure 1.23 Measles Cases by Date of Onset, October 15, 1970–January 16, 1971

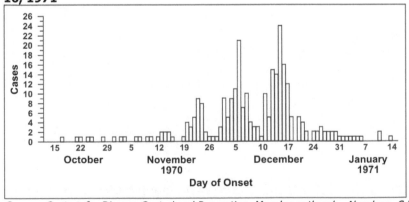

Source: Centers for Disease Control and Prevention. Measles outbreak—Aberdeen, S.D. MMWR 1971;20:26.

Some epidemics have features of both common-source epidemics and propagated epidemics. The pattern of a common-source outbreak followed by secondary person-to-person spread is not uncommon. These are called **mixed epidemics**. For example, a common-source epidemic of shigellosis occurred among a group of 3,000 women attending a national music festival (Figure 1.24). Many developed symptoms after returning home. Over the next few weeks, several state health departments detected subsequent generations of *Shigella* cases propagated by person-to-person transmission from festival attendees.[48]

Figure 1.24 *Shigella* Cases at a Music Festival by Day of Onset, August 1988

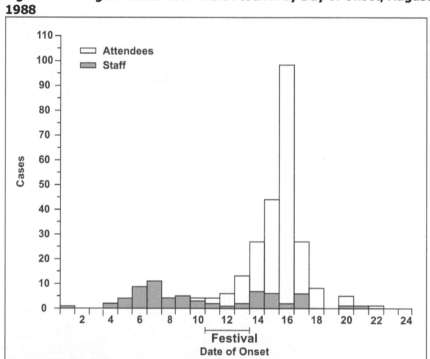

Adapted from: Lee LA, Ostroff SM, McGee HB, Johnson DR, Downes FP, Cameron DN, et al. An outbreak of shigellosis at an outdoor music festival. Am J Epidemiol 1991;133:608–15.

Finally, some epidemics are neither common-source in its usual sense nor propagated from person to person. Outbreaks of zoonotic or vectorborne disease may result from sufficient prevalence of infection in host species, sufficient presence of vectors, and sufficient human-vector interaction. Examples (Figures 1.25 and 1.26) include the epidemic of Lyme disease that emerged in the northeastern United States in the late 1980s (spread from deer to human by deer ticks) and the outbreak of West Nile encephalitis in the Queens section of New York City in 1999 (spread from birds to humans by mosquitoes).[49,50]

**Figure 1.25 Number of Reported Cases of Lyme Disease by Year —
United States, 1992–2003.**

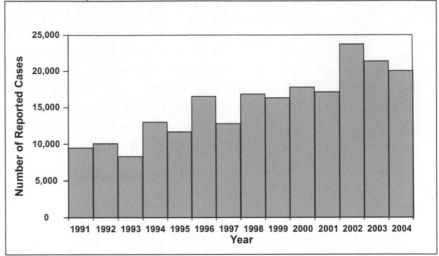

Data Source: Centers for Disease Control and Prevention. Summary of notifiable diseases–
United States, 2003. Published April 22, 2005, for MMWR 2003;52(No. 54):9,17,71–72.

**Figure 1.26 Number of Reported Cases of West Nile Encephalitis — New
York City, 1999**

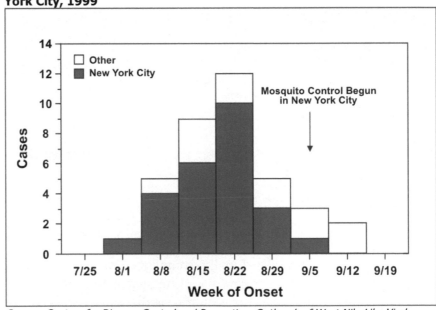

Source: Centers for Disease Control and Prevention. Outbreak of West Nile-Like Viral
Encephalitis–New York, 1999. MMWR 1999;48(38):845–9.

Exercise 1.11

For each of the following situations, identify the type of epidemic spread with which it is most consistent.

A. Point source
B. Intermittent or continuous common source
C. Propagated

_____ 1. 21 cases of shigellosis among children and workers at a day care center over a period of 6 weeks, no external source identified incubation period for shigellosis is usually 1-3 days)

_____ 2. 36 cases of giardiasis over 6 weeks traced to occasional use of a supplementary reservoir (incubation period for giardiasis 3-25 days or more, usually 7-10 days)

_____ 3. 43 cases of norovirus infection over 2 days traced to the ice machine on a cruise ship (incubation period for norovirus is usually 24-48 hours)

 Check your answers on page 1-84

Summary

As the basic science of public health, epidemiology includes the study of the frequency, patterns, and causes of health-related states or events in populations, and the application of that study to address public health issues. Epidemiologists use a systematic approach to assess the What, Who, Where, When, and Why/How of these health states or events. Two essential concepts of epidemiology are population and comparison. Core epidemiologic tasks of a public health epidemiologist include public health surveillance, field investigation, research, evaluation, and policy development. In carrying out these tasks, the epidemiologist is almost always part of the team dedicated to protecting and promoting the public's health.

Epidemiologists look at differences in disease and injury occurrence in different populations to generate hypotheses about risk factors and causes. They generally use cohort or case-control studies to evaluate these hypotheses. Knowledge of basic principles of disease occurrence and spread in a population is essential for implementing effective control and prevention measures.

Exercise Answers

Exercise 1.1

1. B
2. B
3. A
4. A
5. C
6. A

Exercise 1.2

1. Having identified a cluster of cases never before seen in the area, public health officials must seek additional information to assess the community's health. Is the cluster limited to persons who have just returned from traveling where West Nile virus infection is common, or was the infection acquired locally, indicating that the community is truly at risk? Officials could check whether hospitals have seen more patients than usual for encephalitis. If so, officials could document when the increase in cases began, where the patients live or work or travel, and personal characteristics such as age. Mosquito traps could be placed to catch mosquitoes and test for presence of the West Nile virus. If warranted, officials could conduct a serosurvey of the community to document the extent of infection. Results of these efforts would help officials assess the community's burden of disease and risk of infection.

2. West Nile virus infection is spread by mosquitoes. Persons who spend time outdoors, particularly at times such as dusk when mosquitoes may be most active, can make personal decisions to reduce their own risk or not. Knowing that the risk is present but may be small, an avid gardener might or might not decide to curtail the time spent gardening in the evening, or use insect repellent containing DEET, or wear long pants and long-sleeve shirts even though it is August, or empty the bird bath where mosquitoes breed.

3. What proportion of persons infected with West Nile virus actually develops encephalitis? Do some infected people have milder symptoms or no symptoms at all? Investigators could conduct a serosurvey to assess infection, and ask about symptoms and illness. In addition, what becomes of the persons who did develop encephalitis? What proportion survived? Did they recover completely or did some have continuing difficulties?

4. Although the cause and mode of transmission were known (West Nile virus and mosquitoes, respectively), public health officials asked many questions regarding how the virus was introduced (mosquito on an airplane? wayward bird? bioterrorism?), whether the virus had a reservoir in the area (e.g., birds), what types of mosquitoes could transmit the virus, what were the host risk factors for infection or encephalitis, etc.

Exercise 1.3

1. A
2. E
3. F
4. B
5. D
6. C

Exercise 1.4

1. Confirmed
2. Probable
3. Probable
4. Probable
5. Possible

Exercise 1.5

1. Third criterion may be limiting because patient may not be aware of close contact
2. Probably reasonable
3. Criteria do not require sophisticated evaluation or testing, so can be used anywhere in the world
4. Too broad. Most persons with cough and fever returning from Toronto, China, etc., are more likely to have upper respiratory infections than SARS.

Exercise 1.6

The following tables can be created from the data in Tables 1.5 and 1.6:

Table A. Deaths and Death Rates for an Unusual Event, By Sex and Socioeconomic Status

	Female			Male		
	High	Middle	Low	High	Middle	Low
Persons at risk	143	107	212	179	173	499
Survivors	134	94	80	59	25	58
Deaths	9	13	132	120	148	441
Death rate (%)	6.3%	12.1%	62.3%	67.0%	85.5%	88.4%

Table B. Deaths and Death Rates for an Unusual Event, By Sex

	Female	Male	Total
Persons at risk	462	851	1,313
Survivors	308	142	450
Deaths	154	709	863
Death rate (%)	33.3%	83.3%	65.7%

Table C. Deaths and Death Rates for an Unusual Event, By Age Group

	Child	Adult	Total
Persons at risk	83	1,230	1,313
Survivors	52	398	450
Deaths	31	832	863
Death rate (%)	37.3%	67.6%	65.7%

By reviewing the data in these tables, you can see that men (see Table B) and adults (see Table C) were more likely to die than were women and children. Death rates for both women and men declined as socioeconomic status increased (see Table A), but the men in even the highest socioeconomic class were more likely to die than the women in the lowest socioeconomic class. These data, which are consistent with the phrase "Women and children first," represent the mortality experience of passengers on the Titanic.

Data Sources: Passengers on the Titanic [Internet]. StatSci.org; [updated 2002 Dec 29; cited 2005 April]. Available from http://www.statsci.org/data/general/titanic.html.
Victims of the Titanic Disaster [Internet]. Encyclopedia Titanica; [cited 2005 April]. Available from http://www.encyclopedia-titanica.org.

Note:the precise number of passengers, deaths, and class of service are disputed. The Encyclopedia Titanica website includes numerous discussions of these disputed numbers.

Exercise 1.7

1. D
2. B
3. C
4. A

Exercise 1.8

1.
   a. Agent: *Bacillus anthracis*, a bacterium that can survive for years in spore form, is a necessary cause.
   b. Host: People are generally susceptible to anthrax. However, infection can be prevented by vaccination. Cuts or abrasions of the skin may permit entry of the bacteria.
   c. Environment: Persons at risk for naturally acquired infection are those who are likely to be exposed to infected animals or contaminated animal products, such as veterinarians, animal handlers, abattoir workers, and laboratorians. Persons who are potential targets of bioterrorism are also at increased risk.

2.
   a. Component cause
   b. Necessary cause
   c. Component cause
   d. Sufficient cause

Exercise 1.9

Reservoirs: humans and possibly monkeys

Portals of exit: skin (via mosquito bite)

Modes of transmission: indirect transmission to humans by mosquito vector

Portals of entry: through skin to blood (via mosquito bite)

Factors in host susceptibility: except for survivors of dengue infection who are immune to subsequent infection from the same serotype, susceptibility is universal

Exercise 1.10

1. E
2. C
3. D
4. A
5. B

Exercise 1.11

1. C
2. B
3. A

SELF-ASSESSMENT QUIZ

Now that you have read Lesson 1 and have completed the exercises, you should be ready to take the self-assessment quiz. This quiz is designed to help you assess how well you have learned the content of this lesson. You may refer to the lesson text whenever you are unsure of the answer.

Unless instructed otherwise, choose ALL correct answers for each question.

1. In the definition of epidemiology, "distribution" refers to:
   A. Who
   B. When
   C. Where
   D. Why

2. In the definition of epidemiology, "determinants" generally includes:
   A. Agents
   B. Causes
   C. Control measures
   D. Risk factors
   E. Sources

3. Epidemiology, as defined in this lesson, would include which of the following activities?
   A. Describing the demographic characteristics of persons with acute aflatoxin poisoning in District A
   B. Prescribing an antibiotic to treat a patient with community-acquired methicillin-resistant *Staphylococcus aureus* infection
   C. Comparing the family history, amount of exercise, and eating habits of those with and without newly diagnosed diabetes
   D. Recommending that a restaurant be closed after implicating it as the source of a hepatitis A outbreak

4. John Snow's investigation of cholera is considered a model for epidemiologic field investigations because it included a:
   A. Biologically plausible hypothesis
   B. Comparison of a health outcome among exposed and unexposed groups
   C. Multivariate statistical model
   D. Spot map
   E. Recommendation for public health action

5. Public health surveillance includes which of the following activities:
   A. Diagnosing whether a case of encephalitis is actually due to West Nile virus infection
   B. Soliciting case reports of persons with symptoms compatible with SARS from local hospitals
   C. Creating graphs of the number of dog bites by week and neighborhood
   D. Writing a report on trends in seat belt use to share with the state legislature
   E. Disseminating educational materials about ways people can reduce their risk of Lyme disease

6. The hallmark feature of an analytic epidemiologic study is: (Choose one best answer)
   A. Use of an appropriate comparison group
   B. Laboratory confirmation of the diagnosis
   C. Publication in a peer-reviewed journal
   D. Statistical analysis using logistic regression

7. A number of passengers on a cruise ship from Puerto Rico to the Panama Canal have recently developed a gastrointestinal illness compatible with norovirus (formerly called Norwalk-like virus). Testing for norovirus is not readily available in any nearby island, and the test takes several days even where available. Assuming you are the epidemiologist called on to board the ship and investigate this possible outbreak, your case definition should include, at a minimum: (Choose one best answer)
   A. Clinical criteria, plus specification of time, place, and person
   B. Clinical features, plus the exposure(s) you most suspect
   C. Suspect cases
   D. The nationally agreed standard case definition for disease reporting

8. A *specific* case definition is one that:
   A. Is likely to include only (or mostly) true cases
   B. Is considered "loose" or "broad"
   C. Will include more cases than a *sensitive* case definition
   D. May exclude mild cases

9. Comparing numbers and rates of illness in a community, rates are preferred for: (Choose one best answer)
   A. Conducting surveillance for communicable diseases
   B. Deciding how many doses of immune globulin are needed
   C. Estimating subgroups at highest risk
   D. Telling physicians which strain of influenza is most prevalent

10. For the cruise ship scenario described in Question 7, how would you display the time course of the outbreak? (Choose one best answer)
    A. Endemic curve
    B. Epidemic curve
    C. Seasonal trend
    D. Secular trend

11. For the cruise ship scenario described in Question 7, if you suspected that the norovirus may have been transmitted by ice made or served aboard ship, how might you display "place"?
    A. Spot map by assigned dinner seating location
    B. Spot map by cabin
    C. Shaded map of United States by state of residence
    D. Shaded map by whether passenger consumed ship's ice or not

12. Which variables might you include in characterizing the outbreak described in Question 7 by person?
    A. Age of passenger
    B. Detailed food history (what person ate) while aboard ship
    C. Status as passenger or crew
    D. Symptoms

13. When analyzing surveillance data by age, which of the following age groups is preferred? (Choose one best answer)
    A. 1-year age groups
    B. 5-year age groups
    C. 10-year age groups
    D. Depends on the disease

14. A study in which children are randomly assigned to receive either a newly formulated vaccine or the currently available vaccine, and are followed to monitor for side effects and effectiveness of each vaccine, is an example of which type of study?
    A. Experimental
    B. Observational
    C. Cohort
    D. Case-control
    E. Clinical trial

15. The Iowa Women's Health Study, in which researchers enrolled 41,837 women in 1986 and collected exposure and lifestyle information to assess the relationship between these factors and subsequent occurrence of cancer, is an example of which type(s) of study?
    A. Experimental
    B. Observational
    C. Cohort
    D. Case-control
    E. Clinical trial

16. British investigators conducted a study to compare measles-mumps-rubella (MMR) vaccine history among 1,294 children with pervasive development disorder (e.g., autism and Asperger's syndrome) and 4,469 children without such disorders. (They found no association.) This is an example of which type(s) of study?
    A. Experimental
    B. Observational
    C. Cohort
    D. Case-control
    E. Clinical trial

Source: Smeeth L, Cook C, Fombonne E, Heavey L, Rodrigues LC, Smith PG, Hall AJ. MMR vaccination and pervasive developmental disorders. Lancet 2004;364:963–9.

17. A cohort study differs from a case-control study in that:
    A. Subjects are enrolled or categorized on the basis of their exposure status in a cohort study but not in a case-control study
    B. Subjects are asked about their exposure status in a cohort study but not in a case-control study
    C. Cohort studies require many years to conduct, but case-control studies do not
    D. Cohort studies are conducted to investigate chronic diseases, case-control studies are used for infectious diseases

18. A key feature of a cross-sectional study is that:
    A. It usually provides information on prevalence rather than incidence
    B. It is limited to health exposures and behaviors rather than health outcomes
    C. It is more useful for descriptive epidemiology than it is for analytic epidemiology
    D. It is synonymous with survey

19. The epidemiologic triad of disease causation refers to: (Choose one best answer)
    A. Agent, host, environment
    B. Time, place, person
    C. Source, mode of transmission, susceptible host
    D. John Snow, Robert Koch, Kenneth Rothman

20. For each of the following, identify the appropriate letter from the time line in Figure 1.27 representing the natural history of disease.
    _____ Onset of symptoms
    _____ Usual time of diagnosis
    _____ Exposure

Figure 1.27 Natural History of Disease Timeline

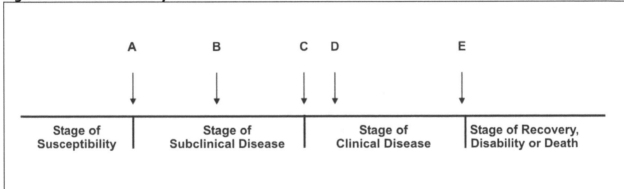

21. A reservoir of an infectious agent can be:
    A. An asymptomatic human
    B. A symptomatic human
    C. An animal
    D. The environment

22. Indirect transmission includes which of the following?
    A. Droplet spread
    B. Mosquito-borne
    C. Foodborne
    D. Doorknobs or toilet seats

23. Disease control measures are generally directed at which of the following?
    A. Eliminating the reservoir
    B. Eliminating the vector
    C. Eliminating the host
    D. Interrupting mode of transmission
    E. Reducing host susceptibility

24. Which term best describes the pattern of occurrence of the three diseases noted below in a single area?
    A. Endemic
    B. Outbreak
    C. Pandemic
    D. Sporadic

    _____   Disease 1: usually 40-50 cases per week; last week, 48 cases
    _____   Disease 2: fewer than 10 cases per year; last week, 1 case
    _____   Disease 3: usually no more than 2-4 cases per week; last week, 13 cases

25. A propagated epidemic is usually the result of what type of exposure?
    A. Point source
    B. Continuous common source
    C. Intermittent common source
    D. Person-to-person

Answers to Self-Assessment Quiz

1. A, B, C. In the definition of epidemiology, "distribution" refers to descriptive epidemiology, while "determinants" refers to analytic epidemiology. So "distribution" covers time (when), place (where), and person (who), whereas "determinants" covers causes, risk factors, modes of transmission (why and how).

2. A, B, D, E. In the definition of epidemiology, "determinants" generally includes the causes (including agents), risk factors (including exposure to sources), and modes of transmission, but does not include the resulting public health action.

3. A, C, D. Epidemiology includes assessment of the distribution (including describing demographic characteristics of an affected population), determinants (including a study of possible risk factors), and the application to control health problems (such as closing a restaurant). It does not generally include the actual treatment of individuals, which is the responsibility of health-care providers.

4. A, B, D, E. John Snow's investigation of cholera is considered a model for epidemiologic field investigations because it included a biologically plausible (but not popular at the time) hypothesis that cholera was water-borne, a spot map, a comparison of a health outcome (death) among exposed and unexposed groups, and a recommendation for public health action. Snow's elegant work predated multivariate analysis by 100 years.

5. B, C, D. Public health surveillance includes collection (B), analysis (C), and dissemination (D) of public health information to help guide public health decision making and action, but it does not include individual clinical diagnosis, nor does it include the actual public health actions that are developed based on the information.

6. A. The hallmark feature of an analytic epidemiologic study is use of an appropriate comparison group.

7. A. A case definition for a field investigation should include clinical criteria, plus specification of time, place, and person. The case definition should be independent of the exposure you wish to evaluate. Depending on the availability of laboratory confirmation, certainty of diagnosis, and other factors, a case definition may or may not be developed for suspect cases. The nationally agreed standard case definition for disease reporting is usually quite specific, and usually does not include suspect or possible cases.

8. A, D. A *specific* or *tight* case definition is one that is likely to include only (or mostly) true cases, but at the expense of excluding milder or atypical cases.

9. C. Rates assess risk. Numbers are generally preferred for identifying individual cases and for resource planning.

10. B. An epidemic curve, with date or time of onset on its x-axis and number of cases on the y-axis, is the classic graph for displaying the time course of an epidemic.

11. A, B, C. "Place" includes location of actual or suspected exposure as well as location of residence, work, school, and the like.

12. A, C. "Person" refers to demographic characteristics. It generally does not include clinical features characteristics or exposures.

13. D. Epidemiologists tailor descriptive epidemiology to best describe the data they have. Because different diseases have different age distributions, epidemiologists use different age breakdowns appropriate for the disease of interest.

14. A, E. A study in which subjects are randomized into two intervention groups and monitored to identify health outcomes is a clinical trial, which is type of experimental study. It is not a cohort study, because that term is limited to observational studies.

15. B, C. A study that assesses (but does not dictate) exposure and follows to document subsequent occurrence of disease is an observational cohort study.

16. B, D. A study in which subjects are enrolled on the basis of having or not having a health outcome is an observational case-control study.
    Source: Smeeth L, Cook C, Fombonne E, Heavey L, Rodrigues LC, Smith PG, Hall AJ. MMR vaccination and pervasive developmental disorders. Lancet 2004;364:963–9.

17. A. The key difference between a cohort and case-control study is that, in a cohort study, subjects are enrolled on the basis of their exposure, whereas in a case-control study subjects are enrolled on the basis of whether they have the disease of interest or not. Both types of studies assess exposure and disease status. While some cohort studies have been conducted over several years, others, particularly those that are outbreak-related, have been conducted in days. Either type of study can be used to study a wide array of health problems, including infectious and non-infectious.

18. A, C, D. A cross-sectional study or survey provides a snapshot of the health of a population, so it assesses prevalence rather than incidence. As a result, it is not as useful as a cohort or case-control study for analytic epidemiology. However, a cross-sectional study can easily measure prevalence of exposures and outcomes.

19. A. The epidemiologic triad of disease causation refers to agent-host-environment.

20. C   Onset of symptoms
    D   Usual time of diagnosis
    A   Exposure

21. A, B, C, D. A reservoir of an infectious agent is the habitat in which an agent normally lives, grows, and multiplies, which may include humans, animals, and the environment.

22. B, C, D. Indirect transmission refers to the transmission of an infectious agent by suspended airborne particles, inanimate objects (vehicles, food, water) or living intermediaries (vectors such as mosquitoes). Droplet spread is generally considered short-distance direct transmission.

23. A, B, D, E. Disease control measures are generally directed at eliminating the reservoir or vector, interrupting transmission, or protecting (but not eliminating!) the host.

24. A. Disease 1: usually 40-50 cases per week; last week, 48 cases
    D. Disease 2: fewer than 10 cases per year; last week, 1 case
    B. Disease 3: usually no more than 2-4 cases per week; last week, 13 cases

25. D. A propagated epidemic is one in which infection spreads from person to person.

References

1. Last JM, editor. Dictionary of epidemiology. 4th ed. New York: Oxford University Press; 2001. p. 61.

2. Cates W. Epidemiology: Applying principles to clinical practice. Contemp Ob/Gyn 1982;20:147–61.

3. Greenwood M. Epidemics and crowd-diseases: an introduction to the study of epidemiology, Oxford University Press; 1935.

4. Thacker SB. Historical development. In: Teutsch SM, Churchill RE, editors. Principles and practice of public health surveillance, 2nd ed. New York: Oxford University Press; 2002. p. 1–16.

5. Snow J. Snow on cholera. London: Humphrey Milford: Oxford University Press; 1936.

6. Doll R, Hill AB. Smoking and carcinoma of the lung. Brit Med J 1950;2:739–48.

7. Kannel WB. The Framingham Study: its 50-year legacy and future promise. J Atheroscler Thromb 2000;6:60–6.

8. Fenner F, Henderson DA, Arita I, Jezek Z, Ladnyi ID. Smallpox and its eradication. Geneva: World Health Organization; 1988.

9. Morris JN. Uses of epidemiology. Edinburgh: Livingstone; 1957.

10. U.S. Department of Health and Human Services (HHS). Healthy people 2000: national health promotion and disease prevention objectives. Washington, DC: HHS, Public Health Service; 1991.

11. U.S. Department of Health and Human Services (HHS). Healthy people 2010. 2nd ed. Washington, DC: U.S. Government Printing Office (GPO); November 2000.

12. U.S. Department of Health and Human Services (HHS). Tracking healthy people 2010. Washington, DC: GPO; November 2000.

13. Eidson M, Philen RM, Sewell CM, Voorhees R, Kilbourne EM. L-tryptophan and eosinophilia-myalgia syndrome in New Mexico. Lancet 1990;335:645–8.

14. Kamps BS, Hoffmann C, editors. SARS Reference, 3rd ed. Flying Publisher, 2003. Available from: http://www.sarsreference.com/index.htm.

15. Murphy TV, Gargiullo PM, Massoudi MS, et al. Intussusception among infants given an oral rotavirus vaccine. N Eng J Med 2001;344:564–72.

16. Fraser DW, Tsai TR, Orenstein W, Parkin WE, Beecham HJ, Sharrar RG, et al. Legionnaires' disease: description of an epidemic of pneumonia. New Engl J Med 1977; 297:1189–97.

17. Tyler CW, Last JM. Epidemiology. In: Last JM, Wallace RB, editors. Maxcy-Rosenau-Last public health and preventive medicine, 14th ed. Norwalk (Connecticut): Appleton & Lange; 1992. p. 11.

18. Orenstein WA, Bernier RH. Surveillance: information for action. Pediatr Clin North Am 1990; 37:709–34.

19. Wagner MM, Tsui FC, Espino JU, Dato VM, Sittig DF, Caruana FA, et al. The emerging science of very early detection of disease outbreaks. J Pub Health Mgmt Pract 2001;6:51–9.

20. Centers for Disease Control and Prevention. Framework for evaluating public health surveillance systems for early detection of outbreaks: recommendations from the CDC Working Group. MMWR May 7, 2004; 53(RR05);1–11.

21. Centers for Disease Control and Prevention. Interim guidance on infection control precautions for patients with suspected severe acute respiratory syndrome (SARS) and close contacts in households. Available from: http://www.cdc.gov/ncidod/sars/ic-closecontacts.htm.

22. Beaglehole R, Bonita R, Kjellstrom T. Basic epidemiology. Geneva: World Health Organization; 1993. p. 133.

23. Centers for Disease Control and Prevention. Updated guidelines for evaluating public health surveillance systems: recommendations from the Guidelines Working Group. MMWR Recommendations and Reports 2001:50(RR13).

24. Rothman KJ. Policy recommendations in epidemiology research papers. Epidemiol 1993; 4: 94–9.

25. Centers for Disease Control and Prevention. Case definitions for infectious conditions under public health surveillance. MMWR Recomm Rep 1997:46(RR-10):1–55.

26. MacDonald P, Boggs J, Whitwam R, Beatty M, Hunter S, MacCormack N, et al. Listeria-associated birth complications linked with homemade Mexican-style cheese, North Carolina, October 2000 [abstract]. 50th Annual Epidemic Intelligence Service Conference; 2001 Apr 23-27; Atlanta, GA.

27. Centers for Disease Control and Prevention. Outbreak of severe acute respiratory syndrome–worldwide, 2003. MMWR 2003: 52:226–8.

28. Centers for Disease Control and Prevention. Revised U.S. surveillance case definition for severe acute respiratory syndrome (SARS) and update on SARS cases–United States and worldwide, December 2003. MMWR 2003:52:1202–6.

29. Centers for Disease Control and Prevention. Indicators for chronic disease surveillance. MMWR Recomm Rep 2004;53(RR-11):1–6.

30. Centers for Disease Control and Prevention. Summary of notifiable diseases–United States, 2001. MMWR 2001;50(53).

31. Arias E, Anderson RN, Hsiang-Ching K, Murphy SL, Kovhanek KD. Deaths: final data for 2001. National vital statistics reports; vol 52, no. 3. Hyattsville (Maryland): National Center for Health Statistics; 2003.

32. Goodman RA, Smith JD, Sikes RK, Rogers DL, Mickey JL. Fatalities associated with farm tractor injuries: an epidemiologic study. Public Health Rep 1985;100:329–33.

33. Heyman DL, Rodier G. Global surveillance, national surveillance, and SARS. Emerg Infect Dis. 2003;10:173–5.

34. American Cancer Society [Internet]. Atlanta: The American Cancer Society, Inc. Available from: http://www.cancer.org/docroot/PRO/content/PRO_1_1_ Cancer_ Statistics_2005_Presentation.asp.

35. Centers for Disease Control and Prevention. Current trends. Lung cancer and breast cancer trends among women–Texas. MMWR 1984;33(MM19):266.

36. Liao Y, Tucker P, Okoro CA, Giles WH, Mokdad AH, Harris VB, et. al. REACH 2010 surveillance for health status in minority communities — United States, 2001–2002. MMWR 2004;53:1–36.

37. Centers for Disease Control and Prevention. Asthma mortality –Illinois, 1979-1994. MMWR. 1997;46(MM37):877–80.

38. Centers for Disease Control and Prevention. Hepatitis A outbreak associated with green onions at a restaurant–Monaca, Pennsylvania, 2003. MMWR 2003; 52(47):1155–7.

39. Knowler WC, Barrett-Connor E, Fowler SE, Hamman RF, Lachin JM, Walker EA, Nathan DM, Diabetes Prevention Program Research Group. Reduction in the incidence of type 2 diabetes with lifestyle intervention or metformin. N Engl J Med 2002;346:393–403.

40. Colditz GA, Manson JE, Hankinson SE. The Nurses' Health Study: 20-year contribution to the understanding of health among women. J Women's Health 1997;49–62.

41. Centers for Disease Control and Prevention. Outbreak of Cyclosporiasis associated with snow peas–Pennsylvania, 2004. MMWR 2004;53:876–8.

42. Rothman KJ. Causes. Am J Epidemiol 1976;104:587–92.

43. Mindel A, Tenant-Flowers M. Natural history and management of early HIV infection. BMJ 2001;332:1290–93.

44. Cobb S, Miller M, Wald N. On the estimation of the incubation period in malignant disease. J Chron Dis 1959;9:385–93.

45. Leavitt JW. Typhoid Mary: captive to the public's health. Boston: Beacon Press; 1996.

46. Remington PL, Hall WN, Davis IH, Herald A, Gunn RA. Airborne transmission of measles in a physician's office. JAMA 1985;253:1575–7.

47. Kelsey JL, Thompson WD, Evans AS. Methods in observational epidemiology. New York: Oxford University Press; 1986. p. 216.

48. Lee LA, Ostroff SM, McGee HB, Jonson DR, Downes FP, Cameron DN, et al. An outbreak of shigellosis at an outdoor music festival. Am J Epidemiol 1991; 133:608–15.

49. White DJ, Chang H-G, Benach JL, Bosler EM, Meldrum SC, Means RG, et al. Geographic spread and temporal increase of the Lyme disease epidemic. JAMA 1991;266:1230–6.

50. Centers for Disease Control and Prevention. Outbreak of West Nile-Like Viral Encephalitis–New York, 1999. MMWR 1999;48(38):845–9.

51. Centers for Disease Control and Prevention. Prevalence of overweight and obesity among adults with diagnosed diabetes–United States, 1988-1994 and 1999-2002.MMWR 2004;53(45):1066–8.

52. National Center for Health Statistics [Internet]. Atlanta: Centers for Disease Control and Prevention [updated 2005 Feb 8]. Available from: http://www.cdc.gov/nchs/products/pubs/pubd/hestats/overwght99.htm

Websites

For more information on:	Visit the following websites:
CDC's Epidemic Intelligence Service	http://www.cdc.gov/eis
CDC's framework for program evaluation in public health	http://www.cdc.gov/mmwr/preview/mmwrhtml/rr4811a1.htm
CDC's program for public health surveillance	http://www.cdc.gov/epo/dphsi
Complete and current list of case definitions for surveillance	http://www.cdc.gov/epo/dphsi/casedef/case_definition.htm
John Snow	http://www.ph.ucla.edu/epi/snow.html

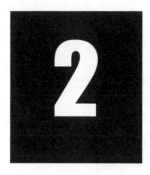

SUMMARIZING DATA

Imagine that you work in a county health department and are faced with two challenges. First, a case of hepatitis B is reported to the health department. The patient, a 40-year-old man, denies having either of the two common risk factors for the disease: he has never used injection drugs and has been in a monogamous relationship with his wife for twelve years. However, he remembers going to the dentist for some bridge work approximately three months earlier. Hepatitis B has occasionally been transmitted between dentist and patients, particularly before dentists routinely wore gloves.

Question: What proportion of other persons with new onset of hepatitis B reported recent exposure to the same dentist, or to any dentist during their likely period of exposure?

Then, in the following week, the health department receives 61 death certificates. A new employee in the Vital Statistics office wonders how many death certificates the health department usually receives each week.

Question: What is the average number of death certificates the health department receives each week? By how much does this number vary? What is the range over the past year?

If you were given the appropriate raw data, would you be able to answer these two questions confidently? The materials in this lesson will allow you do so — and more.

Objectives

After studying this lesson and answering the questions in the exercises, you will be able to:
- *Construct a frequency distribution*
- *Calculate and interpret four measures of central location: mode, median, arithmetic mean, and geometric mean*
- *Apply the most appropriate measure of central location for a frequency distribution*
- *Apply and interpret four measures of spread: range, interquartile range, standard deviation, and confidence interval (for mean)*

Major Sections

Organizing Data

Whether you are conducting routine surveillance, investigating an outbreak, or conducting a study, you must first compile information in an organized manner. One common method is to create a **line list** or **line listing**. Table 2.1 is a typical line listing from an epidemiologic investigation of an apparent cluster of hepatitis A.

The line listing is one type of epidemiologic database, and is organized like a spreadsheet with rows and columns. Typically, each row is called a **record** or **observation** and represents one person or case of disease. Each column is called a **variable** and contains information about one characteristic of the individual, such as race or date of birth. The first column or variable of an epidemiologic database usually contains the person's name, initials, or identification number. Other columns might contain demographic information, clinical details, and exposures possibly related to illness.

A **variable** can be any characteristic that differs from person to person, such as height, sex, smallpox vaccination status, or physical activity pattern. The **value** of a variable is the number or descriptor that applies to a particular person, such as 5'6" (168 cm), female, and never vaccinated.

Table 2.1 Line Listing of Hepatitis A Cases, County Health Department, January — February 2004

ID	Date of Diagnosis	Town	Age (Years)	Sex	Hosp	Jaundice	Outbreak	IV Drugs	IgM Pos	Highest ALT*
01	01/05	B	74	M	Y	N	N	N	Y	232
02	01/06	J	29	M	N	Y	N	Y	Y	285
03	01/08	K	37	M	Y	Y	N	N	Y	3250
04	01/19	J	3	F	N	N	N	N	Y	1100
05	01/30	C	39	M	N	Y	N	N	Y	4146
06	02/02	D	23	M	Y	Y	N	Y	Y	1271
07	02/03	F	19	M	Y	Y	N	N	Y	300
08	02/05	I	44	M	N	Y	N	N	Y	766
09	02/19	G	28	M	Y	N	N	Y	Y	23
10	02/22	E	29	F	N	Y	Y	N	Y	543
11	02/23	A	21	F	Y	Y	Y	N	Y	1897
12	02/24	H	43	M	N	Y	Y	N	Y	1220
13	02/26	B	49	F	N	N	N	N	Y	644
14	02/26	H	42	F	N	N	Y	N	Y	2581
15	02/27	E	59	F	Y	Y	Y	N	Y	2892
16	02/27	E	18	M	Y	N	Y	N	Y	814
17	02/27	A	19	M	N	Y	Y	N	Y	2812
18	02/28	E	63	F	Y	Y	Y	N	Y	4218
19	02/28	E	61	F	Y	Y	Y	N	Y	3410
20	02/29	A	40	M	N	Y	Y	N	Y	4297

* ALT = Alanine aminotransferase

Some epidemiologic databases, such as line listings for a small cluster of disease, may have only a few rows (records) and a limited number of columns (variables). Such small line listings are sometimes maintained by hand on a single sheet of paper. Other databases, such as birth or death records for the entire country, might have thousands of records and hundreds of variables and are best handled with a computer. However, even when records are computerized, a line listing with key variables is often printed to facilitate review of the data.

Icon of the Epi Info computer software developed at CDC

One computer software package that is widely used by epidemiologists to manage data is Epi Info, a free package developed at CDC. Epi Info allows the user to design a questionnaire, enter data right into the questionnaire, edit the data, and analyze the data. Two versions are available:

Epi Info 3 (formerly Epi Info 2000 or Epi Info 2002) is Windows-based, and continues to be supported and upgraded. It is the recommended version and can be downloaded from the CDC website: http://www.cdc.gov/epiinfo/downloads.htm.

Epi Info 6 is DOS-based, widely used, but being phased out.

This lesson includes Epi Info commands for creating frequency distributions and calculating some of the measures of central location and spread described in the lesson. Since Epi Info 3 is the recommended version, only commands for this version are provided in the text; corresponding commands for Epi Info 6 are offered at the end of the lesson.

Types of Variables

Look again at the variables (columns) and values (individual entries in each column) in Table 2.1. If you were asked to summarize these data, how would you do it?

First, notice that for certain variables, the values are **numeric**; for others, the values are **descriptive**. The type of values influence the way in which the variables can be summarized. Variables can be classified into one of four types, depending on the type of scale used to characterize their values (Table 2.2).

Table 2.2 Types of Variables

Scale		Example	Values
Nominal	\ "categorical" or	disease status	yes / no
Ordinal	/ "qualitative"	ovarian cancer	Stage I, II, III, or IV
Interval	\ "continuous" or	date of birth	any date from recorded time to current
Ratio	/ "quantitative"	tuberculin skin test	0 – ??? of induration

- A **nominal-scale variable** is one whose values are categories without any numerical ranking, such as county of residence. In epidemiology, nominal variables with only two categories are very common: alive or dead, ill or well, vaccinated or unvaccinated, or did or did not eat the potato salad. A nominal variable with two mutually exclusive categories is sometimes called a dichotomous variable.
- An **ordinal-scale variable** has values that can be ranked but are not necessarily evenly spaced, such as stage of cancer (see Table 2.3).
- An **interval-scale variable** is measured on a scale of equally spaced units, but without a true zero point, such as date of birth.
- A **ratio-scale variable** is an interval variable with a true zero point, such as height in centimeters or duration of illness.

Nominal- and ordinal-scale variables are considered **qualitative** or **categorical** variables, whereas interval- and ratio-scale variables are considered **quantitative** or **continuous** variables. Sometimes the same variable can be measured using both a nominal scale and a ratio scale. For example, the tuberculin skin tests of a group of persons potentially exposed to a co-worker with tuberculosis can be measured as "positive" or "negative" (nominal scale) or in millimeters of induration (ratio scale).

Table 2.3 Example of Ordinal-Scale Variable: Stages of Breast Cancer*

Stage	Tumor Size	Lymph Node Involvement	Metastasis (Spread)
I	Less than 2 cm	No	No
II	Between 2 and 5 cm	No or in same side of breast	No
III	More than 5 cm	Yes, on same side of breast	No
IV	Not applicable	Not applicable	Yes

* This table describes the stages of breast cancer. Note that each stage is more extensive than the previous one and generally carries a less favorable prognosis, but you cannot say that the difference between Stages 1 and 3 is the same as the difference between Stages 2 and 4.

Exercise 2.1

For each of the variables listed below from the line listing in Table 2.1, identify what type of variable it is.

A. *Nominal*
B. *Ordinal*
C. *Interval*
D. *Ratio*

_____ 1. Date of diagnosis

_____ 2. Town of residence

_____ 3. Age (years)

_____ 4. Sex

_____ 5. Highest alanine aminotransferase (ALT)

 Check your answers on page 2-59

Frequency Distributions

Look again at the data in Table 2.1. How many of the cases (or case-patients) are male?

When a database contains only a limited number of records, you can easily pick out the information you need directly from the raw data. By scanning the 5th column, you can see that 12 of the 20 case-patients are male.

With larger databases, however, picking out the desired information at a glance becomes increasingly difficult. To facilitate the task, the variables can be summarized into tables called **frequency distributions**.

A frequency distribution displays the values a variable can take and the number of persons or records with each value. For example, suppose you have data from a study of women with ovarian cancer and wish to look at parity, that is, the number of times each woman has given birth. To construct a frequency distribution that displays these data:

- First, list all the values that the variable *parity* can take, from the lowest possible value to the highest.
- Then, for each value, record the number of women who had that number of births (twins and other multiple-birth pregnancies count only once).

Table 2.4 displays what the resulting frequency distribution would look like. Notice that the frequency distribution includes all values of parity between the lowest and highest observed, even though there were no women for some values. Notice also that each column is clearly labeled, and that the total is given in the bottom row.

Table 2.4 Distribution of Case-Subjects by Parity (Ratio-Scale Variable), Ovarian Cancer Study, CDC

Parity	Number of Cases
0	45
1	25
2	43
3	32
4	22
5	8
6	2
7	0
8	1
9	0
10	1
Total	179

Data Sources: Lee NC, Wingo PA, Gwinn ML, Rubin GL, Kendrick JS, Webster LA, Ory HW. The reduction in risk of ovarian cancer associated with oral contraceptive use. N Engl J Med 1987;316: 650–5.
Centers for Disease Control Cancer and Steroid Hormone Study. Oral contraceptive use and the risk of ovarian cancer. JAMA 1983;249:1596–9.

To create a frequency distribution from a data set in Analysis Module:

Select **frequencies**, then choose variable.

Table 2.4 displays the frequency distribution for a continuous variable. Continuous variables are often further summarized with measures of central location and measures of spread. Distributions for ordinal and nominal variables are illustrated in Tables 2.5 and 2.6, respectively. Categorical variables are usually further summarized as ratios, proportions, and rates (discussed in Lesson 3).

Table 2.5 Distribution of Cases by Stage of Disease (Ordinal-Scale Variable), Ovarian Cancer Study, CDC

Stage	CASES	
	Number	Percent
I	45	20
II	11	5
III	104	58
IV	30	17
Total	179	100

Data Sources: Lee NC, Wingo PA, Gwinn ML, Rubin GL, Kendrick JS, Webster LA, Ory HW. The reduction in risk of ovarian cancer associated with oral contraceptive use. N Engl J Med 1987;316: 650–5.
Centers for Disease Control Cancer and Steroid Hormone Study. Oral contraceptive use and the risk of ovarian cancer. JAMA 1983;249:1596–9.

Table 2.6 Distribution of Cases by Enrollment Site (Nominal-Scale Variable), Ovarian Cancer Study, CDC

| | CASES | |
Enrollment Site	Number	Percent
Atlanta	18	10
Connecticut	39	22
Detroit	35	20
Iowa	30	17
New Mexico	7	4
San Francisco	33	18
Seattle	9	5
Utah	8	4
Total	179	100

Data Sources: Lee NC, Wingo PA, Gwinn ML, Rubin GL, Kendrick JS, Webster LA, Ory HW. The reduction in risk of ovarian cancer associated with oral contraceptive use. N Engl J Med 1987;316: 650–5.
Centers for Disease Control Cancer and Steroid Hormone Study. Oral contraceptive use and the risk of ovarian cancer. JAMA 1983;249:1596–9.

Epi Info Demonstration: Creating a Frequency Distribution

Scenario: In Oswego, New York, numerous people became sick with gastroenteritis after attending a church picnic. To identify all who became ill and to determine the source of illness, an epidemiologist administered a questionnaire to almost all of the attendees. The data from these questionnaires have been entered into an Epi Info file called Oswego.

Question: In the outbreak that occurred in Oswego, how many of the participants became ill?

Answer: In Epi Info:
Select Analyzing Data.
Select Read (Import). The default data set should be Sample.mdb. Under Views, scroll down to view OSWEGO, and double click, or click once and then click OK.
Select Frequencies. Then click on the down arrow beneath Frequency of, scroll down and select ILL, then click OK.

The resulting frequency distribution should indicate 46 ill persons, and 29 persons not ill.

Your Turn: How many of the Oswego picnic attendees drank coffee? [Answer: 31]

Exercise 2.2

At an influenza immunization clinic at a retirement community, residents were asked in how many previous years they had received influenza vaccine. The answers from the first 19 residents are listed below. Organize these data into a frequency distribution.

2, 0, 3, 1, 0, 1, 2, 2, 4, 8, 1, 3, 3, 12, 1, 6, 2, 5, 1

 Check your answers on page 2-59

Properties of Frequency Distributions

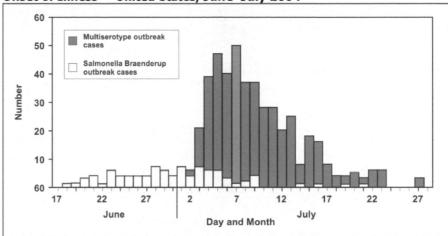

The data in a frequency distribution can be graphed. We call this type of graph a histogram. Figure 2.1 is a graph of the number of outbreak-related salmonellosis cases by date of illness onset.

Figure 2.1 Number of Outbreak-Related Salmonellosis Cases by Date of Onset of Illness — United States, June–July 2004

Source: Centers for Disease Control and Prevention. Outbreaks of Salmonella infections associated with eating Roma tomatoes–United States and Canada, 2004. MMWR 54;325–8.

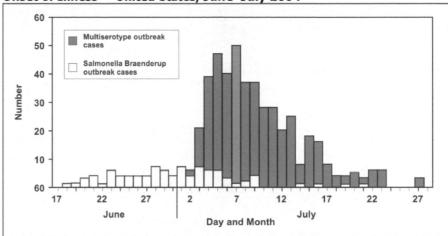

Even a quick look at this graph reveals three features:
- Where the distribution has its peak (**central location**),
- How widely dispersed it is on both sides of the peak (**spread**), and
- Whether it is more or less symmetrically distributed on the two sides of the peak

Central location

Note that the data in Figure 2.1 seem to cluster around a central value, with progressively fewer persons on either side of this central value. This type of symmetric distribution, as illustrated in Figure 2.2, is the classic bell-shaped curve — also known as a normal distribution. The clustering at a particular value is known as the **central location** or **central tendency** of a frequency distribution. The central location of a distribution is one of its most important properties. Sometimes it is cited as a single value that summarizes the entire distribution. Figure 2.3 illustrates the graphs of three frequency distributions identical in shape but with different central locations.

Graphing will be covered in Lesson 4

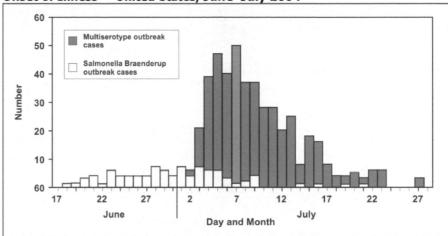

Figure 2.2 Bell-Shaped Curve

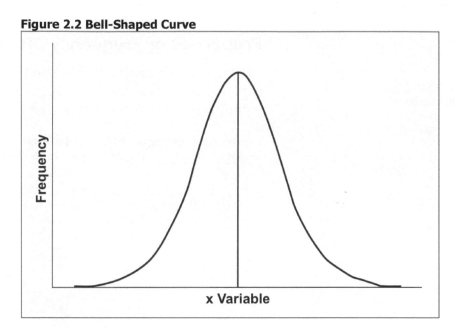

Figure 2.3 Three Identical Curves with Different Central Locations

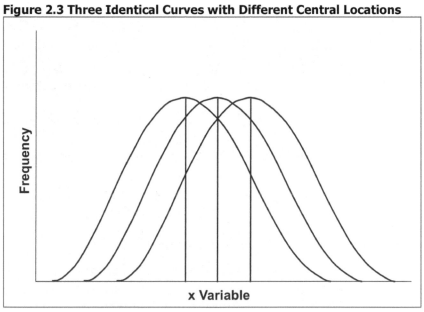

Three measures of central location are commonly used in epidemiology: **arithmetic mean**, **median**, and **mode**. Two other measures that are used less often are the **midrange** and **geometric mean**. All of these measures will be discussed later in this lesson.

Depending on the shape of the frequency distribution, all measures of central location can be identical or different. Additionally, measures of central location can be in the middle or off to one side or the other.

Spread

A second property of frequency distribution is **spread** (also called variation or dispersion). Spread refers to the distribution out from a central value. Two measures of spread commonly used in epidemiology are **range** and **standard deviation**. For most distributions seen in epidemiology, the spread of a frequency distribution is independent of its central location. Figure 2.4 illustrates three theoretical frequency distributions that have the same central location but different amounts of spread. Measures of spread will be discussed later in this lesson.

Figure 2.4 Three Distributions with Same Central Location but Different Spreads

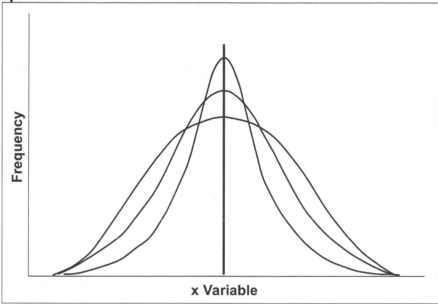

Shape

Skewness refers to the **tail**, not the **hump**. So a distribution that is skewed to the left has a long left tail.

A third property of a frequency distribution is its **shape**. The graphs of the three theoretical frequency distributions in Figure 2.4 were completely **symmetrical**. Frequency distributions of some characteristics of human populations tend to be symmetrical. On the other hand, the data on parity in Figure 2.5 are **asymmetrical** or more commonly referred to as **skewed**.

Figure 2.5 Distribution of Case-Subjects by Parity, Ovarian Cancer Study, CDC

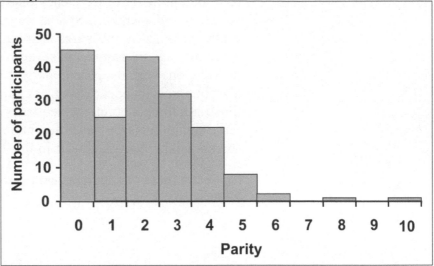

Data Sources: Lee NC, Wingo PA, Gwinn ML, Rubin GL, Kendrick JS, Webster LA, Ory HW. The reduction in risk of ovarian cancer associated with oral contraceptive use. N Engl J Med 1987;316: 650–5.
Centers for Disease Control Cancer and Steroid Hormone Study. Oral contraceptive use and the risk of ovarian cancer. JAMA 1983;249:1596–9.

A distribution that has a central location to the left and a tail off to the right is said to be **positively skewed** or **skewed to the right**. In Figure 2.6, distribution A is skewed to the right. A distribution that has a central location to the right and a tail to the left is said to be **negatively skewed** or **skewed to the left**. In Figure 2.6, distribution C is skewed to the left.

Figure 2.6 Three Distributions with Different Skewness

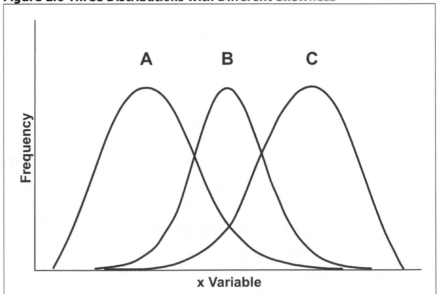

Question: How would you describe the parity data in Figure 2.5?

Answer: Figure 2.5 is skewed to the right. Skewing to the right is common in distributions that begin with zero, such as number of servings consumed, number of sexual partners in the past month, and number of hours spent in vigorous exercise in the past week.

One distribution deserves special mention — the **Normal** or **Gaussian distribution**. This is the classic symmetrical bell-shaped curve like the one shown in Figure 2.2. It is defined by a mathematical equation and is very important in statistics. Not only do the mean, median, and mode coincide at the central peak, but the area under the curve helps determine measures of spread such as the standard deviation and confidence interval covered later in this lesson.

Methods for Summarizing Data

Knowing the type of variable helps you decide how to summarize the data. Table 2.7 displays the ways in which different variables might be summarized.

Table 2.7 Methods for Summarizing Different Types of Variables

Scale	Ratio or Proportion	Measure of Central Location	Measure of Spread
Nominal	yes	no	no
Ordinal	yes	no	no
Interval	yes, but might need to group first	yes	yes
Ratio	yes, but might need to group first	yes	yes

Measures of Central Location

A measure of central location provides a single value that summarizes an entire distribution of data. Suppose you had data from an outbreak of gastroenteritis affecting 41 persons who had recently attended a wedding. If your supervisor asked you to describe the ages of the affected persons, you could simply list the ages of each person. Alternatively, your supervisor might prefer one summary number — a measure of **central location**. Saying that the mean (or average) age was 48 years rather than reciting 41 ages is certainly more efficient, and most likely more meaningful.

Measures of central location include the **mode, median, arithmetic mean, midrange**, and **geometric mean**. Selecting the best measure to use for a given distribution depends largely on two factors:
- The **shape or skewness** of the distribution, and
- The intended **use** of the measure.

Each measure — what it is, how to calculate it, and when best to use it — is described in this section.

Mode

Definition of mode
The mode is the value that occurs most often in a set of data. It can be determined simply by tallying the number of times each value occurs. Consider, for example, the number of doses of diphtheria-pertussis-tetanus (DPT) vaccine each of seventeen 2-year-old children in a particular village received:

$$0, 0, 1, 1, 2, 2, 2, 3, 3, 3, 3, 3, 3, 4, 4, 4, 4$$

Two children received no doses; two children received 1 dose; three received 2 doses; six received 3 doses; and four received all 4 doses. Therefore, the mode is 3 doses, because more children received 3 doses than any other number of doses.

Method for identifying the mode

Step 1. Arrange the observations into a frequency distribution, indicating the values of the variable and the frequency with which each value occurs. (Alternatively, for a data set with only a few values, arrange the actual values in ascending order, as was done with the DPT vaccine doses above.)

Step 2. Identify the value that occurs most often.

EXAMPLES: Identifying the Mode

Example A: *Table 2.8 (on page 2-17) provides data from 30 patients who were hospitalized and received antibiotics. For the variable "length of stay" (LOS) in the hospital, identify the mode.*

Step 1. Arrange the data in a frequency distribution.

LOS	Frequency	LOS	Frequency	LOS	Frequency
0	1	10	5	20	0
1	0	11	1	21	0
2	1	12	3	22	1
3	1	13	1	.	0
4	1	14	1	.	0
5	2	15	0	27	1
6	1	16	1	.	0
7	1	17	0	.	0
8	1	18	2	49	1
9	3	19	1		

Alternatively, arrange the values in ascending order.

0, 2, 3, 4, 5, 5, 6, 7, 8, 9,
9, 9, 10, 10, 10, 10, 10, 11, 12, 12,
12, 13, 14, 16, 18, 18, 19, 22, 27, 49

Step 2. Identify the value that occurs most often.

Most values appear once, but the distribution includes two 5s, three 9s, five 10s, three 12s, and two 18s. Because 10 appears most frequently, the mode is 10.

Example B: *Find the mode of the following incubation periods for hepatitis A: 27, 31, 15, 30, and 22 days.*

Step 1. Arrange the values in ascending order.

15, 22, 27, 30, and 31 days

Step 2. Identify the value that occurs most often.

None

Note: When no value occurs more than once, the distribution is said to have no mode.

Example C: *Find the mode of the following incubation periods for Bacillus cereus food poisoning:*
2, 3, 3, 3, 3, 3, 4, 4, 5, 6, 7, 9, 10, 11, 11, 12, 12, 12, 12, 12, 14, 14, 15, 17, 18, 20, 21 hours

Step 1. Arrange the values in ascending order.

Done

Step 2. Identify the values that occur most often.

Five 3s and five 12s

Example C illustrates the fact that a frequency distribution can have more than one mode. When this occurs, the distribution is said to be **bi-modal**. Indeed, *Bacillus cereus* is known to cause two syndromes with different incubation periods: a short-incubation-period (1–6 hours) syndrome characterized by vomiting; and a long-incubation-period (6–24 hours) syndrome characterized by diarrhea.

Table 2.8 Sample Data from the Northeast Consortium Vancomycin Quality Improvement Project

ID	Admission Date	Discharge Date	LOS	DOB (mm/dd)	DOB (year)	Age	Sex	ESRD	No. Days Vancomycin	Vancomycin OK?
1	1/01	1/10	9	11/18	1928	66	M	Y	3	N
2	1/08	1/30	22	01/21	1916	78	F	N	10	Y
3	1/16	3/06	49	04/22	1920	74	F	N	32	Y
4	1/23	2/04	12	05/14	1919	75	M	N	5	Y
5	1/24	2/01	8	08/17	1929	65	M	N	4	N
6	1/27	2/14	18	01/11	1918	77	M	N	6	Y
7	2/06	2/16	10	01/09	1920	75	F	N	2	Y
8	2/12	2/22	10	06/12	1927	67	M	N	1	N
9	2/22	3/04	10	05/09	1915	79	M	N	8	N
10	2/22	3/08	14	04/09	1920	74	F	N	10	N
11	2/25	3/04	7	07/28	1915	79	F	N	4	N
12	3/02	3/14	12	04/24	1928	66	F	N	8	N
13	3/11	3/17	6	11/09	1925	69	M	N	3	N
14	3/18	3/23	5	04/08	1924	70	F	N	2	N
15	3/19	3/28	9	09/13	1915	79	F	N	1	Y
16	3/27	4/01	5	01/28	1912	83	F	N	4	Y
17	3/31	4/02	2	03/14	1921	74	M	N	2	Y
18	4/12	4/24	12	02/07	1927	68	F	N	3	N
19	4/17	5/06	19	03/04	1921	74	F	N	11	Y
20	4/29	5/26	27	02/23	1921	74	F	N	14	N
21	5/11	5/15	4	05/05	1923	72	M	N	4	Y
22	5/14	5/14	0	01/03	1911	84	F	N	1	N
23	5/20	5/30	10	11/11	1922	72	F	N	9	Y
24	5/21	6/08	18	08/08	1912	82	M	N	14	Y
25	5/26	6/05	10	09/28	1924	70	M	Y	5	N
26	5/27	5/30	3	05/14	1899	96	F	N	2	N
27	5/28	6/06	9	07/22	1921	73	M	N	1	Y
28	6/07	6/20	13	12/30	1896	98	F	N	3	N
29	6/07	6/23	16	08/31	1906	88	M	N	1	N
30	6/16	6/27	11	07/07	1917	77	F	N	7	Y

To identify the mode from a data set in Analysis Module:

Epi Info does not have a Mode command. Thus, the best way to identify the mode is to create a histogram and look for the tallest column(s).

Select **graphs**, then choose histogram under **Graph Type.**

The tallest column(s) is(are) the mode(s).

NOTE: The Means command provides a mode, but only the lowest value if a distribution has more than one mode.

Properties and uses of the mode

The mode is the easiest measure of central location to understand and explain. It is also the easiest to identify, and requires no calculations.

- The mode is the preferred measure of central location for addressing which value is the most popular or the most common. For example, the mode is used to describe which day of the week people most prefer to come to the influenza vaccination clinic, or the "typical" number of doses of DPT the children in a particular community have received by their second birthday.

- As demonstrated, a distribution can have a single mode. However, a distribution has more than one mode if two or more values tie as the most frequent values. It has no mode if no value appears more than once.

- The mode is used almost exclusively as a "descriptive" measure. It is almost never used in statistical manipulations or analyses.

- The mode is not typically affected by one or two extreme values (outliers).

Exercise 2.3

Using the same vaccination data as in Exercise 2.2, find the mode. (If you answered Exercise 2.2, find the mode from your frequency distribution.)

2, 0, 3, 1, 0, 1, 2, 2, 4, 8, 1, 3, 3, 12, 1, 6, 2, 5, 1

 Check your answers on page 2-59

Median

Definition of median

The median is the middle value of a set of data that has been put into rank order. Similar to the median on a highway that divides the road in two, the statistical median is the value that divides the data into two halves, with one half of the observations being smaller than the median value and the other half being larger. The median is also the 50th percentile of the distribution. Suppose you had the following ages in years for patients with a particular illness:

$$4, 23, 28, 31, 32$$

The median age is 28 years, because it is the middle value, with two values smaller than 28 and two values larger than 28.

Method for identifying the median

Step 1. Arrange the observations into increasing or decreasing order.

Step 2. Find the middle position of the distribution by using the following formula:

$$\text{Middle position} = (n + 1) / 2$$

a. If the number of observations (n) is **odd**, the middle position falls on a single observation.

b. If the number of observations is **even**, the middle position falls between two observations.

Step 3. Identify the value at the middle position.

a. If the number of observations (n) is **odd** and the middle position falls on a single observation, the median equals the value of that observation.

b. If the number of observations is **even** and the middle position falls between two observations, the median equals the average of the two values.

epi Info

To identify the median from a data set in Analysis Module:

Click on the **Means** command under the Statistics folder.
In the **Means Of** drop-down box, select the variable of interest
→ Select **Variable**
Click **OK**
→ You should see the list of the frequency by the variable you selected. Scroll down until you see the Median among other data.

EXAMPLES: Identifying the Median

Example A: Odd Number of Observations
Find the median of the following incubation periods for hepatitis A: 27, 31, 15, 30, and 22 days.

Step 1. Arrange the values in ascending order.

15, 22, 27, 30, and 31 days

Step 2. Find the middle position of the distribution by using (n + 1) / 2.

Middle position = (5 + 1) / 2 = 6 / 2 = 3

Therefore, the median will be the value at the third observation.

Step 3. Identify the value at the middle position.

Third observation = 27 days

Example B: Even Number of Observations
Suppose a sixth case of hepatitis was reported. Now find the median of the following incubation periods for hepatitis A: 27, 31, 15, 30, 22 and 29 days.

Step 1. Arrange the values in ascending order.

15, 22, 27, 29, 30, and 31 days

Step 2. Find the middle position of the distribution by using (n + 1) / 2.

Middle location = 6 + 1 / 2 = 7 / 2 = 3½

Therefore, the median will be a value halfway between the values of the third and fourth observations.

Step 3. Identify the value at the middle position.

The median equals the average of the values of the third (value = 27) and fourth (value = 29) observations:

Median = (27 + 29) / 2 = 28 days

Epi Info Demonstration: Finding the Median

Question: In the data set named SMOKE, what is the median number of cigarettes smoked per day?

Answer: In Epi Info:
Select Analyze Data.
Select Read (Import). The default data set should be Sample.mdb. Under Views, scroll down to view SMOKE, and double click, or click once and then click OK.
Select Means. Then click on the down arrow beneath Means of, scroll down and select NUMCIGAR, then click OK.

The resulting output should indicate a median of 20 cigarettes smoked per day.

Your Turn: What is the median height of the participants in the smoking study? (Note: The variable is coded as feet-inch-inch, so 5'1" is coded as 501.) [Answer: 503]

Properties and uses of the median

- The median is a good descriptive measure, particularly for data that are skewed, because it is the central point of the distribution.

- The median is relatively easy to identify. It is equal to either a single observed value (if odd number of observations) or the average of two observed values (if even number of observations).

- The median, like the mode, is not generally affected by one or two extreme values (outliers). For example, if the values on the previous page had been 4, 23, 28, 31, and 131 (instead of 31), the median would still be 28.

- The median has less-than-ideal statistical properties. Therefore, it is not often used in statistical manipulations and analyses.

Exercise 2.4

Determine the median for the same vaccination data used in Exercises 2.2. and 2.3.

2, 0, 3, 1, 0, 1, 2, 2, 4, 8, 1, 3, 3, 12, 1, 6, 2, 5, 1

 Check your answers on page 2-59

Arithmetic mean

Definition of mean

The arithmetic mean is a more technical name for what is more commonly called the **mean** or **average**. The arithmetic mean is the value that is closest to all the other values in a distribution.

Method for calculating the mean

Step 1. Add all of the observed values in the distribution.

Step 2. Divide the sum by the number of observations.

EXAMPLE: Finding the Mean

Find the mean of the following incubation periods for hepatitis A: 27, 31, 15, 30, and 22 days.

Step 1. Add all of the observed values in the distribution.

$$27 + 31 + 15 + 30 + 22 = 125$$

Step 2. Divide the sum by the number of observations.

$$125 / 5 = 25.0$$

Therefore, the mean incubation period is 25.0 days.

Properties and uses of the arithmetic mean

- The mean has excellent statistical properties and is commonly used in additional statistical manipulations and analyses. One such property is called the **centering property of the mean**. When the mean is subtracted from each observation in the data set, the sum of these differences is zero (i.e., the negative sum is equal to the positive sum). For the data in the previous hepatitis A example:

Value	minus	Mean	Difference
15	–	25.0	-10.0
22	–	25.0	-3.0
27	–	25.0	+ 2.0
30	–	25.0	+ 5.0
31	–	25.0	+ 6.0
125	–	125.0 = 0	+ 13.0 - 13.0 = 0

To identify the mean from a data set in Analysis Module:

Click on the **Means** command under the Statistics folder
In the **Means Of** drop-down box, select the variable of interest
→ Select **Variable**
Click **OK**
→ You should see the list of the frequency by the variable you selected. Scroll down until you see the Mean among other data.

Mean: the center of gravity of the distribution

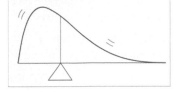

This demonstrates that the mean is the arithmetic center of the distribution.

- Because of this centering property, the mean is sometimes called the **center of gravity** of a frequency distribution. If the frequency distribution is plotted on a graph, and the graph is balanced on a fulcrum, the point at which the distribution would balance would be the mean.

- The arithmetic mean is the best descriptive measure for data that are normally distributed.

- On the other hand, the mean is not the measure of choice for data that are severely skewed or have extreme values in one direction or another. Because the arithmetic mean uses all of the observations in the distribution, it is affected by any extreme value. Suppose that the last value in the previous distribution was 131 instead of 31. The mean would be 225 / 5 = 45.0 rather than 25.0. As a result of one extremely large value, the mean is much larger than all values in the distribution except the extreme value (the "outlier").

Epi Info Demonstration: Finding the Mean

Question: In the data set named SMOKE, what is the mean weight of the participants?

Answer: In Epi Info:
Select Analyze Data.
  Select Read (Import). The default data set should be Sample.mdb. Under Views, scroll down to view SMOKE, and double click, or click once and then click OK. Note that 9 persons have a weight of 777, and 10 persons have a weight of 999. These are code for "refused" and "missing." To delete these records, enter the following commands:
  Click on Select. Then type in the *weight < 770,* or select weight from available values, then type < 750, and click on OK.
Select Means. Then click on the down arrow beneath Means of, scroll down and select WEIGHT, then click OK.

The resulting output should indicate a mean weight of 158.116 pounds.

Your Turn: What is the mean number of cigarettes smoked per day? [Answer: 17]

Exercise 2.5

Determine the mean for the same set of vaccination data.

2, 0, 3, 1, 0, 1, 2, 2, 4, 8, 1, 3, 3, 12, 1, 6, 2, 5, 1

 Check your answers on page 2-60

The midrange (midpoint of an interval)

Definition of midrange

The midrange is the half-way point or the midpoint of a set of observations. The midrange is usually calculated as an intermediate step in determining other measures.

Method for identifying the midrange

Step 1.   Identify the smallest (minimum) observation and the largest (maximum) observation

Step 2.   Add the minimum plus the maximum, then divide by two.

Exception: Age differs from most other variables because age does not follow the usual rules for rounding to the nearest integer. Someone who is 17 years and 360 days old cannot claim to be 18 year old for at least 5 more days. Thus, to identify the midrange for age (in years) data, you must add the smallest (minimum) observation plus the largest (maximum) observation plus 1, then divide by two.

Midrange (most types of data) = (minimum + maximum) / 2
Midrange (age data) = (minimum + maximum + 1) / 2

Consider the following example:

In a particular pre-school, children are assigned to rooms on the basis of age on September 1. Room 2 holds all of the children who were at least 2 years old but not yet 3 years old as of September 1. In other words, every child in room 2 was 2 years old on September 1. What is the midrange of ages of the children in room 2 on September 1?

For descriptive purposes, a reasonable answer is 2. However, recall that the midrange is usually calculated as an intermediate step in other calculations. Therefore, more precision is necessary.

Consider that children born in August have just turned 2 years old. Others, born in September the previous year, are almost but not quite 3 years old. Ignoring seasonal trends in births and assuming a very large room of children, birthdays are expected to be uniformly distributed throughout the year. The youngest child, born on September 1, is exactly 2.000 years old. The oldest child, whose birthday is September 2 of the previous year, is 2.997 years old. For statistical purposes, the mean and midrange of this theoretical group of 2-year-olds are both 2.5 years.

Properties and uses of the midrange

- The midrange is not commonly reported as a measure of central location.

- The midrange is more commonly used as an intermediate step in other calculations, or for plotting graphs of data collected in intervals.

EXAMPLES: Identifying the Midrange

Example A: *Find the midrange of the following incubation periods for hepatitis A: 27, 31, 15, 30, and 22 days.*

Step 1. Identify the minimum and maximum values.

$$Minimum = 15, maximum = 31$$

Step 2. Add the minimum plus the maximum, then divide by two.

$$Midrange = 15 + 31 / 2 = 46 / 2 = 23 days$$

Example B: *Find the midrange of the grouping 15–24 (e.g., number of alcoholic beverages consumed in one week).*

Step 1. Identify the minimum and maximum values.

$$Minimum = 15, maximum = 24$$

Step 2. Add the minimum plus the maximum, then divide by two.

$$Midrange = 15 + 24 / 2 = 39 / 2 = 19.5$$

This calculation assumes that the grouping 15–24 really covers 14.50–24.49…. Since the midrange of 14.50–24.49… = 19.49…, the midrange can be reported as 19.5.

Example C: *Find the midrange of the age group 15–24 years.*

Step 1. Identify the minimum and maximum values.

$$Minimum = 15, maximum = 24$$

Step 2. Add the minimum plus the maximum plus 1, then divide by two.

$$Midrange = (15 + 24 + 1) / 2 = 40 / 2 = 20 years$$

Age differs from the majority of other variables because age does not follow the usual rules for rounding to the nearest integer. For most variables, 15.99 can be rounded to 16. However, an adolescent who is 15 years and 360 days old cannot claim to be 16 years old (and hence get his driver's license or learner's permit) for at least 5 more days. Thus, the interval of 15–24 years really spans 15.0–24.99… years. The midrange of 15.0 and 24.99… = 19.99… = 20.0 years.

Geometric mean

To calculate the geometric mean, you need a scientific calculator with log and y^x keys.

Definition of geometric mean

The geometric mean is the mean or average of a set of data measured on a logarithmic scale. The geometric mean is used when the logarithms of the observations are distributed normally (symmetrically) rather than the observations themselves. The geometric mean is particularly useful in the laboratory for data from serial dilution assays (1/2, 1/4, 1/8, 1/16, etc.) and in environmental sampling data.

More About Logarithms

A logarithm is the power to which a base is raised.

To what power would you need to raise a base of 10 to get a value of 100?
Because 10 times 10 or 10^2 equals 100, the log of 100 at base 10 equals 2. Similarly, the log of 16 at base 2 equals 4, because $2^4 = 2 \times 2 \times 2 \times 2 = 16$.

$2^0 = 1$ (anything raised to the 0 power is 1) $10^0 = 1$ (Anything raised to the 0 power equals 1)
$2^1 = 2 = 2$ $10^1 = 10$
$2^2 = 2 \times 2 = 4$ $10^2 = 100$
$2^3 = 2 \times 2 \times 2 = 8$ $10^3 = 1,000$
$2^4 = 2 \times 2 \times 2 \times 2 = 16$ $10^4 = 10,000$
$2^5 = 2 \times 2 \times 2 \times 2 \times 2 = 32$ $10^5 = 100,000$
$2^6 = 2 \times 2 \times 2 \times 2 \times 2 \times 2 = 64$ $10^6 = 1,000,000$
$2^7 = 2 \times 2 \times 2 \times 2 \times 2 \times 2 \times 2 = 128$ $10^7 = 10,000,000$
and so on.   and so on.

An antilog raises the base to the power (logarithm). For example, the antilog of 2 at base 10 is 10^2, or 100. The antilog of 4 at base 2 is 2^4, or 16. The majority of titers are reported as multiples of 2 (e.g., 2, 4, 8, etc.); therefore, base 2 is typically used when dealing with titers.

Method for calculating the geometric mean

There are two methods for calculating the geometric mean.

Method A

Step 1.   Take the logarithm of each value.

Step 2.   Calculate the mean of the log values by summing the log values, then dividing by the number of observations.

Step 3.   Take the antilog of the mean of the log values to get the geometric mean.

Method B

Step 1.   Calculate the product of the values by multiplying all of the values together.

Step 2.   Take the nth root of the product (where n is the number of observations) to get the geometric mean.

EXAMPLES: Calculating the Geometric Mean

Example A: Using Method A
Calculate the geometric mean from the following set of data.

10, 10, 100, 100, 100, 100, 10,000, 100,000, 100,000, 1,000,000

Because these values are all multiples of 10, it makes sense to use logs of base 10.

Step 1. Take the log (in this case, to base 10) of each value.

$$\log10(x_i) = 1, 1, 2, 2, 2, 2, 4, 5, 5, 6$$

Step 2. Calculate the mean of the log values by summing and dividing by the number of observations (in this case, 10).

$$\text{Mean of } \log10(x_i) = (1+1+2+2+2+2+4+5+5+6) / 10 = 30 / 10 = 3$$

Step 3. Take the antilog of the mean of the log values to get the geometric mean.

$$\text{Antilog}10(3) = 10^3 = 1,000.$$

The geometric mean of the set of data is 1,000.

Example B: Using Method B
Calculate the geometric mean from the following 95% confidence intervals of an odds ratio: 1.0, 9.0

Step 1. Calculate the product of the values by multiplying all values together.

$$1.0 \times 9.0 = 9.0$$

Step 2. Take the square root of the product.

The geometric mean = square root of 9.0 = 3.0.

Properties and uses of the geometric mean

The geometric mean is the average of logarithmic values, converted back to the base. The geometric mean tends to dampen the effect of extreme values and is always smaller than the corresponding arithmetic mean. In that sense, the geometric mean is less sensitive than the arithmetic mean to one or a few extreme values.

- The geometric mean is the measure of choice for variables measured on an exponential or logarithmic scale, such as dilutional titers or assays.
- The geometric mean is often used for environmental samples, when levels can range over several orders of magnitude. For example, levels of coliforms in samples taken from a body of water can range from less than 100 to more than 100,000.

Exercise 2.6

Using the dilution titers shown below, calculate the geometric mean titer of convalescent antibodies against tularemia among 10 residents of Martha's Vineyard. [Hint: Use only the second number in the ratio, i.e., for 1:640, use 640.]

ID #	Acute	Convalescent
1	1:16	1:512
2	1:16	1:512
3	1:32	1:128
4	not done	1:512
5	1:32	1:1024
6	"negative"	1:1024
7	1:256	1:2048
8	1:32	1:128
9	"negative"	1:4096
10	1:16	1:1024

✔ **Check your answers on page 2-60**

Selecting the appropriate measure

Measures of central location are single values that summarize the observed values of a distribution. The mode provides the most common value, the median provides the central value, the arithmetic mean provides the average value, the midrange provides the midpoint value, and the geometric mean provides the logarithmic average.

The mode and median are useful as descriptive measures. However, they are not often used for further statistical manipulations. In contrast, the mean is not only a good descriptive measure, but it also has good statistical properties. The mean is used most often in additional statistical manipulations.

While the arithmetic mean is the measure of choice when data are normally distributed, the median is the measure of choice for data that are not normally distributed. Because epidemiologic data tend not to be normally distributed (incubation periods, doses, ages of patients), the median is often preferred. The geometric mean is used most commonly with laboratory data, particularly dilution titers or assays and environmental sampling data.

The arithmetic mean uses all the data, which makes it sensitive to outliers. Although the geometric mean also uses all the data, it is not as sensitive to outliers as the arithmetic mean. The midrange, which is based on the minimum and maximum values, is more sensitive to outliers than any other measures. The mode and median tend not to be affected by outliers.

In summary, each measure of central location — mode, median, mean, midrange, and geometric mean — is a single value that is used to represent all of the observed values of a distribution. Each measure has its advantages and limitations. The selection of the most appropriate measure requires judgment based on the characteristics of the data (e.g., normally distributed or skewed, with or without outliers, arithmetic or log scale) and the reason for calculating the measure (e.g., for descriptive or analytic purposes).

Exercise 2.7

For each of the variables listed below from the line listing in Table 2.9, identify which measure of central location is best for representing the data.

A. Mode
B. Median
C. Mean
D. Geometric mean
E. No measure of central location is appropriate

_____ 1. Year of diagnosis

_____ 2. Age (years)

_____ 3. Sex

_____ 4. Highest IFA titer

_____ 5. Platelets x 10^6/L

_____ 6. White blood cell count x 10^9/L

Table 2.9 Line Listing for 12 Patients with Human Monocytotropic Ehrlichiosis — Missouri, 1998–1999

Patient ID	Year of Diagnosis	Age (years)	Sex	Highest IFA* Titer	Platelets x 10^6/L	White Blood Cell Count x 10^9/L
01	1999	44	M	1:1024	90	1.9
02	1999	42	M	1:512	114	3.5
03	1999	63	M	1:2048	83	6.4
04	1999	53	F	1:512	180	4.5
05	1999	77	M	1:1024	44	3.5
06	1999	43	F	1:512	89	1.9
10	1998	22	F	1:128	142	2.1
11	1998	59	M	1:256	229	8.8
12	1998	67	M	1:512	36	4.2
14	1998	49	F	1:4096	271	2.6
15	1998	65	M	1:1024	207	4.3
18	1998	27	M	1:64	246	8.5
Mean:	1998.5	50.92	na	1:976.00	144.25	4.35
Median:	1998.5	51	na	1:512	128	3.85
Geometric Mean:	1998.5	48.08	na	1:574.70	120.84	3.81
Mode:	none	none	M	1:512	none	1.9, 3.5

*Immunofluorescence assay

Data Source: Olano JP, Masters E, Hogrefe W, Walker DH. Human monocytotropic ehrlichiosis, Missouri. Emerg Infect Dis 2003;9:1579-86.

 Check your answers on page 2-60

Measures of Spread

Spread, or dispersion, is the second important feature of frequency distributions. Just as measures of central location describe where the peak is located, measures of spread describe the dispersion (or variation) of values from that peak in the distribution. Measures of spread include the **range**, **interquartile range**, and **standard deviation**.

Range

Definition of range

The range of a set of data is the difference between its largest (maximum) value and its smallest (minimum) value. In the statistical world, the range is reported as a single number and is the result of subtracting the maximum from the minimum value. In the epidemiologic community, the range is usually reported as "from (the minimum) to (the maximum)," that is, as two numbers rather than one.

Method for identifying the range

Step 1. Identify the smallest (minimum) observation and the largest (maximum) observation.

Step 2. Epidemiologically, report the minimum and maximum values. Statistically, subtract the minimum from the maximum value.

EXAMPLE: Identifying the Range

Find the range of the following incubation periods for hepatitis A: 27, 31, 15, 30, and 22 days.

Step 1. Identify the minimum and maximum values.

Minimum = 15, maximum = 31

Step 2. Subtract the minimum from the maximum value.

Range = 31–15 = 16 days

For an epidemiologic or lay audience, you could report that "incubation periods ranged from 15 to 31 days." Statistically, that range is 16 days.

Percentiles

Percentiles divide the data in a distribution into 100 equal parts. The Pth percentile (P ranging from 0 to 100) is the value that has P percent of the observations falling at or below it. In other words, the 90th percentile has 90% of the observations at or below it. The median, the halfway point of the distribution, is the 50th percentile. The maximum value is the 100th percentile, because all values fall at or below the maximum.

Quartiles

Sometimes, epidemiologists group data into four equal parts, or quartiles. Each quartile includes 25% of the data. The cut-off for the first quartile is the 25th percentile. The cut-off for the second quartile is the 50th percentile, which is the median. The cut-off for the third quartile is the 75th percentile. And the cut-off for the fourth quartile is the 100th percentile, which is the maximum.

Interquartile range

The interquartile range is a measure of spread used most commonly with the median. It represents the central portion of the distribution, from the 25th percentile to the 75th percentile. In other words, the interquartile range includes the second and third quartiles of a distribution. The interquartile range thus includes approximately one half of the observations in the set, leaving one quarter of the observations on each side.

Method for determining the interquartile range

Step 1.   Arrange the observations in increasing order.

Step 2.   Find the position of the 1st and 3rd quartiles with the following formulas. Divide the sum by the number of observations.

Position of 1st quartile (Q_1) = 25th percentile = $(n + 1) / 4$
Position of 3rd quartile (Q_3) = 75th percentile = $3(n + 1) / 4 = 3 \times Q_1$

Step 3.   Identify the value of the 1st and 3rd quartiles.

    a.   If a quartile lies **on an observation** (i.e., if its position is a whole number), the value of the quartile is the value of that observation. For example, if the position of a quartile is 20, its value is the value of the 20th observation.

    b.   If a quartile lies **between observations**, the value of the quartile is the value of the lower observation plus the specified fraction of the difference between the observations. For example, if the position of a quartile is 20¼, it lies between the 20th and 21st observations, and its value is the value of the 20th observation, plus ¼ the difference between the value of the 20th and 21st observations.

Step 4. Epidemiologically, report the values at Q_1 and Q_3. Statistically, calculate the interquartile range as Q_3 minus Q_1.

Figure 2.7 The Middle Half of the Observations in a Frequency Distribution Lie within the Interquartile Range

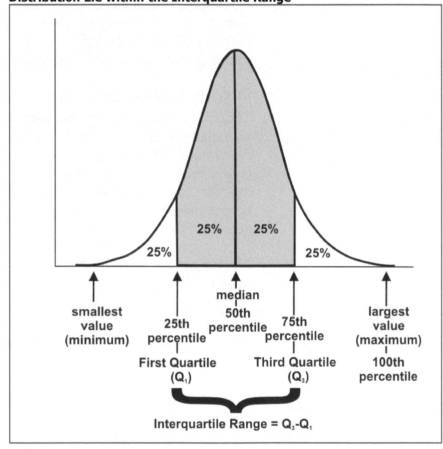

EXAMPLE: Finding the Interquartile Range

Find the interquartile range for the length of stay data in Table 2.8 on page 2-17.

Step 1. Arrange the observations in increasing order.

$$0, \quad 2, \quad 3, \quad 4, \quad 5, \quad 5, \quad 6, \quad 7, \quad 8, \quad 9,$$
$$9, \quad 9, \quad 10, \quad 10, \quad 10, \quad 10, \quad 10, \quad 11, \quad 12, \quad 12,$$
$$12, \quad 13, \quad 14, \quad 16, \quad 18, \quad 18, \quad 19, \quad 22, \quad 27, \quad 49$$

Step 2. Find the position of the 1st and 3rd quartiles. Note that the distribution has 30 observations.

$$\text{Position of Q1} = (n + 1) / 4 = (30 + 1) / 4 = 7.75$$

$$\text{Position of Q3} = 3(n + 1) / 4 = 3(30 + 1) / 4 = 23.25$$

Thus, Q_1 lies ¾ of the way between the 7th and 8th observations, and Q_3 lies ¼ of the way between the 23rd and 24th observations.

Step 3. Identify the value of the 1st and 3rd quartiles (Q_1 and Q_3).

Value of Q_1: The position of Q_1 is 7¾; therefore, the value of Q_1 is equal to the value of the 7th observation plus ¾ of the difference between the values of the 7th and 8th observations:

Value of the 7th observation: 6
Value of the 8th observation: 7

$$Q_1 = 6 + ¾(7 - 6) = 6 + ¾(1) = 6.75$$

Value of Q_3: The position of Q_3 was 23¼; thus, the value of Q_3 is equal to the value of the 23rd observation plus ¼ of the difference between the value of the 23rd and 24th observations:

Value of the 23rd observation: 14
Value of the 24th observation: 16

$$Q_3 = 14 + ¼(16 - 14) = 14 + ¼(2) = 14 + (2 / 4) = 14.5$$

Step 4. Calculate the interquartile range as Q_3 minus Q_1.

$$Q_3 = 14.5$$
$$Q_1 = 6.75$$
$$\text{Interquartile range} = 14.5 - 6.75 = 7.75$$

As indicated above, the median for the length of stay data is 10. Note that the distance between Q_1 and the median is $10 - 6.75 = 3.25$. The distance between Q_3 and the median is $14.5 - 10 = 4.5$. This indicates that the length of stay data is skewed slightly to the right (to the longer lengths of stay).

Epi Info Demonstration: Finding the Interquartile Range

Question: In the data set named SMOKE, what is the interquartile range for the weight of the participants?

Answer: In Epi Info:
Select **Analyze Data**.
Select **Read (Import).** The default data set should be Sample.mdb. Under Views, scroll down to **view SMOKE**, and double click, or click once and then click **OK**.
Click on **Select**. Then type in *weight < 770*, or select weight from available values, then type < 770, and click on **OK**.
Select **Means**. Then click on the down arrow beneath **Means of**, scroll down and select **WEIGHT**, then click **OK**.
Scroll to the bottom of the output to find the first quartile (25% = 130) and the third quartile (75% = 180). So the interquartile range runs from 130 to 180 pounds, for a range of 50 pounds.

Your Turn: What is the interquartile range of height of study participants? [Answer: 506 to 777]

Properties and uses of the interquartile range

- The interquartile range is generally used in conjunction with the median. Together, they are useful for characterizing the central location and spread of any frequency distribution, but particularly those that are skewed.
- For a more complete characterization of a frequency distribution, the 1st and 3rd quartiles are sometimes used with the minimum value, the median, and the maximum value to produce a five-number summary of the distribution. For example, the five-number summary for the length of stay data is:
  Minimum value = 0,
  $Q_1 = 6.75$,
  Median = 10,
  $Q_3 = 14.5$, and
  Maximum value = 49.
- Together, the five values provide a good description of the center, spread, and shape of a distribution. These five values can be used to draw a graphical illustration of the data, as in the boxplot in Figure 2.8.

Figure 2.8 Interquartile Range from Cumulative Frequencies

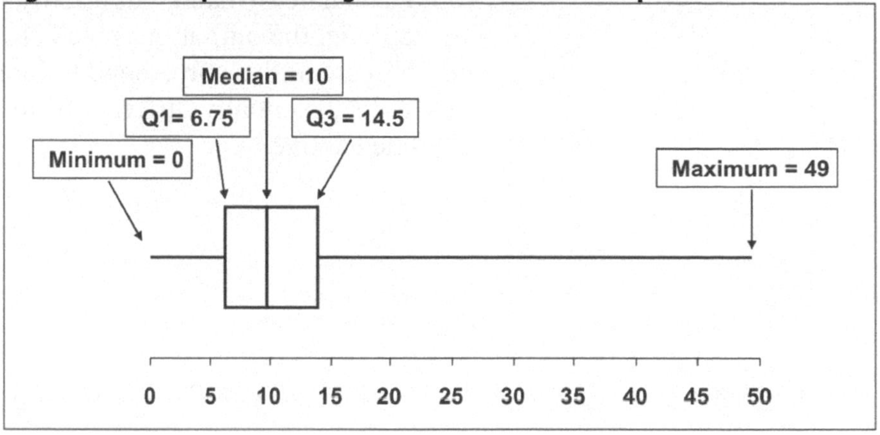

Some statistical analysis software programs such as Epi Info produce frequency distributions with three output columns: the number or count of observations for each value of the distribution, the percentage of observations for that value, and the cumulative percentage. The cumulative percentage, which represents the percentage of observations at or below that value, gives you the percentile (see Table 2.10).

Table 2.10 Frequency Distribution of Length of Hospital Stay, Sample Data, Northeast Consortium Vancomycin Quality Improvement Project

Length of Stay (Days)	Frequency	Percent	Cumulative Percent
0	1	3.3	3.3
2	1	3.3	6.7
3	1	3.3	10.0
4	1	3.3	13.3
5	2	6.7	20.0
6	1	3.3	23.3
7	1	3.3	26.7
8	1	3.3	30.0
9	3	10.0	40.0
10	5	16.7	56.7
11	1	3.3	60.0
12	3	10.0	70.0
13	1	3.3	73.3
14	1	3.3	76.7
16	1	3.3	80.0
18	2	6.7	86.7
19	1	3.3	90.0
22	1	3.3	93.3
27	1	3.3	96.7
49	1	3.3	100.0
Total	**30**		**100.0**

A shortcut to calculating Q_1, the median, and Q_3 by hand is to look at the tabular output from these software programs and note which values include 25%, 50%, and 75% of the data, respectively. This shortcut method gives slightly different results than those you would calculate by hand, but usually the differences are minor. For example, the output in Table 2.10 indicates that the 25th, 50th, and 75th percentiles correspond to lengths of stay of 7, 10 and 14 days, not substantially different from the 6.75, 10 and 14.5 days calculated above.

Exercise 2.8

Determine the first and third quartiles and interquartile range for the same vaccination data as in the previous exercises.

2, 0, 3, 1, 0, 1, 2, 2, 4, 8, 1, 3, 3, 12, 1, 6, 2, 5, 1

 Check your answers on page 2-60

Standard deviation

Definition of standard deviation

The standard deviation is the measure of spread used most commonly with the arithmetic mean. Earlier, the centering property of the mean was described — subtracting the mean from each observation and then summing the differences adds to 0. This concept of subtracting the mean from each observation is the basis for the standard deviation. However, the difference between the mean and each observation is squared to eliminate negative numbers. Then the average is calculated and the square root is taken to get back to the original units.

Method for calculating the standard deviation

Step 1. Calculate the arithmetic mean.

Step 2. Subtract the mean from each observation. Square the difference.

Step 3. Sum the squared differences.

Step 4. Divide the sum of the squared differences by n – 1.

Step 5. Take the square root of the value obtained in Step 4. The result is the **standard deviation**.

Properties and uses of the standard deviation

- The numeric value of the standard deviation does not have an easy, non-statistical interpretation, but similar to other measures of spread, the standard deviation conveys how widely or tightly the observations are distributed from the center. From the previous example, the mean incubation period was 25 days, with a standard deviation of 6.6 days. If the standard deviation in a second outbreak had been 3.7 days (with the same mean incubation period of 25 days), you could say that the incubation periods in the second outbreak showed less variability than did the incubation periods of the first outbreak.

- Standard deviation is usually calculated only when the data are more-or-less "normally distributed," i.e., the data fall into a typical bell-shaped curve. For normally distributed data, the arithmetic mean is the recommended measure of central location, and the standard deviation is the recommended measure of spread. In fact, means should never be reported without their associated standard deviation.

To calculate the standard deviation from a data set in Analysis Module:

Click on the **Means** command under the Statistics folder
In the **Means Of** drop-down box, select the variable of interest
→ Select **Variable**
Click **OK**
→ You should see the list of the frequency by the variable you selected. Scroll down until you see the Standard Deviation (Std Dev) and other data.

EXAMPLE: Calculating the Standard Deviation

Find the mean of the following incubation periods for hepatitis A: 27, 31, 15, 30, and 22 days.

Step 1. Calculate the arithmetic mean.

Mean = (27 + 31 + 15 + 30 + 22) / 5 = 125 / 5 = 25.0

Step 2. Subtract the mean from each observation. Square the difference.

Value	Minus	Mean	Difference	Difference Squared
27	–	25.0	+ 2.0	4.0
31	–	25.0	+ 6.0	36.0
15	–	25.0	−10.0	100.0
30	–	25.0	+ 5.0	25.0
22	–	25.0	− 3.0	9.0

Step 3. Sum the squared differences.

Sum = 4 + 36 + 100 + 25 + 9 = 174

Step 4. Divide the sum of the squared differences by (n − 1). This is the variance.

Variance = 174 / (5 − 1) = 174 / 4 = 43.5 days squared

Step 5. Take the square root of the variance. The result is the standard deviation.

Standard deviation = square root of 43.5 = 6.6 days

Areas included in normal distribution:

±1 SD includes 68.3%

±1.96 SD includes 95.0%

±2 SD includes 95.5%

±3 SD includes 99.7%

Consider the normal curve illustrated in Figure 2.9. The mean is at the center, and data are equally distributed on either side of this mean. The points that show ±1, 2, and 3 standard deviations are marked on the x axis. For normally distributed data, approximately two-thirds (68.3%, to be exact) of the data fall within one standard deviation of either side of the mean; 95.5% of the data fall within two standard deviations of the mean; and 99.7% of the data fall within three standard deviations. Exactly 95.0% of the data fall within 1.96 standard deviations of the mean.

Figure 2.9 Area Under Normal Curve within 1, 2 and 3 Standard Deviations

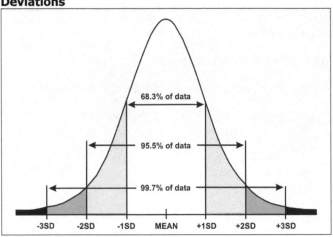

Exercise 2.9

Calculate the standard deviation for the same set of vaccination data.

2, 0, 3, 1, 0, 1, 2, 2, 4, 8, 1, 3, 3, 12, 1, 6, 2, 5, 1

 Check your answers on page 2-61

Standard error of the mean

Definition of standard error

The standard deviation is sometimes confused with another measure with a similar name — the standard error of the mean. However, the two are not the same. The standard deviation describes variability in a set of data. The standard error of the mean refers to variability we might expect in the arithmetic means of repeated samples taken from the same population.

The standard error assumes that the data you have is actually a sample from a larger population. According to the assumption, your sample is just one of an infinite number of possible samples that could be taken from the source population. Thus, the mean for your sample is just one of an infinite number of other sample means. The standard error quantifies the variation in those sample means.

Method for calculating the standard error of the mean

Step 1.   Calculate the standard deviation.

Step 2.   Divide the standard deviation by the square root of the number of observations (n).

Properties and uses of the standard error of the mean

- The primary practical use of the standard error of the mean is in calculating confidence intervals around the arithmetic mean. (Confidence intervals are addressed in the next section.)

EXAMPLE: Finding the Standard Error of the Mean

Find the standard error of the mean for the length-of-stay data in Table 2.10, given that the standard deviation is 9.1888.

Step 1. Calculate the standard deviation.

$$\text{Standard deviation (given)} = 9.188$$

Step 2. Divide the standard deviation by the square root of n.

$$n = 30$$

$$\text{Standard error of the mean} = 9.188 / \sqrt{30} = 9.188 / 5.477 = 1.67$$

Confidence limits (confidence interval)

Definition of a confidence interval

Often, epidemiologists conduct studies not only to measure characteristics in the subjects studied, but also to make generalizations about the larger population from which these subjects came. This process is called inference. For example, political pollsters use samples of perhaps 1,000 or so people from across the country to make inferences about which presidential candidate is likely to win on Election Day. Usually, the inference includes some consideration about the precision of the measurement. (The results of a political poll may be reported to have a margin of error of, say, plus or minus three points.) In epidemiology, a common way to indicate a measurement's precision is by providing a confidence interval. A narrow confidence interval indicates high precision; a wide confidence interval indicates low precision.

Confidence intervals are calculated for some but not all epidemiologic measures. The two measures covered in this lesson for which confidence intervals are often presented are the mean and the geometric mean. Confidence intervals can also be calculated for some of the epidemiologic measures covered in Lesson 3, such as a proportion, risk ratio, and odds ratio.

The confidence interval for a mean is based on the mean itself and some multiple of the standard error of the mean. Recall that the standard error of the mean refers to the variability of means that might be calculated from repeated samples from the same population. Fortunately, regardless of how the data are distributed, means (particularly from large samples) tend to be normally distributed. (This is from an argument known as the Central Limit Theorem). So we can use Figure 2.9 to show that the range from the mean minus one standard deviation to the mean plus one standard deviation includes 68.3% of the area under the curve.

Consider a population-based sample survey in which the mean total cholesterol level of adult females was 206, with a standard error of the mean of 3. If this survey were repeated many times, 68.3% of the means would be expected to fall between the mean minus 1 standard error and the mean plus 1 standard error, i.e., between 203 and 209. One might say that the investigators are 68.3% confident those limits contain the actual mean of the population.

In public health, investigators generally want to have a greater level of confidence than that, and usually set the confidence level at 95%. Although the statistical definition of a confidence interval is that 95% of the confidence intervals from an infinite number of similarly conducted samples would include the true population values, this definition has little meaning for a single study. More commonly, epidemiologists interpret a 95% confidence interval as the range of values consistent with the data from their study.

Method for calculating a 95% confidence interval for a mean

Step 1.   Calculate the mean and its standard error.

Step 2.   Multiply the standard error by 1.96.

Step 3.   Lower limit of the 95% confidence interval = mean minus 1.96 x standard error.
Upper limit of the 95% confidence interval = mean plus 1.96 x standard error.

EXAMPLE: Calculating a 95% Confidence Interval for a Mean

Find the 95% confidence interval for a mean total cholesterol level of 206, standard error of the mean of 3.

Step 1. Calculate the mean and its error.

Mean = 206, standard error of the mean = 3 (both given)

Step 2. Multiply the standard error by 1.96.

3 x 1.96 = 5.88

Step 3. Lower limit of the 95% confidence interval = mean minus 1.96 x standard error.

206 − 5.88 = 200.12

Upper limit of the 95% confidence interval = mean plus 1.96 x standard error.

206 + 5.88 = 211.88

Rounding to one decimal, the 95% confidence interval is 200.1 to 211.9. In other words, this study's best estimate of the true population mean is 206, but is consistent with values ranging from as low as 200.1 and as high as 211.9. Thus, the confidence interval indicates how precise the estimate is. (This confidence interval is narrow, indicating that the sample mean of 206 is fairly precise.) It also indicates how confident the researchers should be in drawing inferences from the sample to the entire population.

Properties and uses of confidence intervals

- The mean is not the only measure for which a confidence interval can or should be calculated. Confidence intervals are also commonly calculated for proportions, rates, risk ratios, odds ratios, and other epidemiologic measures when the purpose is to draw inferences from a sample survey or study to the larger population.

- Most epidemiologic studies are not performed under the ideal conditions required by the theory behind a confidence interval. As a result, most epidemiologists take a common-sense approach rather than a strict statistical approach to the interpretation of a confidence interval, i.e., the confidence interval represents the range of values consistent with the data from a study, and is simply a guide to the variability in a study.

- Confidence intervals for means, proportions, risk ratios, odds ratios, and other measures all are calculated using different formulas. The formula for a confidence interval of the mean is well accepted, as is the formula for a confidence interval for a proportion. However, a number of different formulas are available for risk ratios and odds ratios. Since different formulas can sometimes give different results, this supports interpreting a confidence interval as a guide rather than as a strict range of values.

- Regardless of the measure, the interpretation of a confidence interval is the same: the narrower the interval, the more precise the estimate; and the range of values in the interval is the range of population values most consistent with the data from the study.

Demonstration: Using Confidence Intervals

Imagine you are going to Las Vegas to bet on the true mean total cholesterol level among adult women in the United States.

Question: On what number are you going to bet?

Answer: On 206, since that is the number found in the sample. The mean you calculated from your sample is your best guess of the true population mean.

Question: How does a confidence interval help?

Answer: It tells you how much to bet! If the confidence interval is narrow, your best guess is relatively precise, and you might feel comfortable (confident) betting more. But if the confidence interval is wide, your guess is relatively imprecise, and you should bet less on that one number, or perhaps not bet at all!

Exercise 2.10

When the serum cholesterol levels of 4,462 men were measured, the mean cholesterol level was 213, with a standard deviation of 42. Calculate the standard error of the mean for the serum cholesterol level of the men studied.

 Check your answers on page 2-62

Choosing the Right Measure of Central Location and Spread

Measures of central location and spread are useful for summarizing a distribution of data. They also facilitate the comparison of two or more sets of data. However, not every measure of central location and spread is well suited to every set of data. For example, because the normal distribution (or bell-shaped curve) is perfectly symmetrical, the mean, median, and mode all have the same value (as illustrated in Figure 2.10). In practice, however, observed data rarely approach this ideal shape. As a result, the mean, median, and mode usually differ.

Figure 2.10 Effect of Skewness on Mean, Median, and Mode

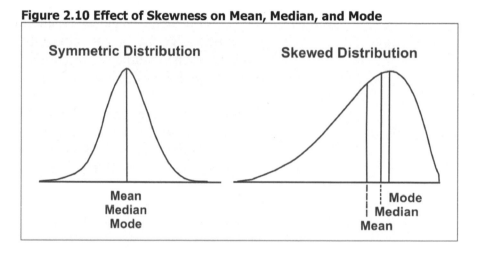

How, then, do you choose the most appropriate measures? A partial answer to this question is to select the measure of central location on the basis of how the data are distributed, and then use the corresponding measure of spread. Table 2.11 summarizes the recommended measures.

Table 2.11 Recommended Measures of Central Location and Spread by Type of Data

Type of Distribution	Measure of Central Location	Measure of Spread
Normal	Arithmetic mean	Standard deviation
Asymmetrical or skewed	Median	Range or interquartile range
Exponential or logarithmic	Geometric mean	Geometric standard

In statistics, the arithmetic mean is the most commonly used measure of central location, and is the measure upon which the majority of statistical tests and analytic techniques are based. The standard deviation is the measure of spread most commonly used with the mean. But as noted previously, one disadvantage of the mean is that it is affected by the presence of one or a few observations with extremely high or low values. The mean is "pulled" in the direction of the extreme values. You can tell the direction in which the data are skewed by comparing the values of the mean and the median; the mean is pulled away from the median in the direction of the extreme values. If the mean is higher than the median, the distribution of data is skewed to the right. If the mean is lower than the median, as in the right side of Figure 2.10, the distribution is skewed to the left.

The advantage of the median is that it is not affected by a few extremely high or low observations. Therefore, when a set of data is skewed, the median is more representative of the data than is the mean. For descriptive purposes, and to avoid making any assumption that the data are normally distributed, many epidemiologists routinely present the median for incubation periods, duration of illness, and age of the study subjects.

Two measures of spread can be used in conjunction with the median: the range and the interquartile range. Although many statistics books recommend the interquartile range as the preferred measure of spread, most practicing epidemiologists use the simpler range instead.

The mode is the least useful measure of central location. Some sets of data have no mode; others have more than one. The most common value may not be anywhere near the center of the distribution. Modes generally cannot be used in more elaborate statistical calculations. Nonetheless, even the mode can be helpful when one is interested in the most common value or most popular choice.

The geometric mean is used for exponential or logarithmic data such as laboratory titers, and for environmental sampling data whose values can span several orders of magnitude. The measure of spread used with the geometric mean is the geometric standard deviation. Analogous to the geometric mean, it is the antilog of the standard deviation of the log of the values.

The geometric standard deviation is substituted for the standard deviation when incorporating logarithms of numbers. Examples include describing environmental particle size based on mass, or variability of blood lead concentrations.[1]

Sometimes, a combination of these measures is needed to adequately describe a set of data.

EXAMPLE: Summarizing Data

Consider the smoking histories of 200 persons (Table 2.12) and summarize the data.

Table 2.12 Self-Reported Average Number of Cigarettes Smoked Per Day, Survey of Students (n = 200)

Number of Cigarettes Smoked Per Day

0	0	0	0	0	0	0	0	0	0	0	0
0	0	0	0	0	0	0	0	0	0	0	0
0	0	0	0	0	0	0	0	0	0	0	0
0	0	0	0	0	0	0	0	0	0	0	0
0	0	0	0	0	0	0	0	0	0	0	0
0	0	0	0	0	0	0	0	0	0	0	0
0	0	0	0	0	0	0	0	0	0	0	0
0	0	0	0	0	0	0	0	0	0	0	0
0	0	0	0	0	0	0	0	0	0	0	0
0	0	0	0	0	0	0	0	0	0	0	0
0	0	0	0	0	0	0	0	0	0	0	0
0	0	0	0	0	0	0	0	0	0	2	3
4	6	7	7	8	8	9	10	12	12	13	13
14	15	15	15	15	15	16	17	17	18	18	18
18	19	19	20	20	20	20	20	20	20	20	20
20	20	21	21	22	22	23	24	25	25	26	28
29	30	30	30	30	32	35	40				

Analyzing all 200 observations yields the following results:

Mean = 5.4
Median = 0
Mode = 0
Minimum value = 0
Maximum value = 40
Range = 0–40
Interquartile range = 8.8 (0.0–8.8)
Standard deviation = 9.5

These results are correct, but they do not summarize the data well. Almost three-fourths of the students, representing the mode, do not smoke at all. Separating the 58 smokers from the 142 nonsmokers yields a more informative summary of the data. Among the 58 (29%) who do smoke:

Mean = 18.5
Median = 19.5
Mode = 20
Minimum value = 2
Maximum value = 40
Range = 2–40
Interquartile range = 8.5 (13.7–22.25)
Standard deviation = 8.0

Thus, a more informative summary of the data might be "142 (71%) of the students do not smoke at all. Of the 58 students (29%) who do smoke, mean consumption is just under a pack* a day (mean = 18.5, median = 19.5). The range is from 2 to 40 cigarettes smoked per day, with approximately half the smokers smoking from 14 to 22 cigarettes per day."

* a typical pack contains 20 cigarettes

Exercise 2.11

The data in Table 2.13 (on page 2-57) are from an investigation of an outbreak of severe abdominal pain, persistent vomiting, and generalized weakness among residents of a rural village. The cause of the outbreak was eventually identified as flour unintentionally contaminated with lead dust.

1. Summarize the blood level data with a frequency distribution.

2. Calculate the arithmetic mean. [Hint: Sum of known values = 2,363]

3. Identify the median and interquartile range.

4. Calculate the standard deviation. [Hint: Sum of squares = 157,743]

5. Calculate the geometric mean using the log lead levels provided. [Hint: Sum of log lead levels = 68.45]

 Check your answers on page 2-62

Table 2.13 Age and Blood Lead Levels (BLLs) of Ill Villagers and Family Members — Country X, 1996

ID	Age (Years)	BLL[†]	Log₁₀BLL	ID	Age (Years)	BLL	Log₁₀BLL
1	3	69	1.84	22	33	103	2.01
2	4	45	1.66	23	33	46	1.66
3	6	49	1.69	24	35	78	1.89
4	7	84	1.92	25	35	50	1.70
5	9	48	1.68	26	36	64	1.81
6	10	58	1.77	27	36	67	1.83
7	11	17	1.23	28	38	79	1.90
8	12	76	1.88	29	40	58	1.76
9	13	61	1.79	30	45	86	1.93
10	14	78	1.89	31	47	76	1.88
11	15	48	1.68	32	49	58	1.76
12	15	57	1.76	33	56	?	?
13	16	68	1.83	34	60	26	1.41
14	16	?	?	35	65	104	2.02
15	17	26	1.42	36	65	39	1.59
16	19	78	1.89	37	65	35	1.54
17	19	56	1.75	38	70	72	1.86
18	20	54	1.73	39	70	57	1.76
19	22	73	1.86	40	76	38	1.58
20	26	74	1.87	41	78	44	1.64
21	27	63	1.80				

† Blood lead levels measured in micrograms per deciliter (mcg/dL)
? Missing value

Data Source: Nasser A, Hatch D, Pertowski C, Yoon S. Outbreak investigation of an unknown illness in a rural village, Egypt (case study). Cairo: Field Epidemiology Training Program, 1999.

Summary

Frequency distributions, measures of central location, and measures of spread are effective tools for summarizing numerical variables including:
- Physical characteristics such as height and diastolic blood pressure,
- Illness characteristics such as incubation period, and
- Behavioral characteristics such as number of lifetime sexual partners.

Some characteristics, such as IQ, follow a normal or symmetrical bell-shaped distribution in the population. Other characteristics have distributions that are skewed to the right (tail toward higher values) or skewed to the left (tail toward lower values). Some characteristics are mostly normally distributed, but have a few extreme values or outliers. Some characteristics, particularly laboratory dilution assays, follow a logarithmic pattern. Finally, other characteristics follow other patterns (such as a uniform distribution) or appear to follow no apparent pattern at all. The distribution of the data is the most important factor in selecting an appropriate measure of central location and spread.

Measures of central location are single values that represent the center of the observed distribution of values. The different measures of central location represent the center in different ways. The arithmetic mean represents the balance point for all the data. The median represents the middle of the data, with half the observed values below the median and half the observed values above it. The mode represents the peak or most prevalent value. The geometric mean is comparable to the arithmetic mean on a logarithmic scale.

Measures of spread describe the spread or variability of the observed distribution. The range measures the spread from the smallest to the largest value. The standard deviation, usually used in conjunction with the arithmetic mean, reflects how closely clustered the observed values are to the mean. For normally distributed data, 95% of the data fall in the range from −1.96 standard deviations to +1.96 standard deviations. The interquartile range, used in conjunction with the median, includes data in the range from the 25th percentile to the 75th percentile, or approximately the middle 50% of the data.

Data that are normally distributed are usually summarized with the arithmetic mean and standard deviation. Data that are skewed or have a few extreme values are usually summarized with the median and range, or with the median and interquartile range. Data that follow a logarithmic scale and data that span several orders of magnitude are usually summarized with the geometric mean.

Exercise Answers

Exercise 2.1

1. C
2. A
3. D
4. A
5. D

Exercise 2.2

Previous Years	Frequency
0	2
1	5
2	4
3	3
4	1
5	1
6	1
7	0
8	1
9	0
10	0
11	0
12	1
Total	**19**

Exercise 2.3

1. Create frequency distribution (done in Exercise 2.2, above)

2. Identify the value that occurs most often.
   Most common value is 1, so mode is 1 previous vaccination.

Exercise 2.4

1. Arrange the observations in increasing order.
   0, 0, 1, 1, 1, 1, 1, 2, 2, 2, 2, 3, 3, 3, 4, 5, 6, 8, 12

2. Find the middle position of the distribution with 19 observations.
   Middle position = (19 + 1) / 2 = 10

3. Identify the value at the middle position.
   0, 0, 1, 1, 1, 1, 1, 2, 2, *2*, 2, 3, 3, 3, 4, 5, 6, 8, 12

Counting from the left or right to the 10th position, the value is 2. So the median = 2 previous vaccinations.

Exercise 2.5

1. Add all of the observed values in the distribution.
   $2 + 0 + 3 + 1 + 0 + 1 + 2 + 2 + 4 + 8 + 1 + 3 + 3 + 12 + 1 + 6 + 2 + 5 + 1 = 57$

2. Divide the sum by the number of observations
   $57 / 19 = 3.0$

   So the mean is 3.0 previous vaccinations

Exercise 2.6

Using Method A:

1. Take the log (in this case, to base 2) of each value.

ID #	Convalescent	Log base 2
1	1:512	9
2	1:512	9
3	1:128	7
4	1:512	9
5	1:1024	10
6	1:1024	10
7	1:2048	11
8	1:128	7
9	1:4096	12
10	1:1024	10

2. Calculate the mean of the log values by summing and dividing by the number of observations (10).
   Mean of $\log_2(x_i) = (9 + 9 + 7 + 9 + 10 + 10 + 11 + 7 + 12 + 10) / 10 = 94 / 10 = 9.4$

3. Take the antilog of the mean of the log values to get the geometric mean.
   $\text{Antilog}_2(9.4) = 2^{9.4} = 675.59$. Therefore, the geometric mean dilution titer is 1:675.6.

Exercise 2.7

1. E or A; equal number of patients in 1999 and 1998.
2. C or B; mean and median are very close, so either would be acceptable.
3. E or A; for a nominal variable, the most frequent category is the mode.
4. D
5. B; mean is skewed, so median is better choice.
6. B; mean is skewed, so median is better choice.

Exercise 2.8

1. Arrange the observations in increasing order.
   0, 0, 1, 1, 1, 1, 1, 2, 2, 2, 2, 3, 3, 3, 4, 5, 6, 8, 12

2. Find the position of the 1st and 3rd quartiles. Note that the distribution has 19 observations.

    Position of $Q_1 = (n + 1) / 4 = (19 + 1) / 4 = 5$
    Position of $Q_3 = 3(n + 1) / 4 = 3(19 + 1) / 4 = 15$

3. Identify the value of the 1st and 3rd quartiles.

    Value at Q_1 (position 5) = 1
    Value at Q_3 (position 15) = 4

4. Calculate the interquartile range as Q_3 minus Q_1.

    Interquartile range = $4 - 1 = 3$

5. The median (at position 10) is 2. Note that the distance between Q_1 and the median is $2 - 1 = 1$. The distance between Q_3 and the median is $4 - 2 = 2$. This indicates that the vaccination data is skewed slightly to the right (tail points to greater number of previous vaccinations).

Exercise 2.9

1. Calculate the arithmetic mean.

    Mean $= (2 + 0 + 3 + 1 + 0 + 1 + 2 + 2 + 4 + 8 + 1 + 3 + 3 + 12 + 1 + 6 + 2 + 5 + 1) / 19$
    $= 57 / 19$
    $= 3.0$

2. Subtract the mean from each observation. Square the difference.

3. Sum the squared differences.

Value minus Mean			Difference	Difference Squared
2	–	3.0	−1.0	1.0
0	–	3.0	−3.0	9.0
3	–	3.0	0.0	0.0
1	–	3.0	−2.0	4.0
0	–	3.0	−3.0	9.0
1	–	3.0	−2.0	4.0
2	–	3.0	−1.0	1.0
2	–	3.0	−1.0	1.0
4	–	3.0	1.0	1.0
8	–	3.0	5.0	25.0
1	–	3.0	−2.0	4.0
3	–	3.0	0.0	0.0
3	–	3.0	0.0	0.0
12	–	3.0	9.0	81.0
1	–	3.0	−2.0	4.0
6	–	3.0	3.0	9.0
2	–	3.0	−1.0	1.0
5	–	3.0	2.0	4.0
1	–	3.0	−2.0	4.0
57	–	57.0 = 0	0.0	162.0

4. Divide the sum of the squared differences by n – 1.

    Variance = $162 / (19 - 1) = 162 / 18 = 9.0$ previous vaccinations squared

5. Take the square root of the variance. This is the standard deviation.

    Standard deviation $= 9.0 = 3.0$ previous vaccinations

Exercise 2.10

Standard error of the mean = 42 divided by the square root of 4,462 = 0.629

Exercise 2.11

1. Summarize the blood level data with a frequency distribution.

Table 2.14 Frequency Distribution (1:g/dL Intervals) of Blood Lead Levels — Rural Village, 1996 (Intervals with No Observations Not Shown)

Blood Lead Level (g/dL)	Frequency	Blood Lead Level (g/dL)	Frequency	Blood Lead Level (g/dL)	Frequency
17	1	57	2	76	2
26	2	58	3	78	3
35	1	61	1	79	1
38	1	63	1	84	1
39	1	64	1	86	1
44	1	67	1	103	1
45	1	68	1	104	1
46	1	69	1	Unknown	48
49	1	72	1		
50	1	73	1		
54	1	74	1		
56	1				

To summarize the data further you could use intervals of 5, 10, or perhaps even 20 mcg/dL. Table 2.15 below uses 10 mcg/dL intervals.

Table 2.15 Frequency Distribution (10 mcg/dL Intervals) of Blood Lead Levels — Rural Village, 1996

Blood Lead Level (g/dL)	Frequency
0–9	0
10–19	1
20–29	2
30–39	3
40–49	6
50–59	8
60–69	6
70–79	9
80–89	2
90–99	0
100–110	2
Total	39

2. Calculate the arithmetic mean.
   Arithmetic mean = sum / n = 2,363 / 39 = 60.6 mcg/dL

3. Identify the median and interquartile range.
   Median at (39 + 1) / 2 = 20th position. Median = value at 20th position = 58
   Q_1 at (39 + 1) / 4 = 10th position. Q_1 = value at 10th position = 48
   Q_3 at 3 x Q_1 position = 30th position. Q_3 = value at 30th position – 76

4. Calculate the standard deviation.
   Square of sum $= 2,363^2 = 5,583,769$
   Sum of squares x n $= 157,743$ x $39 = 6,157,977$
   Difference $= 6,151,977 - 5,583,769 = 568,208$
   Variance $= 568,208 / (39$ x $38) = 383.4062$
   Standard deviation $=$ square root $(383.4062) = 19.58$ mcg/dL

5. Calculate the geometric mean using the log lead levels provided.
   Geometric mean $= 10^{(68.45 / 39)} = 10^{(1.7551)} = 56.9$ mcg/dL

SELF-ASSESSMENT QUIZ

Now that you have read Lesson 2 and have completed the exercises, you should be ready to take the self-assessment quiz. This quiz is designed to help you assess how well you have learned the content of this lesson. You may refer to the lesson text whenever you are unsure of the answer.

Unless instructed otherwise, choose ALL correct answers for each question.

Use Table 2.16 for Questions 1 and 2, and for Questions 10–13.

Table 2.16 Admitting Clinical Characteristics of Patients with Severe Acute Respiratory Syndrome — Singapore, March–May, 2003

ID	Date of Diagnosis	Sex	Age (Years)	How Acquired	Symptoms[†]	Temp (°C)	Lymphocyte Count (x 10⁻⁹/L)[‡]	Outcome
01	*	Female	71	Community	F, confusion	38.7	0.78	Survived
02	3/16	Female	43	Community	C,D,S,H,F,G	38.9	0.94	Died
03	3/29	Male	40	HCW¶	C,H,M,F	36.8	0.71	Survived
04	*	Female	78	Community	D	36.0	1.02	Died
05	*	Female	53	Community	C,D,F	39.6	0.53	Died
06	4/6	Male	63	Community	C,M,F,dizziness	35.1	0.63	Died
07	*	Male	84	Inpatient	D,F	38.0	0.21	Died
08	*	Male	63	Inpatient	F	38.5	0.83	Survived
09	*	Female	74	Inpatient	F	38.0	1.34	Died
10	*	Male	72	Inpatient	F	38.5	1.04	Survived
11	*	Female	28	HCW	H,M,F	38.2	0.30	Survived
12	*	Female	24	HCW	M,F	38.0	0.84	Survived
13	*	Female	28	HCW	M,F	38.5	1.13	Survived
14	*	Male	21	HCW	H,M,F	38.8	0.97	Survived

* Date of onset not provided in manuscript
† C=cough, D=dyspnea, F=fever, H=headache, M=myalgia, S=sore throat
‡ Normal > 1.50 x 10⁻⁹/L
¶ HCW = health-care worker

Data Source: Singh K, Hsu L-Y, Villacian JS, Habib A, Fisher D, Tambyah PA. Severe acute respiratory syndrome: lessons from Singapore. Emerg Infect Dis 2003;9:1294–8.

1. Table 2.16 is an example of a/an _____.

2. For each of the following variables included in Table 2.16, identify if it is:
   A. Categorical   E. Ordinal
   B. Continuous   F. Qualitative
   C. Interval   G. Quantitative
   D. Nominal   H. Ratio

   _____ Sex
   _____ Age
   _____ Lymphocyte Count

3. Which of the following best describes the similarities and differences in the three distributions shown in Figure 2.11?
   A. Same mean, median, mode; different standard deviation
   B. Same mean, median, mode; same standard deviation
   C. Different mean, median, mode; different standard deviation
   D. Different mean, median, mode; same standard deviation

Figure 2.11

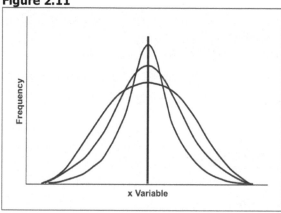

4. Which of the following terms accurately describe the distribution shown in Figure 2.12?
   A. Negatively skewed
   B. Positively skewed
   C. Skewed to the right
   D. Skewed to the left
   E. Asymmetrical

Figure 2.12

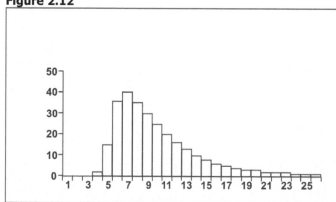

5. What is the likely relationship between mean, median, and mode of the distribution shown in Figure 2.12?
   A. Mean < median < mode
   B. Mean = median = mode
   C. Mean > median > mode
   D. Mode < mean and median, but cannot tell relationship between mean and median

6. The mode is the value that:
   A. Is midway between the lowest and highest value
   B. Occurs most often
   C. Has half the observations below it and half above it
   D. Is statistically closest to all of the values in the distribution

7. The median is the value that:
   A. Is midway between the lowest and highest value
   B. Occurs most often
   C. Has half the observations below it and half above it
   D. Is statistically closest to all of the values in the distribution

8. The mean is the value that:
   A. Is midway between the lowest and highest value
   B. Occurs most often
   C. Has half the observations below it and half above it
   D. Is statistically closest to all of the values in the distribution

9. The geometric mean is the value that:
   A. Is midway between the lowest and highest value on a log scale
   B. Occurs most often on a log scale
   C. Has half the observations below it and half above it on a log scale
   D. Is statistically closest to all of the values in the distribution on a log scale

Use Table 2.16 for Questions 10–13. Note that the sum of the 14 temperatures listed in Table 2.16 is 531.6.

10. The mode of the temperatures listed in Table 2.16 is:
    A. 37.35°C
    B. 37.9°C
    C. 38.0°C
    D. 38.35°C
    E. 38.5°C

11. The median of the temperatures listed in Table 2.16 is:
    A. 37.35°C
    B. 37.9°C
    C. 38.0°C
    D. 38.35°C
    E. 38.5°C

12. The mean of the temperatures listed in Table 2.16 is:
    A. 37.35°C
    B. 37.9°C
    C. 38.0°C
    D. 38.35°C
    E. 38.5°C

13. The midrange of the temperatures listed in Table 2.16 is:
    A. 37.35°C
    B. 37.9°C
    C. 38.0°C
    D. 38.35°C
    E. 38.5°C

14. In epidemiology, the measure of central location generally preferred for summarizing skewed data such as incubation periods is the:
    A. Mean
    B. Median
    C. Midrange
    D. Mode

15. The measure of central location generally preferred for additional statistical analysis is the:
    A. Mean
    B. Median
    C. Midrange
    D. Mode

16. Which of the following are considered measures of spread?
    A. Interquartile range
    B. Percentile
    C. Range
    D. Standard deviation

The measure of spread **most** affected by one extreme value is the:
    A. Interquartile range
    B. Range
    C. Standard deviation
    D. Mean

17. The interquartile range covers what proportion of a distribution?
    A. 25%
    B. 50%
    C. 75%
    D. 100%

18. The measure of central location most commonly used with the interquartile range is the:
    A. Arithmetic mean
    B. Geometric mean
    C. Median
    D. Midrange
    E. Mode

19. The measure of central location most commonly used with the standard deviation is the:
    A. Arithmetic mean
    B. Median
    C. Midrange
    D. Mode

20. The algebraic relationship between the variance and standard deviation is that:
    A. The standard deviation is the square root of the variance
    B. The variance is the square root of the standard deviation
    C. The standard deviation is the variance divided by the square root of n
    D. The variance is the standard deviation divided by the square root of n

21. Before calculating a standard deviation, one should ensure that:
    A. The data are somewhat normally distributed
    B. The total number of observations is at least 50
    C. The variable is an interval-scale or ratio-scale variable
    D. The calculator or software has a square-root function

23. Simply by scanning the values in each distribution below, identify the distribution with the largest standard deviation.
    A. 1, 10, 15, 18, 20, 20, 22, 25, 30, 39
    B. 1, 3, 8, 10, 20, 20, 30, 32, 37, 39
    C. 1, 15, 17, 19, 20, 20, 21, 23, 25, 39
    D. 41, 42, 43, 44, 45, 45, 46, 47, 48, 49

24. Given the area under a normal curve, which two of the following ranges are the same? (Circle the TWO that are the same.)
    A. From the 2.5^{th} percentile to the 97.5^{th} percentile
    B. From the 5th percentile to the 95th percentile
    C. From the 25th percentile to the 75th percentile
    D. From 1 standard deviation below the mean to 1 standard deviation above the mean
    E. From 1.96 standard deviations below the mean to 1.96 standard deviations above the mean

25. The primary use of the standard error of the mean is in calculating the:
    A. confidence interval
    B. error rate
    C. standard deviation
    D. variance

Answers to Self-Assessment Quiz

1. Line list or line listing. A line listing is a table in which each row typically represents one person or case of disease, and each column represents a variable such as ID, age, sex, etc.

2. Sex   A, D, F
   Age   B, G, H
   Lymphocyte count   B, G, H
   Sex is a nominal variable, meaning that its categories have names but not numerical value. Nominal variables are qualitative or categorical variables.
   Age and *lymphocyte count* are ratio variables because they are both numeric variable with true zero points. Ratio variables are continuous and quantitative variables.

3. A. Because the centers of each distribution line up, they have the same measure of central location. But because each distribution is spread differently, they have different measures of spread.

4. B, C, E. Right/left skewness refers to the tail of a distribution. Because the "hump" of this distribution is on the left and the tail is on the right, it is said to be skewed positively to the right. A skewed distribution is not symmetrical.

5. C. For a distribution such as that shown in Figure 2.12, with its hump to the left, the mode will be smaller than either the median or the mean. The long tail to the right will pull the mean upward, so that the sequence will be mode < median < mean.

6. B. The mode is the value that occurs most often.

7. C. The median is the value that has half the observations below it and half above it.

8. D. The mean is the value that is statistically closest to all of the values in the distribution

9. D. The geometric mean is the value that is statistically closest to all of the values in the distribution on a log scale.

10. C, E. The mode is the value that occurs most often. A distribution can have one mode, more than one mode, or no mode. In this distribution, both 38.0°C and 38.5°C appear 3 times.

11. D. The median is the value that has half the observations below it and half above it. For a distribution with an even number of values, the median falls between 2 observations, in this situation between the 7th and 8th values. The 7th value is 38.2°C and the 8th value is 38.5°C, so the median is the average of those two values, i.e., 38.35°C.

12. C. The mean is the average of all the values. Given 14 temperatures that sum to 531.6, the mean is calculated as 531.6 / 14, which equals 37.97°C, which should be rounded to 38.0°C.

13. A. The midrange is halfway between the smallest and largest values. Since the lowest and

highest temperatures are 35.1°C and 39.6°C , the midrange is calculated as 35.1 + 39.6 / 2, or 37.35°C.

14. B. In epidemiology, the measure of central location generally preferred for summarizing skewed data such as incubation periods is the median.

15. A. The measure of central location generally preferred for additional statistical analysis is the mean, which is the only measure that has good statistical properties.

16. A, C, D, E. Interquartile range, range, standard deviation, and variance are all measures of spread. A percentile identifies a particular place on the distribution, but is not a measure of spread.

17. B. The range is the difference between the extreme values on either side, so it is most directly affected by those values.

18. B. The interquartile range covers the central 50% of a distribution.

19. C. The interquartile range usually accompanies the median, since both are based on percentiles. The interquartile range covers from the 25th to the 75th percentile, while the median marks the 50th percentile.

20. A. The standard deviation usually accompanies the arithmetic mean.

21. A. The standard deviation is the square root of the variance.

22. A, D. Use of the mean and standard deviation are usually restricted to data that are more-or-less normally distributed. Calculation of the standard deviation requires squaring differences and then taking the square root, so you need a calculator that has a square-root function.

23. B. Distributions A, B, and C all range from 1 to 39 and have two central values of 20. Considering the eight values other than the smallest and largest, distribution C has values close to 20 (from 15 to 25), Distribution A has values from 10 to 30, and Distribution B has values from 3 to 37. So Distribution B has the broadest spread among the first 3 distributions. Distribution D has larger values than the first 3 distributions (41-49 rather than 1-39), but they cluster rather tightly around the central value of 45.

24. A and E. The area from the 2.5th percentile to the 97.5th percentile includes 95% of the area below the curve, which corresponds to ± 1.96 standard deviations along the x-axis.

25. A. The primary use of the standard error of the mean is in calculating a confidence interval.

References

1. Griffin S., Marcus A., Schulz T., Walker S. Calculating the interindividual geometric standard deviation of r use in the integrated exposure uptake biokinetic model for lead in children. Environ Health Perspect 1999;107:481–7.

Instructions for Epi Info 6 (DOS)

To download:
    Go to http://www.cdc.gov/epiinfo/Epi6/ei6.htm and click on "Downloads."

To get a complete installation package:
    Download and run all three self-expanding, compressed files to a temporary directory.
        EPI604_1.EXE (File Size = 1,367,649 bytes)
        EPI604_2.EXE (File Size = 1,341,995 bytes)
        EPI604_3.EXE (File Size = 1,360,925 bytes)
    Then run INSTALL.EXE to install the software.

To create a frequency distribution from a data set in Analysis Module:
    EpiInfo6: >freq *variable*.

To identify the mode from a data set in Analysis Module:
    Epi Info does not have a Mode command. Thus, the best way to identify the mode is to create a histogram and look for the tallest column(s).
    EpiInfo6: >histogram *variable*.

To identify the median from a data set in Analysis Module:
    EpiInfo6: >means *variable*. Output indicates median.

To identify the mean from a data set in Analysis Module:
    EpiInfo6: >means *variable*. Output indicates median.

To calculate the standard deviation from a data set in Analysis Module:
    EpiInfo6: >means *variable*. Output indicates standard deviation, abbreviated as Std Dev.

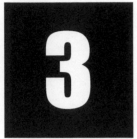

MEASURES OF RISK

Lesson 2 described measures of central location and spread, which are useful for summarizing continuous variables. However, many variables used by field epidemiologists are categorical variables, some of which have only two categories — exposed yes/no, test positive/negative, case/control, and so on. These variables have to be summarized with frequency measures such as ratios, proportions, and rates. Incidence, prevalence, and mortality rates are three frequency measures that are used to characterize the occurrence of health events in a population.

Objectives

After studying this lesson and answering the questions in the exercises, you will be able to:
- *Calculate and interpret the following epidemiologic measures:*
  - *Ratio*
  - *Proportion*
  - *Incidence proportion (attack rate)*
  - *Incidence rate*
  - *Prevalence*
  - *Mortality rate*
- *Choose and apply the appropriate measures of association and measures of public health impact*

Major Sections

Frequency Measures

Numerator = upper
portion of a fraction

Denominator = lower
portion of a fraction

A measure of central location provides a single value that summarizes an entire distribution of data. In contrast, a frequency measure characterizes only part of the distribution. Frequency measures compare one part of the distribution to another part of the distribution, or to the entire distribution. Common frequency measures are **ratios**, **proportions**, and **rates**. All three frequency measures have the same basic form:

$$\frac{numerator}{denominator} \; x \; 10^n$$

Recall that:

$10^0 = 1$ (anything raised to the 0 power equals 1)
$10^1 = 10$ (anything raised to the 1st power is the value itself)
$10^2 = 10 \times 10 = 100$
$10^3 = 10 \times 10 \times 10 = 1{,}000$

So the fraction of (numerator/denominator) can be multiplied by 1, 10, 100, 1000, and so on. This multiplier varies by measure and will be addressed in each section.

Ratio

Definition of ratio

A ratio is the relative magnitude of two quantities or a comparison of any two values. It is calculated by dividing one interval- or ratio-scale variable by the other. The numerator and denominator need not be related. Therefore, one could compare apples with oranges or apples with number of physician visits.

Method for calculating a ratio

$$\frac{Number \; or \; rate \; of \; events, \; items, \; persons, \; etc. \; in \; one \; group}{Number \; or \; rate \; of \; events, \; items, \; persons, \; etc. \; in \; another \; group}$$

After the numerator is divided by the denominator, the result is often expressed as the result "to one" or written as the result ":1."

Note that in certain ratios, the numerator and denominator are different categories of the same variable, such as males and females, or persons 20–29 years and 30–39 years of age. In other ratios, the numerator and denominator are completely different variables, such as the number of hospitals in a city and the size of the population living in that city.

EXAMPLE: Calculating a Ratio — Different Categories of Same Variable

Between 1971 and 1975, as part of the National Health and Nutrition Examination Survey (NHANES), 7,381 persons ages 40–77 years were enrolled in a follow-up study.[1] At the time of enrollment, each study participant was classified as having or not having diabetes. During 1982–1984, enrollees were documented either to have died or were still alive. The results are summarized as follows.

	Original Enrollment (1971–1975)	Dead at Follow-Up (1982–1984)
Diabetic men	189	100
Nondiabetic men	3,151	811
Diabetic women	218	72
Nondiabetic women	3,823	511

Of the men enrolled in the NHANES follow-up study, 3,151 were nondiabetic and 189 were diabetic. Calculate the ratio of non-diabetic to diabetic men.

Ratio = 3,151 / 189 x 1 = 16.7:1

Properties and uses of ratios

*   Ratios are common descriptive measures, used in all fields. In epidemiology, ratios are used as both descriptive measures and as analytic tools. As a descriptive measure, ratios can describe the male-to-female ratio of participants in a study, or the ratio of controls to cases (e.g., two controls per case). As an analytic tool, ratios can be calculated for occurrence of illness, injury, or death between two groups. These ratio measures, including risk ratio (relative risk), rate ratio, and odds ratio, are described later in this lesson.

*   As noted previously, the numerators and denominators of a ratio can be related or unrelated. In other words, you are free to use a ratio to compare the number of males in a population with the number of females, or to compare the number of residents in a population with the number of hospitals or dollars spent on over-the-counter medicines.

*   Usually, the values of both the numerator and denominator of a ratio are divided by the value of one or the other so that either the numerator or the denominator equals 1.0. So the ratio of non-diabetics to diabetics cited in the previous example is more likely to be reported as 16.7:1 than 3,151:189.

EXAMPLES: Calculating Ratios for Different Variables

Example A: *A city of 4,000,000 persons has 500 clinics. Calculate the ratio of clinics per person.*

$$500 / 4{,}000{,}000 \times 10n = 0.000125 \text{ clinics per person}$$

To get a more easily understood result, you could set $10n = 104 = 10{,}000$. Then the ratio becomes:

$$0.000125 \times 10{,}000 = 1.25 \text{ clinics per 10,000 persons}$$

You could also divide each value by 1.25, and express this ratio as 1 clinic for every 8,000 persons.

Example B: *Delaware's infant mortality rate in 2001 was 10.7 per 1,000 live births.[2] New Hampshire's infant mortality rate in 2001 was 3.8 per 1,000 live births. Calculate the ratio of the infant mortality rate in Delaware to that in New Hampshire.*

$$10.7 / 3.8 \times 1 = 2.8{:}1$$

Thus, Delaware's infant mortality rate was 2.8 times as high as New Hampshire's infant mortality rate in 2001.

A commonly used epidemiologic ratio: death-to-case ratio

Death-to-case ratio is the number of deaths attributed to a particular disease during a specified period divided by the number of new cases of that disease identified during the same period. It is used as a measure of the severity of illness: the death-to-case ratio for rabies is close to 1 (that is, almost everyone who develops rabies dies from it), whereas the death-to-case ratio for the common cold is close to 0.

For example, in the United States in 2002, a total of 15,075 new cases of tuberculosis were reported.[3] During the same year, 802 deaths were attributed to tuberculosis. The tuberculosis death-to-case ratio for 2002 can be calculated as 802 / 15,075. Dividing both numerator and denominator by the numerator yields 1 death per 18.8 new cases. Dividing both numerator and denominator by the denominator (and multiplying by $10^n = 100$) yields 5.3 deaths per 100 new cases. Both expressions are correct.

Note that, presumably, many of those who died had initially contracted tuberculosis years earlier. Thus many of the 802 in the numerator are not among the 15,075 in the denominator. Therefore, the death-to-case ratio is a ratio, but not a proportion.

Proportion

Definition of proportion

A proportion is the comparison of a part to the whole. It is a type of ratio in which the numerator is included in the denominator. You might use a proportion to describe what fraction of clinic patients tested positive for HIV, or what percentage of the population is younger than 25 years of age. A proportion may be expressed as a decimal, a fraction, or a percentage.

Method for calculating a proportion

$$\frac{\textit{Number of persons or events with a particular characteristic}}{\textit{Total number of persons or events, of which the numerator is a subset}} \times 10^n$$

For a proportion, 10^n is usually 100 (or $n = 2$) and is often expressed as a percentage.

EXAMPLE: Calculating a Proportion

Example A: *Calculate the proportion of men in the NHANES follow-up study who were diabetics.*

   Numerator   = 189 diabetic men
   Denominator = Total number of men = 189 + 3,151 = 3,340

   Proportion = (189 / 3,340) x 100 = 5.66%

Example B: *Calculate the proportion of deaths among men.*

   Numerator   = deaths in men
                 = 100 deaths in diabetic men + 811 deaths in nondiabetic men
                 = 911 deaths in men

Notice that the numerator (911 deaths in men) is a subset of the denominator.

   Denominator = all deaths
                 = 911 deaths in men + 72 deaths in diabetic women + 511 deaths in nondiabetic women
                 = 1,494 deaths

   Proportion = 911 / 1,494 = 60.98% = 61%

Your Turn: What proportion of all study participants were men? (Answer = 45.25%)

Properties and uses of proportions

- Proportions are common descriptive measures used in all fields. In epidemiology, proportions are used most often as descriptive measures. For example, one could calculate the proportion of persons enrolled in a study among all those eligible ("participation rate"), the proportion of children in a village vaccinated against measles, or the proportion of persons who developed illness among all passengers of a cruise ship.

- Proportions are also used to describe the amount of disease that can be attributed to a particular exposure. For example, on the basis of studies of smoking and lung cancer, public health officials have estimated that greater than 90% of the lung cancer cases that occur are attributable to cigarette smoking.

- In a proportion, the numerator must be included in the denominator. Thus, the number of apples divided by the number of oranges is not a proportion, but the number of apples divided by the total number of fruits of all kinds is a proportion. Remember, the numerator is always a subset of the denominator.

- A proportion can be expressed as a fraction, a decimal, or a percentage. The statements "one fifth of the residents became ill" and "twenty percent of the residents became ill" are equivalent.

- Proportions can easily be converted to ratios. If the numerator is the number of women (179) who attended a clinic and the denominator is all the clinic attendees (341), the proportion of clinic attendees who are women is 179 / 341, or 52% (a little more than half). To convert to a ratio, subtract the numerator from the denominator to get the number of clinic patients who are not women, i.e., the number of men (341 – 179 = 162 men.)Thus, ratio of women to men could be calculated from the proportion as:

$$\text{Ratio} = 179 / (341 - 179) \times 1$$
$$= 179 / 162$$
$$= 1.1 \text{ to } 1 \text{ female-to-male ratio}$$

Conversely, if a ratio's numerator and denominator together make up a whole population, the ratio can be converted to a proportion. You would add the ratio's numerator and denominator to form the denominator of the proportion, as illustrated in the NHANES follow-up study examples (provided earlier in this lesson).

A specific type of epidemiologic proportion: proportionate mortality

Proportionate mortality is the proportion of deaths in a specified population during a period of time that are attributable to different causes. Each cause is expressed as a percentage of all deaths, and the sum of the causes adds up to 100%. These proportions are not rates because the denominator is all deaths, not the size of the population in which the deaths occurred. Table 3.1 lists the primary causes of death in the United States in 2003 for persons of all ages and for persons aged 25–44 years, by number of deaths, proportionate mortality, and rank.

Table 3.1 Number, Proportionate Mortality, and Ranking of Deaths for Leading Causes of Death, All Ages and 25–44 Year Age Group — United States, 2003

	All Ages			Ages 25–44 Years		
	Number	Percentage	Rank	Number	Percentage	Rank
All causes	2,443,930	100.0		128,924	100.0	
Diseases of heart	684,462	28.0	1	16,283	12.6	3
Malignant neoplasms	554,643	22.7	2	19,041	14.8	2
Cerebrovascular disease	157,803	6.5	3	3,004	2.3	8
Chronic lower respiratory diseases	126,128	5.2	4	401	0.3	*
Accidents (unintentional injuries)	105,695	4.3	5	27,844	21.6	1
Diabetes mellitus	73,965	3.0	6	2,662	2.1	9
Influenza & pneumonia	64,847	2.6	7	1,337	1.0	10
Alzheimer's disease	63,343	2.6	8	0	0.0	*
Nephritis, nephrotic syndrome, nephrosis	33,615	1.4	9	305	0.2	*
Septicemia	34,243	1.4	10	328	0.2	*
Intentional self-harm (suicide)	30,642	1.3	11	11,251	8.7	4
Chronic liver disease and cirrhosis	27,201	1.1	12	3,288	2.6	7
Assault (homicide)	17,096	0.7	13	7,367	5.7	5
HIV disease	13,544	0.5	*	6,879	5.3	6
All other	456,703	18.7		29,480	22.9	

* Not among top ranked causes

Data Sources: Centers for Disease Control and Prevention. Summary of notifiable diseases, United States, 2003. MMWR 2005;2(No. 54).
Hoyert DL, Kung HC, Smith BL. Deaths: Preliminary data for 2003. National Vital Statistics Reports; vol. 53 no 15. Hyattsville, MD: National Center for Health Statistics 2005: p. 15, 27.

As illustrated in Table 3.1, the proportionate mortality for HIV was 0.5% among all age groups, and 5.3% among those aged 25–44 years. In other words, HIV infection accounted for 0.5% of all deaths, and 5.3% of deaths among 25–44 year olds.

Rate

Definition of rate

In epidemiology, a rate is a measure of the frequency with which an event occurs in a defined population over a specified period of time. Because rates put disease frequency in the perspective of the size of the population, rates are particularly useful for comparing disease frequency in different locations, at different times, or among different groups of persons with potentially different sized populations; that is, a rate is a measure of risk.

To a non-epidemiologist, rate means how fast something is happening or going. The speedometer of a car indicates the car's speed or rate of travel in miles or kilometers per hour. This rate is always reported per some unit of time. Some epidemiologists restrict use of the term rate to similar measures that are expressed per unit of time. For these epidemiologists, a rate describes how quickly disease occurs in a population, for example, 70 new cases of breast cancer per 1,000 women per year. This measure conveys a sense of the speed with which disease occurs in a population, and seems to imply that this pattern has occurred and will continue to occur for the foreseeable future. This rate is an *incidence rate*, described in the next section, starting on page 3-13.

Other epidemiologists use the term rate more loosely, referring to proportions with case counts in the numerator and size of population in the denominator as rates. Thus, an **attack rate** is the proportion of the population that develops illness during an outbreak. For example, 20 of 130 persons developed diarrhea after attending a picnic. (An alternative and more accurate phrase for attack rate is **incidence proportion**.) A **prevalence rate** is the proportion of the population that has a health condition at a point in time. For example, 70 influenza case-patients in March 2005 reported in County A. A **case-fatality rate** is the proportion of persons with the disease who die from it. For example, one death due to meningitis among County A's population. All of these measures are proportions, and none is expressed per units of time. Therefore, these measures are not considered "true" rates by some, although use of the terminology is widespread.

Table 3.2 summarizes some of the common epidemiologic measures as ratios, proportions, or rates.

Table 3.2 Epidemiologic Measures Categorized as Ratio, Proportion, or Rate

Condition	Ratio	Proportion	Rate
Morbidity (Disease)	Risk ratio (Relative risk) Rate ratio Odds ratio Period prevalence	Attack rate (Incidence proportion) Secondary attack rate Point prevalence Attributable proportion	Person-time incidence rate
Mortality (Death)	Death-to-case ratio	Proportionate mortality	Crude mortality rate Case-fatality rate Cause-specific mortality rate Age-specific mortality rate Maternal mortality rate Infant mortality rate
Natality (Birth)			Crude birth rate Crude fertility rate

Exercise 3.1

For each of the fractions shown below, indicate whether it is a ratio, a proportion, a rate, or none of the three.

A. *Ratio*
B. *Proportion*
C. *Rate*
D. *None of the above*

_____ 1. number of women in State A who died from heart disease in 2004 / number of women in State A who died in 2004

_____ 2. number of women in State A who died from heart disease in 2004 / estimated number of women living in State A on July 1, 2004

_____ 3. number of women in State A who died from heart disease in 2004 / number of women in State A who died from cancer in 2004

_____ 4. number of women in State A who died from lung cancer in 2004 / number of women in State A who died from cancer (all types) in 2004

_____ 5. number of women in State A who died from lung cancer in 2004 / estimated revenue (in dollars) in State A from cigarette sales in 2004

 Check your answers on page 3-52

Morbidity Frequency Measures

Morbidity has been defined as any departure, subjective or objective, from a state of physiological or psychological well-being. In practice, morbidity encompasses disease, injury, and disability. In addition, although for this lesson the term refers to the number of persons who are ill, it can also be used to describe the periods of illness that these persons experienced, or the duration of these illnesses.[4]

Measures of morbidity frequency characterize the number of persons in a population who become ill (incidence) or are ill at a given time (prevalence). Commonly used measures are listed in Table 3.3.

Table 3.3 Frequently Used Measures of Morbidity

Measure	Numerator	Denominator
Incidence proportion (or attack rate or risk)	Number of new cases of disease during specified time interval	Population at start of time interval
Secondary attack rate	Number of new cases among contacts	Total number of contacts
Incidence rate (or person-time rate)	Number of new cases of disease during specified time interval	Summed person-years of observation or average population during time interval
Point prevalence	Number of current cases (new and preexisting) at a specified point in time	Population at the same specified point in time
Period prevalence	Number of current cases (new and preexisting) over a specified period of time	Average or mid-interval population

Incidence refers to the occurrence of new cases of disease or injury in a population over a specified period of time. Although some epidemiologists use incidence to mean the number of new cases in a community, others use incidence to mean the number of new cases per unit of population.

Two types of incidence are commonly used — **incidence proportion** and **incidence rate**.

Incidence proportion or risk

Definition of incidence proportion

Synonyms for incidence proportion
- Attack rate
- Risk
- Probability of developing disease
- Cumulative incidence

Incidence proportion is the proportion of an initially disease-free population that develops disease, becomes injured, or dies during a specified (usually limited) period of time. Synonyms include attack rate, risk, probability of getting disease, and cumulative incidence. Incidence proportion is a proportion because the persons in the numerator, those who develop disease, are all included in the denominator (the entire population).

Method for calculating incidence proportion (risk)

$$\frac{\textit{Number of new cases of disease or injury during specified period}}{\textit{Size of population at start of period}}$$

EXAMPLES: Calculating Incidence Proportion (Risk)

Example A: *In the study of diabetics, 100 of the 189 diabetic men died during the 13-year follow-up period. Calculate the risk of death for these men.*

    Numerator = 100 deaths among the diabetic men
    Denominator = 189 diabetic men
    $10^n = 10^2 = 100$

        Risk = (100 / 189) x 100 = 52.9%

Example B: *In an outbreak of gastroenteritis among attendees of a corporate picnic, 99 persons ate potato salad, 30 of whom developed gastroenteritis. Calculate the risk of illness among persons who ate potato salad.*

    Numerator = 30 persons who ate potato salad and developed gastroenteritis
    Denominator = 99 persons who ate potato salad
    $10^n = 10^2 = 100$

        Risk = "Food-specific attack rate" = (30 / 99) x 100 = 0.303 x 100 = 30.3%

Properties and uses of incidence proportions

- Incidence proportion is a measure of the risk of disease or the probability of developing the disease during the specified period. As a measure of incidence, it includes only new cases of disease in the numerator. The denominator is the number of persons in the population at the start of the observation period. Because all of the persons with new cases of disease (numerator) are also represented in the denominator, a risk is also a proportion.

- In the outbreak setting, the term **attack rate** is often used as a synonym for risk. It is the risk of getting the disease during a specified period, such as the duration of an outbreak. A variety of attack rates can be calculated.

  Overall attack rate is the total number of new cases divided by the total population.

  A **food-specific attack rate** is the number of persons who ate a specified food and became ill divided by the total number of persons who ate that food, as illustrated in the previous potato salad example.

  A **secondary attack rate** is sometimes calculated to document the difference between community transmission of illness versus transmission of illness in a household, barracks, or other closed population. It is calculated as:

$$\frac{\textit{Number of cases among contacts of primary cases}}{\textit{Total number of contacts}} \; x \; 10^n$$

Often, the total number of contacts in the denominator is calculated as the total population in the households of the primary cases, minus the number of primary cases. For a secondary attack rate, 10^n usually is 100%.

EXAMPLE: Calculating Secondary Attack Rates

Consider an outbreak of shigellosis in which 18 persons in 18 different households all became ill. If the population of the community was 1,000, then the overall attack rate was 18 / 1,000 x 100% = 1.8%. One incubation period later, 17 persons in the same households as these "primary" cases developed shigellosis. If the 18 households included 86 persons, calculate the secondary attack rate.

Secondary attack rate = (17 / (86 - 18)) x 100% = (17 / 68) x 100% = 25.0%

Incidence rate or person-time rate

Definition of incidence rate

Incidence rate or person-time rate is a measure of incidence that incorporates time directly into the denominator. A person-time rate is generally calculated from a long-term cohort follow-up study, wherein enrollees are followed over time and the occurrence of new cases of disease is documented. Typically, each person is observed from an established starting time until one of four "end points" is reached: onset of disease, death, migration out of the study ("lost to follow-up"), or the end of the study. Similar to the incidence proportion, the numerator of the incidence rate is the number of new cases identified during the period of observation. However, the denominator differs. The denominator is the sum of the time each person was observed, totaled for all persons. This denominator represents the total time the population was at risk of and being watched for disease. Thus, the incidence rate is the ratio of the number of cases to the total time the population is at risk of disease.

Method for calculating incidence rate

$$\frac{\textit{Number of new cases of disease or injury during specified period}}{\textit{Time each person was observed, totaled for all persons}}$$

In a long-term follow-up study of morbidity, each study participant may be followed or observed for several years. One person followed for 5 years without developing disease is said to contribute 5 person-years of follow-up.

What about a person followed for one year before being lost to follow-up at year 2? Many researchers assume that persons lost to follow-up were, on average, disease-free for half the year, and thus contribute ½ year to the denominator. Therefore, the person followed for one year before being lost to follow-up contributes 1.5 person-years. The same assumption is made for participants diagnosed with the disease at the year 2 examination — some may have developed illness in month 1, and others in months 2 through 12. So, on average, they developed illness halfway through the year. As a result, persons diagnosed with the disease contribute ½ year of follow-up during the year of diagnosis.

The denominator of the person-time rate is the sum of all of the person-years for each study participant. So, someone lost to follow-up in year 3, and someone diagnosed with the disease in year 3, each contributes 2.5 years of disease-free follow-up to the denominator.

Properties and uses of incidence rates

- An incidence rate describes how quickly disease occurs in a population. It is based on person-time, so it has some advantages over an incidence proportion. Because person-time is calculated for each subject, it can accommodate persons coming into and leaving the study. As noted in the previous example, the denominator accounts for study participants who are lost to follow-up or who die during the study period. In addition, it allows enrollees to enter the study at different times. In the NHANES follow-up study, some participants were enrolled in 1971, others in 1972, 1973, 1974, and 1975.

- Person-time has one important drawback. Person-time assumes that the probability of disease during the study period is constant, so that 10 persons followed for one year equals one person followed for 10 years. Because the risk of many chronic diseases increases with age, this assumption is often not valid.

- Long-term cohort studies of the type described here are not very common. However, epidemiologists far more commonly calculate incidence rates based on a numerator of cases observed or reported, and a denominator based on the mid-year population. This type of incident rate turns out to be comparable to a person-time rate.

- Finally, if you report the incidence rate of, say, the heart disease study as 2.5 per 1,000 person-years, epidemiologists might understand, but most others will not. Person-time is epidemiologic jargon. To convert this jargon to something understandable, simply replace "person-years" with "persons per year." Reporting the results as 2.5 new cases of heart disease per 1,000 persons per year sounds like English rather than jargon. It also conveys the sense of the incidence rate as a dynamic process, the speed at which new cases of disease occur in the population.

EXAMPLES: Calculating Incidence Rates

Example A: *Investigators enrolled 2,100 women in a study and followed them annually for four years to determine the incidence rate of heart disease. After one year, none had a new diagnosis of heart disease, but 100 had been lost to follow-up. After two years, one had a new diagnosis of heart disease, and another 99 had been lost to follow-up. After three years, another seven had new diagnoses of heart disease, and 793 had been lost to follow-up. After four years, another 8 had new diagnoses with heart disease, and 392 more had been lost to follow-up.*

The study results could also be described as follows: No heart disease was diagnosed at the first year. Heart disease was diagnosed in one woman at the second year, in seven women at the third year, and in eight women at the fourth year of follow-up. One hundred women were lost to follow-up by the first year, another 99 were lost to follow-up after two years, another 793 were lost to follow-up after three years, and another 392 women were lost to follow-up after 4 years, leaving 700 women who were followed for four years and remained disease free.

Calculate the incidence rate of heart disease among this cohort. Assume that persons with new diagnoses of heart disease and those lost to follow-up were disease-free for half the year, and thus contribute ½ year to the denominator.

Numerator	= number of new cases of heart disease
	= 0 + 1 + 7 + 8 = 16
Denominator	= person-years of observation
	= (2,000 + ½ × 100) + (1,900 + ½ × 1 + ½ × 99) + (1,100 + ½ × 7 + ½ × 793) + (700 + ½ × 8 + ½ × 392)
	= 6,400 person-years of follow-up
	or
Denominator	= person-years of observation
	= (1 × 1.5) + (7 × 2.5) + (8 × 3.5) + (100 × 0.5) + (99 × 1.5) + (793 × 2.5) + (392 × 3.5) + (700 × 4)
	= 6,400 person-years of follow-up
Person-time rate	= <u>Number of new cases of disease or injury during specified period</u>
	Time each person was observed, totaled for all persons
	= 16 / 6,400
	= .0025 cases per person-year
	= 2.5 cases per 1,000 person-years

In contrast, the incidence proportion can be calculated as 16 / 2,100 = 7.6 cases per 1,000 population during the four-year period, or an average of 1.9 cases per 1,000 per year (7.6 divided by 4 years). The incidence proportion underestimates the true rate because it ignores persons lost to follow-up, and assumes that they remained disease-free for all four years.

Example B: *The diabetes follow-up study included 218 diabetic women and 3,823 nondiabetic women. By the end of the study, 72 of the diabetic women and 511 of the nondiabetic women had died. The diabetic women were observed for a total of 1,862 person years; the nondiabetic women were observed for a total of 36,653 person years. Calculate the incidence rates of death for the diabetic and non-diabetic women.*

For diabetic women, numerator = 72 and denominator = 1,862
       Person-time rate = 72 / 1,862
                    = 0.0386 deaths per person-year
                    = 38.6 deaths per 1,000 person-years

For nondiabetic women, numerator = 511 and denominator = 36,653
       Person-time rate = 511 / 36,653 = 0.0139 deaths per person-year
                    = 13.9 deaths per 1,000 person-years

Prevalence

Definition of prevalence

Prevalence, sometimes referred to as **prevalence rate**, is the proportion of persons in a population who have a particular disease or attribute at a specified point in time or over a specified period of time. Prevalence differs from incidence in that prevalence includes all cases, both new and preexisting, in the population at the specified time, whereas incidence is limited to new cases only.

Point prevalence refers to the prevalence measured at a particular point in time. It is the proportion of persons with a particular disease or attribute on a particular date.

Period prevalence refers to prevalence measured over an interval of time. It is the proportion of persons with a particular disease or attribute at any time during the interval.

Method for calculating prevalence of disease

$$\frac{\text{All new and pre-existing cases during a given time period}}{\text{Population during the same time period}} \ x \ 10^n$$

Method for calculating prevalence of an attribute

$$\frac{\text{Persons having a particular attribute during a given time period}}{\text{Population during the same time period}} \ x \ 10^n$$

The value of 10^n is usually 1 or 100 for common attributes. The value of 10^n might be 1,000, 100,000, or even 1,000,000 for rare attributes and for most diseases.

EXAMPLE: Calculating Prevalence

In a survey of 1,150 women who gave birth in Maine in 2000, a total of 468 reported taking a multivitamin at least 4 times a week during the month before becoming pregnant.[7] Calculate the prevalence of frequent multivitamin use in this group.

Numerator   = 468 multivitamin users
Denominator = 1,150 women

Prevalence   = (468 / 1,150) x 100 = 0.407 x 100 = 40.7%

Properties and uses of prevalence

- Prevalence and incidence are frequently confused. Prevalence refers to proportion of persons who *have* a condition at or during a particular time period, whereas incidence refers to the proportion or rate of persons who *develop* a condition during a particular time period. So prevalence and incidence are similar, but prevalence includes new and pre-existing cases whereas incidence includes new cases only. The key difference is in their numerators.

  Numerator of incidence = new cases that occurred during a given time period

  Numerator of prevalence = all cases present during a given time period

- The numerator of an incidence proportion or rate consists only of persons whose illness began during the specified interval. The numerator for prevalence includes all persons ill from a specified cause during the specified interval **regardless of when the illness began**. It includes not only new cases, but also preexisting cases representing persons who remained ill during some portion of the specified interval.

- Prevalence is based on both incidence and duration of illness. High prevalence of a disease within a population might reflect high incidence or prolonged survival without cure or both. Conversely, low prevalence might indicate low incidence, a rapidly fatal process, or rapid recovery.

- Prevalence rather than incidence is often measured for chronic diseases such as diabetes or osteoarthritis which have long duration and dates of onset that are difficult to pinpoint.

EXAMPLES: Incidence versus Prevalence

Figure 3.1 represents 10 new cases of illness over about 15 months in a population of 20 persons. Each horizontal line represents one person. The down arrow indicates the date of onset of illness. The solid line represents the duration of illness. The up arrow and the cross represent the date of recovery and date of death, respectively.

Figure 3.1 New Cases of Illness from October 1, 2004–September 30, 2005

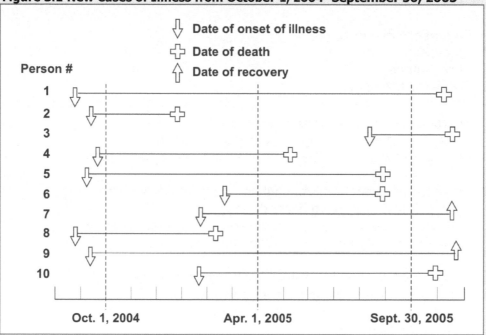

Example A: *Calculate the incidence rate from October 1, 2004, to September 30, 2005, using the midpoint population (population alive on April 1, 2005) as the denominator. Express the rate per 100 population.*

Incidence rate numerator	= number of new cases between October 1 and September 30
	= 4 (the other 6 all had onsets before October 1, and are not included)
Incidence rate denominator	= April 1 population
	= 18 (persons 2 and 8 died before April 1)
Incidence rate	= (4 / 18) x 100
	= 22 new cases per 100 population

Example B: *Calculate the point prevalence on April 1, 2005. Point prevalence is the number of persons ill on the date divided by the population on that date. On April 1, seven persons (persons 1, 4, 5, 7, 9, and 10) were ill.*

Point prevalence	= (7 / 18) x 100
	= 38.89%

Example C: *Calculate the period prevalence from October 1, 2004, to September 30, 2005. The numerator of period prevalence includes anyone who was ill any time during the period. In Figure 3.1, the first 10 persons were all ill at some time during the period.*

Period prevalence	= (10 / 20) x 100
	= 50.0%

Exercise 3.2

For each of the fractions shown below, indicate whether it is an incidence proportion, incidence rate, prevalence, or none of the three.

A. Incidence proportion
B. Incidence rate
C. Prevalence
D. None of the above

_____ 1. number of women in Framingham Study
who have died through last year from heart disease
number of women initially enrolled in Framingham Study

_____ 2. number of women in Framingham Study who have died
through last year from heart disease
number of person-years contributed through last year by
women initially enrolled in Framingham Study

_____ 3. number of women in town of Framingham who reported
having heart disease in recent health survey
estimated number of women residents of Framingham
during same period

_____ 4. number of women in Framingham Study newly diagnosed
with heart disease last year
number of women in Framingham Study without heart disease
at beginning of same year

_____ 5. number of women in State A newly diagnosed with heart disease in 2004
estimated number of women living in State A on July 1, 2004

_____ 6. estimated number of women smokers in State A
according to 2004 Behavioral Risk Factor Survey
estimated number of women living in State A on July 1, 2004

_____ 7. number of women in State A who reported having
heart disease in 2004 health survey
estimated number of women smokers in State A according to
2004 Behavioral Risk Factor Survey

 Check your answers on page 3-52

Mortality Frequency Measures

Mortality rate

A mortality rate is a measure of the frequency of occurrence of death in a defined population during a specified interval. Morbidity and mortality measures are often the same mathematically; it's just a matter of what you choose to measure, illness or death. The formula for the mortality of a defined population, over a specified period of time, is:

$$\frac{\text{Deaths occurring during a given time period}}{\begin{array}{c}\text{Size of the population among which}\\ \text{the deaths occurred}\end{array}} \times 10^n$$

When mortality rates are based on vital statistics (e.g., counts of death certificates), the denominator most commonly used is the size of the population at the middle of the time period. In the United States, values of 1,000 and 100,000 are both used for 10^n for most types of mortality rates. Table 3.4 summarizes the formulas of frequently used mortality measures.

Table 3.4 Frequently Used Measures of Mortality

Measure	Numerator	Denominator	10^n
Crude death rate	Total number of deaths during a given time interval	Mid-interval population	1,000 or 100,000
Cause-specific death rate	Number of deaths assigned to a specific cause during a given time interval	Mid-interval population	100,000
Proportionate mortality	Number of deaths assigned to a specific cause during a given time interval	Total number of deaths from all causes during the same time interval	100 or 1,000
Death-to-case ratio	Number of deaths assigned to a specific cause during a given time interval	Number of new cases of same disease reported during the same time interval	100
Neonatal mortality rate	Number of deaths among children < 28 days of age during a given time interval	Number of live births during the same time interval	1,000
Postneonatal mortality rate	Number of deaths among children 28–364 days of age during a given time interval	Number of live births during the same time interval	1,000
Infant mortality rate	Number of deaths among children < 1 year of age during a given time interval	Number of live births during the same time interval	1,000
Maternal mortality rate	Number of deaths assigned to pregnancy-related causes during a given time interval	Number of live births during the same time interval	100,000

Crude mortality rate (crude death rate)

The crude mortality rate is the mortality rate from all causes of death for a population. In the United States in 2003, a total of 2,419,921 deaths occurred. The estimated population was 290,809,777. The crude mortality rate in 2003 was, therefore, (2,419,921 / 290,809,777) x 100,000, or 832.1 deaths per 100,000 population.[8]

Cause-specific mortality rate

The cause-specific mortality rate is the mortality rate from a specified cause for a population. The numerator is the number of deaths attributed to a specific cause. The denominator remains the size of the population at the midpoint of the time period. The fraction is usually expressed per 100,000 population. In the United States in 2003, a total of 108,256 deaths were attributed to accidents (unintentional injuries), yielding a cause-specific mortality rate of 37.2 per 100,000 population.[8]

Age-specific mortality rate

An age-specific mortality rate is a mortality rate limited to a particular age group. The numerator is the number of deaths in that age group; the denominator is the number of persons in that age group in the population. In the United States in 2003, a total of 130,761 deaths occurred among persons aged 25-44 years, or an age-specific mortality rate of 153.0 per 100,000 25–44 year olds.[8] Some specific types of age-specific mortality rates are neonatal, postneonatal, and infant mortality rates, as described in the following sections.

Infant mortality rate

The infant mortality rate is perhaps the most commonly used measure for comparing health status among nations. It is calculated as follows:

$$\frac{\textit{Number of deaths among children} < \textit{1 year of age reported during a given time period}}{\textit{Number of live births reported during the same time period}} \times \textit{1,000}$$

The infant mortality rate is generally calculated on an annual basis. It is a widely used measure of health status because it reflects the health of the mother and infant during pregnancy and the year thereafter. The health of the mother and infant, in turn, reflects a wide variety of factors, including access to prenatal care, prevalence of prenatal maternal health behaviors (such as alcohol or tobacco use and proper nutrition during pregnancy, etc.), postnatal care and behaviors (including childhood immunizations and proper nutrition), sanitation, and infection control.

Is the infant mortality rate a ratio? Yes. Is it a proportion? No, because some of the deaths in the numerator were among children born the previous year. Consider the infant mortality rate in 2003. That year, 28,025 infants died and 4,089,950 children were born, for an infant mortality rate of 6.951 per 1,000.[8] Undoubtedly, some of the deaths in 2003 occurred among children born in 2002, but the denominator includes only children born in 2003.

Is the infant mortality rate truly a rate? No, because the denominator is not the size of the mid-year population of children < 1 year of age in 2003. In fact, the age-specific death rate for children < 1 year of age for 2003 was 694.7 per 100,000.[8] Obviously the infant mortality rate and the age-specific death rate for infants are very similar (695.1 versus 694.7 per 100,000) and close enough for most purposes. They are not exactly the same, however, because the estimated number of infants residing in the United States on July 1, 2003 was slightly larger than the number of children born in the United States in 2002, presumably because of immigration.

Neonatal mortality rate

The neonatal period covers birth up to but not including 28 days. The numerator of the neonatal mortality rate therefore is the number of deaths among children under 28 days of age during a given time period. The denominator of the neonatal mortality rate, like that of the infant mortality rate, is the number of live births reported during the same time period. The neonatal mortality rate is usually expressed per 1,000 live births. In 2003, the neonatal mortality rate in the United States was 4.7 per 1,000 live births.[8]

Postneonatal mortality rate

The postneonatal period is defined as the period from 28 days of age up to but not including 1 year of age. The numerator of the postneonatal mortality rate therefore is the number of deaths among children from 28 days up to but not including 1 year of age during a given time period. The denominator is the number of live births reported during the same time period. The postneonatal mortality rate is usually expressed per 1,000 live births. In 2003, the postneonatal mortality rate in the United States was 2.3 per 1,000 live births.[8]

Maternal mortality rate

The maternal mortality rate is really a ratio used to measure mortality associated with pregnancy. The numerator is the number of deaths during a given time period among women while pregnant or within 42 days of termination of pregnancy, irrespective of the duration and the site of the pregnancy, from any cause related to or aggravated by the pregnancy or its management, but not from accidental or incidental causes. The denominator is the number of live births reported during the same time period. Maternal mortality rate is usually expressed per 100,000 live births. In 2003, the U.S. maternal mortality rate was 8.9 per 100,000 live births.[8]

Sex-specific mortality rate

A sex-specific mortality rate is a mortality rate among either males or females. Both numerator and denominator are limited to the one sex.

Race-specific mortality rate

A race-specific mortality rate is a mortality rate related to a specified racial group. Both numerator and denominator are limited to the specified race.

Combinations of specific mortality rates

Mortality rates can be further stratified by combinations of cause, age, sex, and/or race. For example, in 2002, the death rate from diseases of the heart among women ages 45–54 years was 50.6 per 100,000.[9] The death rate from diseases of the heart among men in the same age group was 138.4 per 100,000, or more than 2.5 times as high as the comparable rate for women. These rates are a cause-, age-, and sex-specific rates, because they refer to one cause (diseases of the heart), one age group (45–54 years), and one sex (female or male).

EXAMPLE: Calculating Mortality Rates

Table 3.5 provides the number of deaths from all causes and from accidents (unintentional injuries) by age group in the United States in 2002. Review the following rates. Determine what to call each one, then calculate it using the data provided in Table 3.5.

a. Unintentional-injury-specific mortality rate for the entire population

This is a cause-specific mortality rate.

Rate = $\frac{\text{number of unintentional injury deaths in the entire population}}{\text{estimated midyear population}}$ × 100,000

= (106,742 / 288,357,000) × 100,000

= 37.0 unintentional-injury-related deaths per 100,000 population

b. All-cause mortality rate for 25–34 year olds

This is an age-specific mortality rate.

Rate = $\frac{\text{number of deaths from all causes among 25–34 year olds}}{\text{estimated midyear population of 25–34 year olds}}$ × 100,000

= (41,355 / 39,928,000) × 100,000

= 103.6 deaths per 100,000 25–34 year olds

c. All-cause mortality among males

This is a sex-specific mortality rate.

Rate = $\frac{\text{number of deaths from all causes among males}}{\text{estimated midyear population of males}}$ × 100,000

= (1,199,264 / 141,656,000) × 100,000

= 846.6 deaths per 100,000 males

d. Unintentional-injury specific mortality among 25 to 34 year old males

This is a cause-specific, age-specific, and sex-specific mortality rate

Rate = $\frac{\text{number of unintentional injury deaths among 25–34 year old males}}{\text{estimated midyear population of 25–34 year old males}}$ × 100,000

= (9,635 / 20,203,000) × 100,000

= 47.7 unintentional-injury-related deaths per 100,000 25–34 year olds

Table 3.5 All-Cause and Unintentional Injury Mortality and Estimated Population by Age Group, For Both Sexes and For Males Alone — United States, 2002

Age group (years)	All Races, Both Sexes			All Races, Males		
	All Causes	Unintentional Injuries	Estimated Pop. (x 1000)	All Causes	Unintentional Injuries	Estimated Pop. (x 1000)
0–4	32,892	2,587	19,597	18,523	1,577	10,020
5–14	7,150	2,718	41,037	4,198	1713	21,013
15–24	33,046	15,412	40,590	24,416	11,438	20,821
25–34	41,355	12,569	39,928	28,736	9,635	20,203
35–44	91,140	16,710	44,917	57,593	12,012	22,367
45–54	172,385	14,675	40,084	107,722	10,492	19,676
55–64	253,342	8,345	26,602	151,363	5,781	12,784
65+	1,811,720	33,641	35,602	806,431	16,535	14,772
Not stated	357	85	0	282	74	0
Total	2,443,387	106,742	288,357	1,199,264	69,257	141,656

Data Source: Web-based Injury Statistics Query and Reporting System (WISQARS) [online database] Atlanta; National Center for Injury Prevention and Control. Available from: http://www.cdc.gov/ncipc/wisqars.

Exercise 3.3

In 2001, a total of 15,555 homicide deaths occurred among males and 4,753 homicide deaths occurred among females. The estimated 2001 midyear populations for males and females were 139,813,000 and 144,984,000, respectively.

1. Calculate the homicide-related death rates for males and for females.

2. What type(s) of mortality rates did you calculate in Question 1?

3. Calculate the ratio of homicide-mortality rates for males compared to females.

4. Interpret the rate you calculated in Question 3 as if you were presenting information to a policymaker.

 Check your answers on page 3-52

Age-adjusted mortality rates

Mortality rates can be used to compare the rates in one area with the rates in another area, or to compare rates over time. However, because mortality rates obviously increase with age, a higher mortality rate among one population than among another might simply reflect the fact that the first population is older than the second.

Consider that the mortality rates in 2002 for the states of Alaska and Florida were 472.2 and 1,005.7 per 100,000, respectively (see Table 3.6). Should everyone from Florida move to Alaska to reduce their risk of death? No, the reason that Alaska's mortality rate is so much lower than Florida's is that Alaska's population is considerably younger. Indeed, for seven age groups, the age-specific mortality rates in Alaska are actually higher than Florida's.

To eliminate the distortion caused by different underlying age distributions in different populations, statistical techniques are used to adjust or standardize the rates among the populations to be compared. These techniques take a weighted average of the age-specific mortality rates, and eliminate the effect of different age distributions among the different populations. Mortality rates computed with these techniques are **age-adjusted** or **age-standardized mortality rates**. Alaska's 2002 age-adjusted mortality rate (794.1 per 100,000) was higher than Florida's (787.8 per 100,000), which is not surprising given that 7 of 13 age-specific mortality rates were higher in Alaska than Florida.

Death-to-case ratio

Definition of death-to-case ratio

The death-to-case ratio is the number of deaths attributed to a particular disease during a specified time period divided by the number of new cases of that disease identified during the same time period. The death-to-case ratio is a ratio but not necessarily a proportion, because some of the deaths that are counted in the numerator might have occurred among persons who developed disease in an earlier period, and are therefore not counted in the denominator.

Table 3.6 All-Cause Mortality by Age Group — Alaska and Florida, 2002

Age group (years)	ALASKA Population	ALASKA Deaths	ALASKA Death Rate (per 100,000)	FLORIDA Population	FLORIDA Deaths	FLORIDA Death Rate (per 100,000)
<1	9,938	55	553.4	205,579	1,548	753.0
1–4	38,503	12	31.2	816,570	296	36.2
5–9	50,400	6	11.9	1,046,504	141	13.5
10–14	57,216	24	41.9	1,131,068	219	19.4
15–19	56,634	43	75.9	1,073,470	734	68.4
20–24	42,929	63	146.8	1,020,856	1,146	112.3
25–34	84,112	120	142.7	2,090,312	2,627	125.7
35–44	107,305	280	260.9	2,516,004	5,993	238.2
45–54	103,039	427	414.4	2,225,957	10,730	482.0
55–64	52,543	480	913.5	1,694,574	16,137	952.3
65–74	24,096	502	2,083.3	1,450,843	28,959	1,996.0
65–84	11,784	645	5,473.5	1,056,275	50,755	4,805.1
85+	3,117	373	11,966.6	359,056	48,486	13,503.7
Unknown	NA	0	NA	NA	43	NA
Total	3,030	3,030	472.2	16,687,068	167,814	1,005.7
Age-adjusted rate:			794.1			787.8

Data Source: Web-based Injury Statistics Query and Reporting System (WISQARS) [online database] Atlanta; National Center for Injury Prevention and Control. Available from: http://www.cdc.gov/ncipc/wisqars.

Method for calculating death-to-case ratio

$$\frac{\text{Number of deaths attributed to a particular disease during specified period}}{\text{Number of new cases of the disease identified during the specified period}} \times 10^n$$

EXAMPLE: Calculating Death-to-Case Ratios

Between 1940 and 1949, a total of 143,497 incident cases of diphtheria were reported. During the same decade, 11,228 deaths were attributed to diphtheria. Calculate the death-to-case ratio.

Death-to-case ratio = 11,228 / 143,497 x 1 = 0.0783

or

= 11,228 / 143,497 x 100 = 7.83 per 100

Exercise 3.4

Table 3.7 provides the number of reported cases of diphtheria and the number of diphtheria-associated deaths in the United States by decade. Calculate the death-to-case ratio by decade. Describe the data in Table 3.7, including your results.

Table 3.7 Number of Cases and Deaths from Diphtheria by Decade — United States, 1940–1999

Decade	Number of New Cases	Number of Deaths	Death-to-case Ratio (x 100)
1940–1949	143,497	11,228	7.82
1950–1959	23,750	1,710	_____
1960–1969	3,679	390	_____
1970–1979	1,956	90	_____
1980–1989	27	3	_____
1990–1999	22	5	_____

Data Sources: Centers for Disease Control and Prevention. Summary of notifiable diseases, United States, 2001. MMWR 2001;50(No. 53).
Centers for Disease Control and Prevention. Summary of notifiable diseases, United States, 1998. MMWR 1998;47(No. 53).
Centers for Disease Control and Prevention. Summary of notifiable diseases, United States, 1989. MMWR 1989;38 (No. 53).

 Check your answers on page 3-53

Case-fatality rate

The case-fatality rate is the proportion of persons with a particular condition (cases) who die from that condition. It is a measure of the severity of the condition. The formula is:

$$\frac{\text{Number of cause-specific deaths among the incident cases}}{\text{Number of incident cases}} \times 10^n$$

The case-fatality rate is a proportion, so the numerator is restricted to deaths among people included in the denominator. The time periods for the numerator and the denominator do not need to be the same; the denominator could be cases of HIV/AIDS diagnosed during the calendar year 1990, and the numerator, deaths among those diagnosed with HIV in 1990, could be from 1990 to the present.

EXAMPLE: Calculating Case-Fatality Rates

In an epidemic of hepatitis A traced to green onions from a restaurant, 555 cases were identified. Three of the case-patients died as a result of their infections. Calculate the case-fatality rate.

Case fatality rate = (3 / 555) x 100 = 0.5%

The case-fatality rate is a proportion, not a true rate. As a result, some epidemiologists prefer the term **case-fatality ratio**.

The concept behind the case-fatality rate and the death-to-case ratio is similar, but the formulations are different. The death-to-case ratio is simply the number of cause-specific deaths that occurred during a specified time divided by the number of new cases of that disease that occurred during the same time. The deaths included in the numerator of the death-to-case ratio are not restricted to the new cases in the denominator; in fact, for many diseases, the deaths are among persons whose onset of disease was years earlier. In contrast, in the case-fatality rate, the deaths included in the numerator are restricted to the cases in the denominator.

Proportionate mortality

Definition of proportionate mortality

Proportionate mortality describes the proportion of deaths in a specified population over a period of time attributable to different causes. Each cause is expressed as a percentage of all deaths, and the sum of the causes must add to 100%. These proportions are not mortality rates, because the denominator is all deaths rather than the population in which the deaths occurred.

Method for calculating proportionate mortality

For a specified population over a specified period,

$$\frac{\textit{Deaths caused by a particular cause}}{\textit{Deaths from all causes}} \; x \; 100$$

The distribution of primary causes of death in the United States in 2003 for the entire population (all ages) and for persons ages 25–44 years are provided in Table 3.1. As illustrated in that table, accidents (unintentional injuries) accounted for 4.3% of all deaths, but 21.6% of deaths among 25–44 year olds.[8]

Sometimes, particularly in occupational epidemiology, proportionate mortality is used to compare deaths in a population of interest (say, a workplace) with the proportionate mortality in the broader population. This comparison of two proportionate mortalities is called a **proportionate mortality ratio**, or PMR for short. A PMR greater than 1.0 indicates that a particular cause accounts for a greater proportion of deaths in the population of interest than you might expect. For example, construction workers may be more likely to die of injuries than the general population.

However, PMRs can be misleading, because they are not based on mortality rates. A low cause-specific mortality rate in the population of interest can elevate the proportionate mortalities for all of the other causes, because they must add up to 100%. Those workers with a high injury-related proportionate mortality very likely have lower proportionate mortalities for chronic or disabling conditions that keep people out of the workforce. In other words, people who work are more likely to be healthier than the population as a whole — this is known as the healthy worker effect.

Exercise 3.5

Using the data in Table 3.8, calculate the missing proportionate mortalities for persons ages 25-44 years for diseases of the heart and assaults (homicide).

Table 3.8 Number, Proportion (Percentage), and Ranking of Deaths for Leading Causes of Death, All Ages and 25–44 Year Age Group — United States, 2003

	All Ages			Ages 25–44 Years		
	Number	Percentage	Rank	Number	Percentage	Rank
All causes	2,443,930	100.0		128,924	100.0	
Diseases of heart	684,462	28.0	1	16,283	_____	3
Malignant neoplasms	554,643	22.7	2	19,041	14.8	2
Cerebrovascular disease	157,803	6.5	3	3,004	2.3	8
Chronic lower respiratory diseases	126,128	5.2	4	401	0.3	*
Accidents (unintentional injuries)	105,695	4.3	5	27,844	21.6	1
Diabetes mellitus	73,965	3.0	6	2,662	2.1	9
Influenza & pneumonia	64,847	2.6	7	1,337	1.0	10
Alzheimer's disease	63,343	2.6	8	0	0.0	*
Nephritis, nephrotic syndrome, nephrosis	33,615	1.4	9	305	0.2	*
Septicemia	34,243	1.4	10	328	0.2	*
Intentional self-harm (suicide)	30,642	1.3	11	11,251	8.7	4
Chronic liver disease and cirrhosis	27,201	1.1	12	3,288	2.6	7
Assault (homicide)	17,096	0.7	13	7,367	_____	5
HIV disease	13,544	0.5	*	6,879	5.3	6
All other	456,703	18.7		29,480	22.9	

* Not among top ranked causes

Data Sources: CDC. Summary of notifiable diseases, United States, 2003. MMWR 2005;2(No. 54).
Hoyert DL, Kung HC, Smith BL. Deaths: Preliminary data for 2003. National Vital Statistics Reports; vol. 53 no 15. Hyattsville, MD: National Center for Health Statistics 2005: 15, 27.

 Check your answers on page 3-53

Years of potential life lost

Definition of years of potential life lost

Years of potential life lost (YPLL) is one measure of the impact of premature mortality on a population. Additional measures incorporate disability and other measures of quality of life. YPLL is calculated as the sum of the differences between a predetermined end point and the ages of death for those who died before that end point. The two most commonly used end points are age 65 years and average life expectancy.

The use of YPLL is affected by this calculation, which implies a value system in which more weight is given to a death when it occurs at an earlier age. Thus, deaths at older ages are "devalued." However, the YPLL before age 65 ($YPLL_{65}$) places much more emphasis on deaths at early ages than does YPLL based on remaining life expectancy ($YPLL_{LE}$). In 2000, the remaining life expectancy was 21.6 years for a 60-year-old, 11.3 years for a 70-year-old, and 8.6 for an 80-year-old. $YPLL_{65}$ is based on the fewer than 30% of deaths that occur among persons younger than 65. In contrast, YPLL for life expectancy ($YPLL_{LE}$) is based on deaths among persons of all ages, so it more closely resembles crude mortality rates.[10]

YPLL rates can be used to compare YPLL among populations of different sizes. Because different populations may also have different age distributions, YPLL rates are usually age-adjusted to eliminate the effect of differing age distributions.

Method for calculating YPLL from a line listing

Step 1. Decide on end point (65 years, average life expectancy, or other).

Step 2. Exclude records of all persons who died at or after the end point.

Step 3. For each person who died before the end point, calculate that person's YPLL by subtracting the age at death from the end point.

$$YPLL_{individual} = \text{end point} - \text{age at death}$$

Step 4. Sum the individual YPLLs.

$$YPLL = \sum YPLL_{individual}$$

Method for calculating YPLL from a frequency

Step 1. Ensure that age groups break at the identified end point (e.g., 65 years). Eliminate all age groups older than the endpoint.

Step 2. For each age group younger than the end point, identify the midpoint of the age group, where midpoint =

$$\frac{\text{age group's youngest age in years} + \text{oldest age} + 1}{2}$$

Step 3. For each age group younger than the end point, identify that age group's YPLL by subtracting the midpoint from the end point.

Step 4. Calculate age-specific YPLL by multiplying the age group's YPLL times the number of persons in that age group.

Step 5. Sum the age-specific YPLL's.

The **YPLL rate** represents years of potential life lost per 1,000 population below the end-point age, such as 65 years. YPLL rates should be used to compare premature mortality in different populations, because YPLL does not take into account differences in population sizes.

The formula for a YPLL rate is as follows:

$$\frac{\textit{Years of potential life lost}}{\textit{Population under age 65 years}} \; x \; 10^n$$

EXAMPLE: Calculating YPLL and YPLL Rates

Use the data in Tables 3.9 and 3.10 to calculate the leukemia-related mortality rate for all ages, mortality rate for persons under age 65 years, YPLL, and YPLL rate.

1. Leukemia related mortality rate, all ages

$$= (21{,}498 / 288{,}357{,}000) \times 100{,}000 = 7.5 \text{ leukemia deaths per } 100{,}000 \text{ population}$$

2. Leukemia related mortality rate for persons under age 65 years

$$= \frac{125 + 316 + 472 + 471 + 767 + 1{,}459 + 2{,}611}{(19{,}597 + 41{,}037 + 40{,}590 + 39{,}928 + 44{,}917 + 40{,}084 + 26{,}602)} \times 100{,}000$$

$$= 6{,}221 / 252{,}755{,}000 = \times 100{,}000$$

$$= 2.5 \text{ leukemia deaths per } 100{,}000 \text{ persons under age 65 years}$$

3. Leukemia related YPLL

   a. Calculate the midpoint of each age interval. Using the previously shown formula, the midpoint of the age group 0–4 years is (0 + 4 + 1) / 2, or 5 / 2, or 2.5 years. Using the same formula, midpoints must be determined for each age group up to and including the age group 55 to 64 years (see column 3 of Table 3.10).

   b. Subtract the midpoint from the end point to determine the years of potential life lost for a particular age group. For the age group 0–4 years, each death represents 65 minus 2.5, or 62.5 years of potential life lost (see column 4 of Table 3.10).

   c. Calculate age specific years of potential life lost by multiplying the number of deaths in a given age group by its years of potential life lost. For the age group 0–4 years, 125 deaths x 62.5 = 7,812.5 YPLL (see column 5 of Table 3.10).

   d. Total the age specific YPLL. The total YPLL attributed to leukemia in the United States in 2002 was 117,033 years (see Total of column 5, Table 3.10).

4. Leukemia related YPLL rate

$$= \text{YPLL}_{65} \text{ rate}$$
$$= \text{YPLL divided by population to age 65}$$
$$= (117{,}033 / 252{,}755{,}000) \times 1{,}000$$
$$= 0.5 \text{ YPLL per } 1{,}000 \text{ population under age 65}$$

Table 3.9 Deaths Attributed to HIV or Leukemia by Age Group — United States, 2002

Age group (Years)	Population (X 1,000)	Number of HIV Deaths	Number of Leukemia Deaths
0–4	19,597	12	125
5–14	41,037	25	316
15–24	40,590	178	472
25–34	39,928	1,839	471
35–44	44,917	5,707	767
45–54	40,084	4,474	1,459
55–64	26,602	1,347	2,611
65+	35,602	509	15,277
Not stated		4	0
Total	288,357	14,095	21,498

Data Source: Web-based Injury Statistics Query and Reporting System (WISQARS) [online database] Atlanta; National Center for Injury Prevention and Control. Available from: http://www.cdc.gov/ncipc/wisqars.

Table 3.10 Deaths and Years of Potential Life Lost Attributed to Leukemia by Age Group — United States, 2002

Column 1 Age Group (years)	Column 2 Deaths	Column 3 Age Midpoint	Column 4 Years to 65	Column 5 YPLL
0–4	125	2.5	62.5	7,813
5–14	316	10	55	17,380
15–24	472	20	45	21,240
25–34	471	30	35	16,485
35–44	767	40	25	19,175
45–54	1,459	50	15	21,885
55–64	2,611	60	5	13,055
65+	15,277	—	—	—
Not stated	0	—	—	—
Total	21,498			117,033

Data Source: Web-based Injury Statistics Query and Reporting System (WISQARS) [online database] Atlanta; National Center for Injury Prevention and Control. Available from: http://www.cdc.gov/ncipc/wisqars.

Exercise 3.6

Use the HIV data in Table 3.9 to answer the following questions:

1. What is the HIV-related mortality rate, all ages?

2. What is the HIV-related mortality rate for persons under 65 years?

3. What is the HIV-related YPLL before age 65?

4. What is the HIV-related $YPLL_{65}$ rate?

5. Create a table comparing the mortality rates and YPLL for leukemia and HIV. Which measure(s) might you prefer if you were trying to support increased funding for leukemia research? For HIV research?

 Check your answers on page 3-53

Natality (Birth) Measures

Natality measures are population-based measures of birth. These measures are used primarily by persons working in the field of maternal and child health. Table 3.11 includes some of the commonly used measures of natality.

Table 3.11 Frequently Used Measures of Natality

Measure	Numerator	Denominator	10^n
Crude birth rate	Number of live births during a specified time interval	Mid-interval population	1,000
Crude fertility rate	Number of live births during a specified time interval	Number of women ages 15–44 years at mid-interval	1,000
Crude rate of natural increase	Number of live births minus number of deaths during a specified time interval	Mid-interval population	1,000
Low-birth weight ratio	Number of live births <2,500 grams during a specified time interval	Number of live births during the same time interval	100

Measures of Association

The key to epidemiologic analysis is comparison. Occasionally you might observe an incidence rate among a population that seems high and wonder whether it is actually higher than what should be expected based on, say, the incidence rates in other communities. Or, you might observe that, among a group of case-patients in an outbreak, several report having eaten at a particular restaurant. Is the restaurant just a popular one, or have more case-patients eaten there than would be expected? The way to address that concern is by comparing the observed group with another group that represents the expected level.

A measure of association quantifies the relationship between exposure and disease among the two groups. Exposure is used loosely to mean not only exposure to foods, mosquitoes, a partner with a sexually transmissible disease, or a toxic waste dump, but also inherent characteristics of persons (for example, age, race, sex), biologic characteristics (immune status), acquired characteristics (marital status), activities (occupation, leisure activities), or conditions under which they live (socioeconomic status or access to medical care).

The measures of association described in the following section compare disease occurrence among one group with disease occurrence in another group. Examples of measures of association include risk ratio (relative risk), rate ratio, odds ratio, and proportionate mortality ratio.

Risk ratio

Definition of risk ratio

A risk ratio (RR), also called relative risk, compares the risk of a health event (disease, injury, risk factor, or death) among one group with the risk among another group. It does so by dividing the risk (incidence proportion, attack rate) in group 1 by the risk (incidence proportion, attack rate) in group 2 . The two groups are typically differentiated by such demographic factors as sex (e.g., males versus females) or by exposure to a suspected risk factor (e.g., did or did not eat potato salad). Often, the group of primary interest is labeled the exposed group, and the comparison group is labeled the unexposed group.

Method for Calculating risk ratio

The formula for risk ratio (RR) is:

$$\frac{\textit{Risk of disease (incidence proportion, attack rate)}}{\textit{Risk of disease (incidence proportion, attack rate)}}$$

Risk of disease (incidence proportion, attack rate)
in group of primary interest

Risk of disease (incidence proportion, attack rate)
in comparison group

A risk ratio of 1.0 indicates identical risk among the two groups. A risk ratio greater than 1.0 indicates an increased risk for the group in the numerator, usually the exposed group. A risk ratio less than 1.0 indicates a decreased risk for the exposed group, indicating that perhaps exposure actually protects against disease occurrence.

EXAMPLES: Calculating Risk Ratios

Example A: *In an outbreak of tuberculosis among prison inmates in South Carolina in 1999, 28 of 157 inmates residing on the East wing of the dormitory developed tuberculosis, compared with 4 of 137 inmates residing on the West wing.[11] These data are summarized in the two-by-two table so called because it has two rows for the exposure and two columns for the outcome. Here is the general format and notation.*

Table 3.12A General Format and Notation for a Two-by-Two Table

	Ill	Well	Total
Exposed	a	b	$a + b = H_1$
Unexposed	c	d	$c + d = H_0$
Total	$a + c = V_1$	$b + d = V_0$	T

In this example, the exposure is the dormitory wing and the outcome is tuberculosis) illustrated in Table 3.12B. Calculate the risk ratio.

Table 3.12B Incidence of Mycobacterium Tuberculosis Infection Among Congregated, HIV-Infected Prison Inmates by Dormitory Wing — South Carolina, 1999

	Developed tuberculosis?		Total
	Yes	No	
East wing	a = 28	b = 129	$H_1 = 157$
West wing	c = 4	d = 133	$H_0 = 137$
Total	32	262	T = 294

Data source: McLaughlin SI, Spradling P, Drociuk D, Ridzon R, Pozsik CJ, Onorato I. Extensive transmission of Mycobacterium tuberculosis among congregated, HIV-infected prison inmates in South Carolina, United States. Int J Tuberc Lung Dis 2003;7:665–672.

To calculate the risk ratio, first calculate the risk or attack rate for each group. Here are the formulas:

Attack Rate (Risk)
Attack rate for exposed = a / a+b
Attack rate for unexposed = c / c+d

For this example:

Risk of tuberculosis among East wing residents	=	28 / 157	=	0.178	=	17.8%
Risk of tuberculosis among West wing residents	=	4 / 137	=	0.029	=	2.9%

The risk ratio is simply the ratio of these two risks:

Risk ratio = 17.8 / 2.9 = 6.1

Thus, inmates who resided in the East wing of the dormitory were 6.1 times as likely to develop tuberculosis as those who resided in the West wing.

EXAMPLES: Calculating Risk Ratios (Continued)

Example B: *In an outbreak of varicella (chickenpox) in Oregon in 2002, varicella was diagnosed in 18 of 152 vaccinated children compared with 3 of 7 unvaccinated children. Calculate the risk ratio.*

Table 3.13 Incidence of Varicella Among Schoolchildren in 9 Affected Classrooms — Oregon, 2002

	Varicella	Non-case	Total
Vaccinated	a = 18	b = 134	152
Unvaccinated	c = 3	d = 4	7
Total	21	138	159

Data Source: Tugwell BD, Lee LE, Gillette H, Lorber EM, Hedberg K, Cieslak PR. Chickenpox outbreak in a highly vaccinated school population. Pediatrics 2004 Mar;113(3 Pt 1):455–459.

Risk of varicella among vaccinated children = 18 / 152 = 0.118 = 11.8%
Risk of varicella among unvaccinated children = 3 / 7 = 0.429 = 42.9%

Risk ratio = 0.118 / 0.429 = 0.28

The risk ratio is less than 1.0, indicating a decreased risk or protective effect for the exposed (vaccinated) children. The risk ratio of 0.28 indicates that vaccinated children were only approximately one-fourth as likely (28%, actually) to develop varicella as were unvaccinated children.

Rate ratio

A rate ratio compares the incidence rates, person-time rates, or mortality rates of two groups. As with the risk ratio, the two groups are typically differentiated by demographic factors or by exposure to a suspected causative agent. The rate for the group of primary interest is divided by the rate for the comparison group.

$$\text{Rate ratio} = \frac{\text{Rate for group of primary interest}}{\text{Rate for comparison group}}$$

The interpretation of the value of a rate ratio is similar to that of the risk ratio. That is, a rate ratio of 1.0 indicates equal rates in the two groups, a rate ratio greater than 1.0 indicates an increased risk for the group in the numerator, and a rate ratio less than 1.0 indicates a decreased risk for the group in the numerator.

EXAMPLE: Calculating Rate Ratios (Continued)

Public health officials were called to investigate a perceived increase in visits to ships' infirmaries for acute respiratory illness (ARI) by passengers of cruise ships in Alaska in 1998.[13] The officials compared passenger visits to ship infirmaries for ARI during May–August 1998 with the same period in 1997. They recorded 11.6 visits for ARI per 1,000 tourists per week in 1998, compared with 5.3 visits per 1,000 tourists per week in 1997. Calculate the rate ratio.

Rate ratio = 11.6 / 5.3 = 2.2

Passengers on cruise ships in Alaska during May–August 1998 were more than twice as likely to visit their ships' infirmaries for ARI than were passengers in 1997. (Note: Of 58 viral isolates identified from nasal cultures from passengers, most were influenza A, making this the largest summertime influenza outbreak in North America.)

Exercise 3.7

Table 3.14 illustrates lung cancer mortality rates for persons who continued to smoke and for smokers who had quit at the time of follow-up in one of the classic studies of smoking and lung cancer conducted in Great Britain.

Using the data in Table 3.14, calculate the following:

1. Rate ratio comparing current smokers with nonsmokers

2. Rate ratio comparing ex-smokers who quit at least 20 years ago with nonsmokers

3. What are the public health implications of these findings?

Table 3.14 Number and Rate (Per 1,000 Person-years) of Lung Cancer Deaths for Current Smokers and Ex-smokers by Years Since Quitting, Physician Cohort Study — Great Britain, 1951–1961

Cigarette smoking status	Lung cancer deaths	Rate per 1000 person-years	Rate Ratio
Current smokers	133	1.30	_____
For ex-smokers, years since quitting:			
<5 years	5	0.67	9.6
5-9 years	7	0.49	7.0
10-19 years	3	0.18	2.6
20+ years	2	0.19	_____
Nonsmokers	3	0.07	1.0 (reference group)

Data Source: Doll R, Hill AB. Mortality in relation to smoking: 10 years' observation of British doctors. Brit Med J 1964; 1:1399–1410, 1460–1467.

 Check your answers on page 3-54

Odds ratio

An odds ratio (OR) is another measure of association that quantifies the relationship between an exposure with two categories and health outcome. Referring to the four cells in Table 3.15, the odds ratio is calculated as

$$Odds\ ratio\ =\ \left(\frac{a}{b}\right)\left(\frac{c}{d}\right)\ =\ ad\,/\,bc$$

where

a = number of persons exposed and with disease
b = number of persons exposed but without disease
c = number of persons unexposed but with disease
d = number of persons unexposed: and without disease
a+c = total number of persons with disease (case-patients)
b+d = total number of persons without disease (controls)

The odds ratio is sometimes called the **cross-product ratio** because the numerator is based on multiplying the value in cell "a" times the value in cell "d," whereas the denominator is the product of cell "b" and cell "c." A line from cell "a" to cell "d" (for the numerator) and another from cell "b" to cell "c" (for the denominator) creates an x or cross on the two-by-two table.

Table 3.15 Exposure and Disease in a Hypothetical Population of 10,000 Persons

	Disease	No Disease	Total	Risk
Exposed	a = 100	b = 1,900	2,000	5.0%
Not Exposed	c = 80	d = 7,920	8,000	1.0%
Total	180	9,820	10,000	

EXAMPLE: Calculating Odds Ratios

Use the data in Table 3.15 to calculate the risk and odds ratios.

1. Risk ratio

      5.0 / 1.0 = 5.0

2. Odds ratio

      (100 x 7,920) / (1,900 x 80) = 5.2

Notice that the odds ratio of 5.2 is close to the risk ratio of 5.0. That is one of the attractive features of the odds ratio — when the health outcome is uncommon, the odds ratio provides a reasonable approximation of the risk ratio. Another attractive feature is that the odds ratio can be calculated with data from a case-control study, whereas neither a risk ratio nor a rate ratio can be calculated.

In a case-control study, investigators enroll a group of case-patients (distributed in cells a and c of the two-by-two table), and a group of non-cases or controls (distributed in cells b and d).

The odds ratio is the measure of choice in a case-control study (see Lesson 1). A case-control study is based on enrolling a group of persons with disease ("case-patients") and a comparable group without disease ("controls"). The number of persons in the control group is usually decided by the investigator. Often, the size of the population from which the case-patients came is not known. As a result, risks, rates, risk ratios or rate ratios cannot be calculated from the typical case-control study. However, you can calculate an odds ratio and interpret it as an approximation of the risk ratio, particularly when the disease is uncommon in the population.

Exercise 3.8

Calculate the odds ratio for the tuberculosis data in Table 3.12. Would you say that your odds ratio is an accurate approximation of the risk ratio? (Hint: The more common the disease, the further the odds ratio is from the risk ratio.)

 Check your answers on page 3-55

Measures of Public Health Impact

A measure of public health impact is used to place the association between an exposure and an outcome into a meaningful public health context. Whereas a measure of association quantifies the relationship between exposure and disease, and thus begins to provide insight into causal relationships, measures of public health impact reflect the burden that an exposure contributes to the frequency of disease in the population. Two measures of public health impact often used are the attributable proportion and efficacy or effectiveness.

Attributable proportion

Definition of attributable proportion

The attributable proportion, also known as the attributable risk percent, is a measure of the public health impact of a causative factor. The calculation of this measure assumes that the occurrence of disease in the unexposed group represents the baseline or expected risk for that disease. It further assumes that if the risk of disease in the exposed group is higher than the risk in the unexposed group, the difference can be attributed to the exposure. Thus, the attributable proportion is the amount of disease in the exposed group attributable to the exposure. It represents the expected reduction in disease if the exposure could be removed (or never existed).

Appropriate use of attributable proportion depends on a single risk factor being responsible for a condition. When multiple risk factors may interact (e.g., physical activity and age or health status), this measure may not be appropriate.

Method for calculating attributable proportion

Attributable proportion is calculated as follows:

$$\frac{Risk\ for\ exposed\ group - risk\ for\ unexposed\ group}{Risk\ for\ exposed\ group} \; x \; 100\%$$

Attributable proportion can be calculated for rates in the same way.

EXAMPLE: Calculating Attributable Proportion

In another study of smoking and lung cancer, the lung cancer mortality rate among nonsmokers was 0.07 per 1,000 persons per year.[14] The lung cancer mortality rate among persons who smoked 1–14 cigarettes per day was 0.57 lung cancer deaths per 1,000 persons per year. Calculate the attributable proportion.

Attributable proportion = (0.57 − 0.07) / 0.57 x 100% = 87.7%

Given the proven causal relationship between cigarette smoking and lung cancer, and assuming that the groups are comparable in all other ways, one could say that about 88% of the lung cancer among smokers of 1 14 cigarettes per day might be attributable to their smoking. The remaining 12% of the lung cancer cases in this group would have occurred anyway.

Vaccine efficacy or vaccine effectiveness

Vaccine efficacy and vaccine effectiveness measure the proportionate reduction in cases among vaccinated persons. Vaccine efficacy is used when a study is carried out under ideal conditions, for example, during a clinical trial. Vaccine effectiveness is used when a study is carried out under typical field (that is, less than perfectly controlled) conditions.

Vaccine efficacy/effectiveness (VE) is measured by calculating the risk of disease among vaccinated and unvaccinated persons and determining the percentage reduction in risk of disease among vaccinated persons relative to unvaccinated persons. The greater the percentage reduction of illness in the vaccinated group, the greater the vaccine efficacy/effectiveness. The basic formula is written as:

$$\frac{Risk\ among\ unvaccinated\ group - risk\ among\ vaccinated\ group}{Risk\ among\ unvaccinated\ group}$$

OR: *1 − risk ratio*

In the first formula, the numerator (risk among unvaccinated − risk among vaccinated) is sometimes called the risk difference or excess risk.

Vaccine efficacy/effectiveness is interpreted as the proportionate reduction in disease among the vaccinated group. So a VE of 90% indicates a 90% reduction in disease occurrence among the vaccinated group, or a 90% reduction from the number of cases you would expect if they have not been vaccinated.

EXAMPLE: Calculating Vaccine Effectiveness

Calculate the vaccine effectiveness from the varicella data in Table 3.13.

$$VE = (42.9 - 11.8) / 42.9 = 31.1 / 42.9 = 72\%$$

$$Alternatively, VE = 1 - RR = 1 - 0.28 = 72\%$$

So, the vaccinated group experienced 72% fewer varicella cases than they would have if they had not been vaccinated.

Summary

Because many of the variables encountered in field epidemiology are nominal-scale variables, frequency measures are used quite commonly in epidemiology. Frequency measures include ratios, proportions, and rates. Ratios and proportions are useful for describing the characteristics of populations. Proportions and rates are used for quantifying morbidity and mortality. These measures allow epidemiologists to infer risk among different groups, detect groups at high risk, and develop hypotheses about causes — that is, why these groups might be at increased risk.

The two primary measures of morbidity are incidence and prevalence.
- **Incidence** rates reflect the occurrence of new disease in a population.
- **Prevalence** reflects the presence of disease in a population.

A variety of **mortality** rates describe deaths among specific groups, particularly by age or sex or by cause.

The hallmark of epidemiologic analysis is comparison, such as comparison of observed amount of disease in a population with the expected amount of disease. The comparisons can be quantified by using such measures of association as risk ratios, rate ratios, and odds ratios. These measures provide evidence regarding causal relationships between exposures and disease.

Measures of public health impact place the association between an exposure and a disease in a public health context. Two such measures are the attributable proportion and vaccine efficacy.

Exercise Answers

Exercise 3.1

1. B
2. C
3. A
4. B
5. A

Exercise 3.2

1. A; denominator is size of population at start of study, numerator is number of deaths among that population.
2. B; denominator is person-years contributed by participants, numerator is number of death among that population.
3. C; numerator is all existing cases.
4. A; denominator is size of population at risk, numerator is number of new cases among that population.
5. B; denominator is mid-year population, numerator is number of new cases among that population.
6. C; numerator is total number with attribute.
7. D; this is a ratio (heart disease:smokers)

Exercise 3.3

1. Homicide-related death rate (males)
   = (# homicide deaths among males / male population) x 100,000
   = 15,555 / 139,813,000 x 100,000
   = 11.1 homicide deaths / 100,000 population among males

   Homicide-related death rate (females)
   = (# homicide deaths among females / female population) x 100,000
   = 4,753 / 144,984,000 x 100,000
   = 3.3 homicide deaths / 100,000 population among females

2. These are cause- and sex-specific mortality rates.

3. Homicide-mortality rate ratio
   = homicide death rate (males) / homicide death rate (females)
   = 11.1 / 3.3
   = 3.4 to 1

= (see below, which is the answer to question 4).

4. Because the homicide rate among males is higher than the homicide rate among females, specific intervention programs need to target males and females differently.

Exercise 3.4

1940-1949	43,497	11,228	7.82	(Given)
1950-1959	23,750	1,710	7.20	
1960-1969	3,679	390	10.60	
1970-1979	1,956	90	4.60	
1980-1989	27	3	11.11	
1990-1999	22	5	22.72	

The number of new cases and deaths from diphtheria declined dramatically from the 1940s through the 1980s, but remained roughly level at very low levels in the 1990s. The death-to-case ratio was actually higher in the 1980s and 1990s than in 1940s and 1950s. From these data one might conclude that the decline in deaths is a result of the decline in cases, that is, from prevention, rather than from any improvement in the treatment of cases that do occur.

Exercise 3.5

Proportionate mortality for diseases of heart, 25–44 years
    = (# deaths from diseases of heart / # deaths from all causes) x 100
    = 16,283 / 128,294 x 100
    = 12.6%
Proportionate mortality for assault (homicide), 25–44 years
    = (# deaths from assault (homicide) / # deaths from all causes) x 100
    = 7,367 / 128,924 x 100
    = 5.7%

Exercise 3.6

1. HIV-related mortality rate, all ages
    = (# deaths from HIV / estimated population, 2002) x 100,000
    = (14,095 / 288,357,000) x 100,000
    = 4.9 HIV deaths per 100,000 population

2. HIV-related mortality rate for persons under 65 years
    = (# deaths from HIV among <65 years year-olds / estimated population < 65 years, 2002) x 100,000
    = (12 + 25 + 178 + 1,839 + 5,707 + 4,474 + 1,347 / 19,597 + 41,037 + 40,590 +39,928 + 44,917 + 40,084 + 26,602) x 100,000
    = 13,582 / 252,755,000 x 100,000
    = 5.4 HIV deaths per 100,000 persons under age 65 years

3. HIV-related YPLL before age 65

Deaths and years of potential life lost attributed to HIV by age group — United States, 2002

Column 1 Age Group (years)	Column 2 Deaths	Column 3 Age Midpoint	Column 4 Years to 65	Column 5 YPLL
0-4	12	2.5	62.5	750
5-10	25	10	55	1,375
15-24	178	20	45	8,010
25-34	1,839	30	35	64,365
35-44	5,707	40	25	142,675
45-54	4,474	50	15	67,110
55-64	1,347	60	5	6,735
65+	509	-	-	-
Not stated	4	-	-	-
Total	14,095		291,020	

4. HIV-related $YPLL_{65}$ rate
   $YPLL_{65}$ rate = (291,020 / 252,755,000) x 1,000 = 1.2 YPLL per 1,000 population under age 65.

5. Compare mortality rates and YPLL for leukemia and HIV

	Leukemia	HIV
# cause-specific deaths, all ages	21,498	14,095
cause-specific death rate, all ages (per 100,000 pop)	7.5	4.9
# deaths, < 65 years	6,221	13,582
death rate, < 65 years	2.5	5.4
$YPLL_{65}$	117,033	291,020
$YPLL_{65}$ rate	0.5	1.2

An advocate for increased leukemia research funding might use the first two measures, which shows that leukemia is a larger problem in the entire population. An advocate for HIV funding might use the last four measures, since they highlight HIV deaths among younger persons.

Exercise 3.7

1. Rate ratio comparing current smokers with nonsmokers
   = rate among current smokers / rate among non-smokers
   = 1.30 / 0.07
   = 18.6

2. Rate ratio comparing ex-smokers who quit at least 20 years ago with nonsmokers
   = rate among ex-smokers / rate among non-smokers
   = 0.19 / 0.07
   = 2.7

3. The lung cancer rate among smokers is 18 times as high as the rate among non-smokers. Smokers who quit can lower their rate considerably, but it never gets back to the low level seen in never-smokers. So the public health message might be, "If you smoke, quit. But better yet, don't start."

Exercise 3.8

Odds ratio = ad / bc

= (28 x 133) / (129 x 4)

= 7.2

The odds ratio of 7.2 is somewhat larger (18% larger, to be precise) than the risk ratio of 6.1. Whether that difference is "reasonable" or not is a judgment call. The odds ratio of 7.2 and the risk ratio of 6.1 both reflect a very strong association between prison wing and risk of developing tuberculosis.

SELF-ASSESSMENT QUIZ

Now that you have read Lesson 3 and have completed the exercises, you should be ready to take the self-assessment quiz. This quiz is designed to help you assess how well you have learned the content of this lesson. You may refer to the lesson text whenever you are unsure of the answer.

Unless otherwise instructed, choose ALL correct choices for each question.

1. Which of the following are frequency measures?
   A. Birth rate
   B. Incidence
   C. Mortality rate
   D. Prevalence

Use the following choices for Questions 2-4.

   A. Ratio
   B. Proportion
   C. Incidence proportion
   D. Mortality rate

2. _____ $\dfrac{\text{\# women in Country A who died from lung cancer in 2004}}{\text{\# women in Country A who died from cancer in 2004}}$

3. _____ $\dfrac{\text{\# women in Country A who died from lung cancer in 2004}}{\text{\# women in Country A who died from breast cancer in 2004}}$

4. _____ $\dfrac{\text{\# women in Country A who died from lung cancer in 2004}}{\text{estimated \# women living in Country A on July 1, 2004}}$

5. All proportions are ratios, but not all ratios are proportions.
   A. True
   B. False

6. In a state that did not require varicella (chickenpox) vaccination, a boarding school experienced a prolonged outbreak of varicella among its students that began in September and continued through December. To calculate the **probability** or **risk** of illness among the students, which denominator would you use?
   A. Number of susceptible students at the ending of the period (i.e., June)
   B. Number of susceptible students at the midpoint of the period (late October/early November)
   C. Number of susceptible students at the beginning of the period (i.e., September)
   D. Average number of susceptible students during outbreak

7. Many of the students at the boarding school, including 6 just coming down with varicella, went home during the Thanksgiving break. About 2 weeks later, 4 siblings of these 6

students (out of a total of 10 siblings) developed varicella. The secondary attack rate among siblings was, therefore,:

A. 4 / 6
B. 4 / 10
C. 4 / 16
D. 6 / 10

8. Investigators enrolled 100 diabetics without eye disease in a cohort (follow-up) study. The results of the first 3 years were as follows:

Year 1:   0 cases of eye disease detected out of 92; 8 lost to follow-up
Year 2:   2 new cases of eye disease detected out of 80; 2 had died; 10 lost to follow-up
Year 3:   3 new cases of eye disease detected out of 63; 2 more had died; 13 more lost to follow-up

The person-time incidence rate is calculated as:

A. 5 / 100
B. 5 / 63
C. 5 / 235
D. 5 / 250

9. The units for the quantity you calculated in Question 8 could be expressed as:
A. cases per 100 persons
B. percent
C. cases per person-year
D. cases per person per year

10. Use the following choices for the characteristics or features listed below:
A. Incidence
B. Prevalence

_____   Measure of risk
_____   Generally preferred for chronic diseases without clear date of onset
_____   Used in calculation of risk ratio
_____   Affected by duration of illness

Use the following information for Questions 11-15.

Within 10 days after attending a June wedding, an outbreak of cyclosporiasis occurred among attendees. Of the 83 guests and wedding party members, 79 were interviewed; 54 of the 79 met the case definition. The following two-by-two table shows consumption of wedding cake (that had raspberry filling) and illness status.

		Ill	Well	Total
Ate wedding cake?	Yes	50	3	53
	No	4	22	26
	Total	54	25	79

Source: Ho AY, Lopez AS, Eberhart MG, et al. Outbreak of cyclosporiasis associated with imported raspberries, Philadelphia, Pennsylvania, 2000. Emerg Infect Dis 2002;l8:783-6.

11. The fraction 54 / 79 is a/an:
    A. Food-specific attack rate
    B. Attack rate
    C. Incidence proportion
    D. Proportion

12. The fraction 50 / 54 is a/an:
    A. Attack rate
    B. Food-specific attack rate
    C. Incidence proportion
    D. Proportion

13. The fraction 50 / 53 is a/an:
    A. Attack rate
    B. Food-specific attack rate
    C. Incidence proportion
    D. Proportion

14. The best measure of association to use for these data is a/an:
    A. Food-specific attack rate
    B. Odds ratio
    C. Rate ratio
    D. Risk ratio

15. The best estimate of the association between wedding cake and illness is:
    A. 6.1
    B. 7.7
    C. 68.4
    D. 83.7
    E. 91.7
    F. 94.3

16. The attributable proportion for wedding cake is:
    A. 6.1%
    B. 7.7%
    C. 68.4%
    D. 83.7%
    E. 91.7%
    F. 94.3%

Use the following diagram for Questions 17 and 18. Assume that the horizontal lines in the diagram represent duration of illness in 8 different people, out of a community of 700.

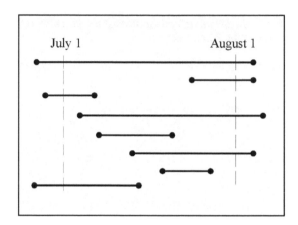

17. What is the prevalence of disease during July?
    A. 3 / 700
    B. 4 / 700
    C. 5 / 700
    D. 8 / 700

18. What is the incidence of disease during July?
    A. 3 / 700
    B. 4 / 700
    C. 5 / 700
    D. 8 / 700

19. What is the following fraction?

    Number of children < 365 days of age who died in Country A in 2004
    ───
            Number of live births in Country A in 2004

    A. Ratio
    B. Proportion
    C. Incidence proportion
    D. Mortality rate

20. Using only the data shown below for deaths attributed to Alzheimer's disease and to pneumonia/influenza, which measure(s) can be calculated?
    A. Proportionate mortality
    B. Cause-specific mortality rate
    C. Age-specific mortality rate
    D. Mortality rate ratio
    E. Years of potential life lost

Table 3.16 Number of Deaths Due to Alzheimer's Disease and Pneumonia/Influenza — United States, 2002

Age Group (years)	Alzheimer's disease	Pneumonia/ Influenza
< 5	0	373
5–14	1	91
15–24	0	167
<34	32	345
35–44	12	971
45–54	52	1,918
55–64	51	2,987
65–74	3,602	6,847
75–84	20,135	19,984
85+	34,552	31,995
Total	58,866	65,681

Source: Kochanek KD, Murphy SL, Anderson RN, Scott C. Deaths: Final data for 2002. National vital statistics reports; vol 53, no 5. Hyattsville, Maryland: National Center for Health Statistics, 2004.

21. Which of the following mortality rates use the estimated total mid-year population as its denominator?
    A. Age-specific mortality rate
    B. Sex-specific mortality rate
    C. Crude mortality rate
    D. Cause-specific mortality rate

22. What is the following fraction?

    <u>Number of deaths due to septicemia among men aged 65-74 years in 2004</u>
    Estimated number of men aged 65-74 years alive on July 1, 2004

    A. Age-specific mortality rate
    B. Age-adjusted mortality rate
    C. Cause-specific mortality rate
    D. Sex-specific mortality rate

23. Vaccine efficacy measures are:
    A. The proportion of vaccinees who do not get the disease
    B. 1 – the attack rate among vaccinees
    C. The proportionate reduction in disease among vaccinees
    D. 1 – disease attributable to the vaccine

24. To study the causes of an outbreak of aflatoxin poisoning in Africa, investigators conducted a case-control study with 40 case-patients and 80 controls. Among the 40 poisoning victims, 32 reported storing their maize inside rather than outside. Among the 80 controls, 20 stored their maize inside. The resulting odds ratio for the association between inside storage of maize and illness is:
    A. 3.2
    B. 5.2
    C. 12.0
    D. 33.3

25. The crude mortality rate in Community A was higher than the crude mortality rate in Community B, but the age-adjusted mortality rate was higher in Community B than in Community A. This indicates that:
    A. Investigators made a calculation error
    B. No inferences can be made about the comparative age of the populations from these data
    C. The population of Community A is, on average, older than that of Community B
    D. The population of Community B is, on average, older than that of Community A

Answers to Self-Assessment Quiz

1. A, B, C, D. Frequency measures of health and disease include those related to birth, death, and morbidity (incidence and prevalence).

2. A, B. All fractions are ratios. This fraction is also a proportion, because all of the deaths from lung cancer in the numerator are included in the denominator. It is not an incidence proportion, because the denominator is not the size of the population at the start of the period. It is not a mortality rate because the denominator is not the estimated midpoint population.

3. A. All fractions are ratios. This fraction is not a proportion, because lung cancer deaths in the numerator are not included in the denominator. It is not an incidence proportion, because the denominator is not the size of the population at the start of the period. It is not a mortality rate because the denominator is not the estimated midpoint population.

4. A, D. All fractions are ratios. This fraction is not a proportion, because some of the deaths occurred before July 1, so those women are not included in the calculation. It is not an incidence proportion, because the denominator is not the size of the population at the start of the period. It is a mortality rate because the denominator is the estimated midpoint population.

5. A. All fractions, including proportions, are ratios. But only ratios in which the numerator is included in the denominator is a proportions.

6. C. Probability or risk are estimated by the incidence proportion, calculated as the number of new cases during a specified period divided by the size of the population at the start of that period.

7. B. The secondary attack rate is calculated as the number of cases among contacts (4) divided by the number of contacts (10).

8. D. During year 1, 92 returning patients contributed 92 person-years; 8 patients lost to follow-up contributed 8 x ½ or 4 years, for a total of 96. During the second year, 78 disease-free patients contributed 78 person-years, plus ½ years for the 2 with newly diagnosed eye disease, the 2 who had died, and the 10 lost to follow-up (all events are assumed to have occurred randomly during the year, or an average, at the half-year point), for a total of 78 + 14 x ½ years, for another 85 years. During the third year, returning healthy patients contributed 60 years; the 3 with eye disease, the 4 who died, and the 11 lost to follow-up contributed 18 x ½ years or 9 years, for a total of 69 years during the 3rd year. The total person-years is therefore 96 + 85 + 69 = 250 person-years.

9. C, D. The person-time rate presented in Question 8 should be reported as 5 cases per 250 person-years. Usually person-time rates are expressed per 1,000 or 10,000 or 100,000, depending on the rarity of the disease, so the rate in Question 8 could be expressed as 2 cases per 100 person-years of follow-up. One could express this more colloquially as 2 new cases of eye disease per 100 diabetics per year.

10. A. Measure of risk

B. Generally preferred for chronic diseases without clear date of onset
A. Used in calculation of risk ratio
B. Affected by duration of illness
Incidence reflects new cases only; incidence proportion is a measure of risk. A risk ratio is simply the ratio of two incidence proportions. Prevalence reflects existing cases at a given point or period of time, so one does not need to know the date of onset. Prevalence is influenced by both incidence and duration of disease — the more cases that occur and the longer the disease lasts, the greater the prevalence at any given time.

		Ill	Well	Total
Ate wedding cake?	Yes	50	3	53
	No	4	22	26
	Total	54	25	79

11. B, C, D. The fraction 54 / 79 (see bottom row of the table) reflects the overall attack rate among persons who attended the wedding and were interviewed. Attack rate is a synonym for incidence proportion.

12. D. The fraction 50 / 54 (under the Ill column) is the proportion of case-patients who ate wedding cake . It is not an attack rate, because the denominator of an attack rate is the size of the population at the start of the period, not all cases.

13. A, B, C, D. The fraction 50 / 53 (see top row of table) is the proportion of wedding cake eaters who became ill, which is a food-specific attack rate. A food-specific attack rate is a type of attack rate, which in turn is synonymous with incidence proportion.

14. C. Investigators were able to interview almost everyone who attended the wedding, so incidence proportions (measure of risk) were calculated. When incidence proportions (risks) can be calculated, the best measure of association to use is the ratio of incidence proportions (risks), i.e., risk ratio.

15. A. The risk ratio is calculated as the attack rate among cake eaters divided by the attack rate among those who did not eat cake, or (50 / 53) / (4 / 26), or 94.3% / 15.4%, which equals 6.1.

16. D. The attributable proportion is calculated as the attack rate among cake eaters minus the attack rate among non-eaters, divided by the attack rate among cake eaters, or 94.3 – 15.4) / 94.3, which equals 83.7%. This attributable proportion means that 83.7% of the illness might be attributable to eating the wedding cake (note that some people got sick without eating cake, so the attributable proportion is not 100%).

17. D. A total of 8 cases are present at some time during the month of July.

18. C. Five new cases occurred during the month of July.

19. A, D. The fraction shown is the infant mortality rate. It is a ratio, because all fractions are ratios. It is not a proportion because some of the children who died in early 2004 may have been born in late 2003, so some of those in the numerator are not in the denominator. Technically, the mortality rate for infants is the number of infants who died

in 2004 divided by the estimated midyear population of infants, so the fraction shown is not a mortality rate in that sense. However, the fraction is known throughout the world as the infant mortality rate, despite the technical inaccuracy.

20. E. The data shown in the table are numbers of deaths. No denominators are provided from which to calculate rates. Neither is the total number of deaths given, so proportionate mortality cannot be calculated. However, calculation of potential life lost need only the numbers of deaths by age, as shown.

21. C, D. Only crude and cause-specific mortality rates use the estimated total mid-year population as its denominator. The denominator for an age-specific mortality rate is the estimated mid-year size of that particular age group. The denominator for a sex-specific mortality rate is the estimated mid-year male or female population.

22. A, C, D. The fraction is the mortality rate due to septicemia (cause) among men (sex) aged 65-74 years (age). Age-specific mortality rates are narrowly defined (in this fraction, limited to 10 years of age), so are generally valid for comparing two populations without any adjustment.

23. C. Vaccine efficacy measures the proportionate reduction in disease among vaccinees.

24. C. The results of this study could be summarized in a two-by-two table as follows:

		Cases	Controls	Total
Stored maize inside?	Yes	a = 32	c = 20	52
	No	b = 8	d = 60	68
	Total	40	80	120

The odds ratio is calculated as ad/bc, or (32 x 60) / (8 x 20), which equals 1,920 / 160 or 12.0.

25. C. The crude mortality rate reflects the mortality experience and the age distribution of a community, whereas the age-adjusted mortality rate eliminates any differences in the age distribution. So if Community A's age-adjusted mortality rate was lower than its crude rate, that indicates that its population is older.

References

1. Kleinman JC, Donahue RP, Harris MI, Finucane FF, Madans JH, Brock DB. Mortality among diabetics in a national sample. Am J Epidemiol 1988;128:389–401.

2. Arias E, Anderson RN, Kung H-C, Murphy SL, Kochanek KD. Deaths: final data for 2001. National vital statistics reports; vol. 52 no. 3. Hyattsville, Maryland: National Center for Health Statistics, 2003; 9:30–3.

3. Centers for Disease Control and Prevention. Reported tuberculosis in the United States, 2003. Atlanta, GA: U.S. Department of Health and Human Services, CDC, September 2004.

4. Last JM. A dictionary of epidemiology, 4th ed. New York: Oxford U. Press; 2001.

5. Hopkins RS, Jajosky RA, Hall PA, Adams DA, Connor FJ, Sharp P, et. al. Summary of notifiable diseases — United States, 2003. MMWR 2003;52(No 54):1–85.

6. U.S. Census Bureau [Internet]. Washington, DC: [updated 11 Jul 2006; cited 2005 Oct 2]. Population Estimates. Available from: http://www.census.gov/popest.

7. Williams LM, Morrow B, Lansky A. Surveillance for selected maternal behaviors and experiences before, during, and after pregnancy: Pregnancy Risk Assessment Monitoring System (PRAMS). In: *Surveillance Summaries*, November 14, 2003. MMWR 2003;52(No. SS-11):1–14.

8. Web-based Injury Statistics Query and Reporting System (WISQARS) [online database] Atlanta; National Center for Injury Prevention and Control. [cited 2006 Feb 1]. Available from: http://www.cdc.gov/ncipc/wisqars.

9. Centers for Disease Control and Prevention. Health, United States, 2004. Hyattsville, MD.; 2004.

10. Wise RP, Livengood JR, Berkelman RL, Goodman RA. Methodologic alternatives for measuring premature mortality. Am J Prev Med 1988;4:268–273.

11. McLaughlin SI, Spradling P, Drociuk D, Ridzon R, Pozsik CJ, Onorato I. Extensive transmission of Mycobacterium tuberculosis among congregated, HIV-infected prison inmates in South Carolina, United States. Int J Tuberc Lung Dis 2003;7:665–72.

12. Tugwell BD, Lee LE, Gillette H, Lorber EM, Hedberg K, Cieslak PR. Chickenpox outbreak in a highly vaccinated school population. Pediatrics 2004 Mar;113(3 Pt 1):455–9.

13. Uyeki TM, Zane SB, Bodnar UR, Fielding KL, Buxton JA, Miller JM, et al. Large summertime Influenza A outbreak among tourists in Alaska and the Yukon Territory. Clin Infect Dis 2003;36:1095–1102.

14. Doll R, Hill AB. Smoking and carcinoma of the lung. Br Med J 1950;1:739–48.

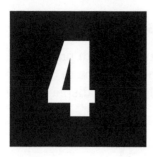

DISPLAYING PUBLIC HEALTH DATA

Imagine that you work in a county or state health department. The department must prepare an annual summary of the individual surveillance reports and other public health data from the year that just ended. This summary needs to display trends and patterns in a concise and understandable manner. You have been selected to prepare this annual summary. What tools might you use to organize and display the data?

Most annual reports use a combination of tables, graphs, and charts to summarize and display data clearly and effectively. Tables and graphs can be used to summarize a few dozen records or a few million. They are used every day by epidemiologists to summarize and better understand the data they or others have collected. They can demonstrate distributions, trends, and relationships in the data that are not apparent from looking at individual records. Thus, tables and graphs are critical tools for descriptive and analytic epidemiology. In addition, remembering the adage that a picture is worth a thousand words, you can use tables and graphs to communicate epidemiologic findings to others efficiently and effectively. This lesson covers tabular and graphic techniques for data display; interpretation was covered in Lessons 2 and 3.

Objectives

After completing this lesson and answering the questions in the exercises, you will be able to:
- *Prepare and interpret one, two, or three variable tables and composite tables (including creating class intervals)*
- *Prepare and interpret arithmetic-scale line graphs, semilogarithmic-scale line graphs, histograms, frequency polygons, bar charts, pie charts, maps, and area maps*
- *State the value and proper use of population pyramids, cumulative frequency graphs, survival curves, scatter diagrams, box plots, dot plots, forest plots, and tree plots*
- *Identify when to use each type of table and graph*

Major Sections

Introduction to Tables and Graphs

Data analysis is an important component of public health practice. In examining data, one must first determine the data type in order to select the appropriate display format. The data to be displayed will be in one of the following categories:

- Nominal
- Ordinal
- Discrete
- Continuous

Nominal measurements have no intrinsic order and the difference between levels of the variable have no meaning. In epidemiology, sex, race, or exposure category (yes/no) are examples of nominal measurements. **Ordinal variables** do have an intrinsic order, but, again, differences between levels are not relevant. Examples of ordinal variables are "low, medium, high" or perhaps categories of other variables (e.g., age ranges). **Discrete variables** have values that are integers (e.g., number of ill persons who were exposed to a risk factor). Finally, **continuous variables** can have any value in a range (e.g., amount of time between meal being served and onset of gastro-intestinal symptoms; infant mortality rate).

Before constructing any display of epidemiologic data, it is important to first determine the point to be conveyed. Are you highlighting a change from past patterns in the data? Are you showing a difference in incidence by geographic area or by some predetermined risk factor? What is the interpretation you want the reader to reach? Your answer to these questions will help to determine the choice of display.

To analyze data effectively, an epidemiologist must become familiar with the data before applying analytic techniques. The epidemiologist may begin by examining individual records such as those contained in a line listing. This review will be followed by production of a table to summarize the data. Sometimes, the resulting tables are the only analysis that is needed, particularly when the amount of data is small and relationships are straightforward.

When the data are more complex, graphs and charts can help the epidemiologist visualize broader patterns and trends and identify variations from those trends. Variations in data may represent important new findings or only errors in typing or coding which need to be corrected. Thus, tables and graphs can be helpful tools to aid in verifying and analyzing the data.

Once an analysis is complete, tables and graphs further serve as useful visual aids for describing the data to others. When preparing tables and graphs, keep in mind that your primary purpose is to communicate information.

Tables and graphs can be presented using a variety of media. In epidemiology, the most common media are print and projection. This lesson will focus on creating effective and attractive tables and graphs for print and will also offer suggestions for projection. At the end, we present tables that summarize all techniques presented and guidelines for use.

Tables

A table is a set of data arranged in rows and columns. Almost any quantitative information can be organized into a table. Tables are useful for demonstrating patterns, exceptions, differences, and other relationships. In addition, tables usually serve as the basis for preparing additional visual displays of data, such as graphs and charts, in which some of the details may be lost.

Tables designed to present data to others should be as simple as possible.[1] Two or three small tables, each focusing on a different aspect of the data, are easier to understand than a single large table that contains many details or variables.

A table in a printed publication should be self-explanatory. If a table is taken out of its original context, it should still convey all the information necessary for the reader to understand the data. To create a table that is self-explanatory, follow the guidelines below.

More About Constructing Tables

- Use a clear and concise title that describes person, place and time — what, where, and when — of the data in the table. Precede the title with a table number.

- Label each row and each column and include the units of measurement for the data (for example, years, mm Hg, mg/dl, rate per 100,000).

- Show totals for rows and columns, where appropriate. If you show percentages (%), also give their total (always 100).

- Identify missing or unknown data either within the table (for example, Table 4.11) or in a footnote below the table.

- Explain any codes, abbreviations, or symbols in a footnote (for example, Syphilis P&S = primary and secondary syphilis).

- Note exclusions in a footnote (e.g., 1 case and 2 controls with unknown family history were excluded from this analysis).

- Note the source of the data below the table or in a footnote if the data are not original.

One-variable tables

In descriptive epidemiology, the most basic table is a simple frequency distribution with only one variable, such as Table 4.1a, which displays number of reported syphilis cases in the United States in 2002 by age group.[2] (Frequency distributions are discussed in Lesson 2.) In this type of frequency distribution table, the first column shows the values or categories of the variable represented by the data, such as age or sex. The second column shows the number of persons or events that fall into each category. In constructing any table, the choice of columns results from the interpretation to be made. In Table 4.1a, the point the analyst wishes to make is the role of age as a risk factor of syphilis. Thus, age group is chosen as column 1 and case count as column 2.

Often, an additional column lists the percentage of persons or events in each category (see Table 4.1b). The percentages shown in Table 4.1b actually add up to 99.9% rather than 100.0% due to rounding to one decimal place. Rounding that results in totals of 99.9% or 100.1% is common in tables that show percentages. Nonetheless, the total percentage should be displayed as 100.0%, and a footnote explaining that the difference is due to rounding should be included.

The addition of percent to a table shows the relative burden of illness; for example, in Table 4.1b, we see that the largest contribution to illness for any single age category is from 35–39 year olds. The subsequent addition of cumulative percent (e.g., Table 4.1c) allows the public health analyst to illustrate the impact of a targeted intervention. Here, any intervention effective at preventing syphilis among young people and young adults (under age 35) would prevent almost half of the cases in this population.

The one-variable table can be further modified to show cumulative frequency and/or cumulative percentage, as in Table 4.1c. From this table, you can see at a glance that 46.7% of the primary and secondary syphilis cases occurred in persons younger than age 35 years, meaning that over half of the syphilis cases occurred in persons age 35 years or older. Note that the choice of age-groupings will affect the interpretation of your data.[3]

To create a frequency distribution from a data set in Analysis Module:

Select **frequencies**, then choose variable under **Frequencies of**.

(Since Epi Info 3 is the recommended version, only commands for this version are provided in the text; corresponding commands for Epi Info 6 are offered at the end of the lesson.)

Table 4.1a Reported Cases of Primary and Secondary Syphilis by Age — United States, 2002

Age Group (years)	Number of Cases
≤14	21
15–19	351
20–24	842
25–29	895
30–34	1,097
35–39	1,367
40–44	1,023
45–54	982
≥55	284
Total	6,862

Data Source: Centers for Disease Control and Prevention. Sexually Transmitted Disease Surveillance 2002. Atlanta: U.S. Department of Health and Human Services; 2003.

Table 4.1b Reported Cases of Primary and Secondary Syphilis by Age — United States, 2002

| Age Group (years) | CASES | |
	Number	Percent
≤14	21	0.3
15–19	351	5.1
20–24	842	12.3
25–29	895	13.0
30–34	1,097	16.0
35–39	1,367	19.9
40–44	1,023	14.9
45–54	982	14.3
≥55	284	4.1
Total	6,862	100.0*

* Actual total of percentages for this table is 99.9% and does not add to 100.0% due to rounding error.

Data Source: Centers for Disease Control and Prevention. Sexually Transmitted Disease Surveillance 2002. Atlanta: U.S. Department of Health and Human Services; 2003.

Table 4.1c Reported Cases of Primary and Secondary Syphilis by Age — United States, 2002

| Age Group (years) | CASES | | Cumulative Percent |
	Number	Percent	
≤14	21	0.3	0.3
15–19	351	5.1	5.4
20–24	842	12.3	17.7
25–29	895	13.0	30.7
30–34	1,097	16.0	46.7
35–39	1,367	19.9	66.6
40–44	1,023	14.9	81.6
45–54	982	14.3	95.9
≥55	284	4.1	100.0
Total	6,862	100.0*	100.0*

* Percentages do not add to 100.0% due to rounding error.

Data Source: Centers for Disease Control and Prevention. Sexually Transmitted Disease Surveillance 2002. Atlanta: U.S. Department of Health and Human Services; 2003.

Two- and three-variable tables

Tables 4.1a, 4.1b, and 4.1c show case counts (frequency) by a single variable, e.g., age. Data can also be cross-tabulated to show counts by an additional variable. Table 4.2 shows the number of syphilis cases cross-classified by both age group and sex of the patient.

Table 4.2 Reported Cases of Primary and Secondary Syphilis by Age and Sex — United States, 2002

Age Group (years)	NUMBER OF CASES		Total
	Male	Female	
≤14	9	12	21
15–19	135	216	351
20–24	533	309	842
25–29	668	227	895
30–34	877	220	1,097
35–39	1,121	246	1,367
40–44	845	178	1,023
45–54	825	157	982
≥55	255	29	284
Total	5,268	1,594	6,862

Data Source: Centers for Disease Control and Prevention. Sexually Transmitted Disease Surveillance 2002. Atlanta: U.S. Department of Health and Human Services; 2003.

To create a two-variable table from a data set in Analysis Module:

Select **frequencies**, then choose variable under **Frequencies of**. Output shows table with row and column percentages, plus chi-square and p-value. For a two-by-two table, output also provides odds ratio, risk ratio, risk difference and confidence intervals. Note that for a cohort study, the row percentage in cells of ill patients is the attack proportion, sometimes called the attack rate.

A two-variable table with data categorized jointly by those two variables is known as a **contingency table**. Table 4.3 is an example of a special type of contingency table, in which each of the two variables has two categories. This type of table is called a two-by-two table and is a favorite among epidemiologists. Two-by-two tables are convenient for comparing persons with and without the exposure and those with and without the disease. From these data, epidemiologists can assess the relationship, if any, between the exposure and the disease. Table 4.3 is a two-by-two table that shows one of the key findings from an investigation of carbon monoxide poisoning following an ice storm and prolonged power failure in Maine.[4] In the table, the exposure variable, location of power generator, has two categories — inside or outside the home. Similarly the outcome variable, carbon monoxide poisoning, has two categories — cases (number of persons who became ill) and controls (number of persons who did not become ill).

Table 4.3 Generator Location and Risk of Carbon Monoxide Poisoning After an Ice Storm — Maine, 1998

		NUMBER OF		Total
		Cases	Controls	
Generator location	Inside home or attached structure	23	23	46
	Outside home	4	139	143
	Total	27	162	189

Data Source: Daley RW, Smith A, Paz-Argandona E, Mallilay J, McGeehin M. An outbreak of carbon monoxide poisoning after a major ice storm in Maine. J Emerg Med 2000;18:87–93.

Table 4.4 illustrates a generic format and standard notation for a two-by-two table. Disease status (e.g., ill versus well, sometimes denoted cases vs. controls if a case-control study) is usually designated along the top of the table, and exposure status (e.g., exposed versus not exposed) is designated along the side. The letters $a, b, c,$ and d within the 4 cells of the two-by-two table refer to the number of persons with the disease status indicated above and the exposure status indicated to its left. For example, in Table 4.4, "c" represents the number of persons in the study who are ill but who did not have the exposure being studied. Note that the "H_i" represents horizontal totals; H_1 and H_0 represent the total number of exposed and unexposed persons, respectively. The "V_i" represents vertical totals; V_1 and V_0 represent the total number of ill and well persons (or cases and controls), respectively. The total number of subjects included in the two-by-two table is represented by the letter T (or N).

Table 4.4 General Format and Notation for a Two-by-Two Table

	Ill	Well	Total	Attack Rate (Risk)
Exposed	a	b	$a + b = H_1$	$a / a+b$
Unexposed	c	d	$c + d = H_0$	$c / c+d$
Total	$a + c = V_1$	$b + d = V_0$	T	V_1 / T

When producing a table to display either in print or projection, it is best, generally, to limit the number of variables to one or two. One exception to this rule occurs when a third variable modifies the effect (technically, produces an interaction) of the first two. Table 4.5 is intended to convey the way in which race/ethnicity may modify the effect of age and sex on incidence of syphilis. Because three-way tables are often hard to understand, they should be used only when ample explanation and discussion is possible.

Table 4.5 Number of Reported Cases of Primary and Secondary Syphilis, by Race/Ethnicity, Age, and Sex — United States, 2002

Race/ethnicity	Age Group (years)	Male	Female	Total
American Indian/	≤14	1	0	1
Alaskan Native	15–19	0	1	1
	20–24	5	3	8
	25–29	3	1	4
	30–34	1	2	3
	35–39	3	5	8
	40–44	4	3	7
	45–54	8	8	16
	≥55	2	1	3
	Total	27	24	51
Asian/Pacific Islander	≤14	1	1	2
	15–19	0	2	2
	20–24	9	4	13
	25–29	16	1	17
	30–34	21	1	22
	35–39	14	1	15
	40–44	14	1	15
	45–54	8	0	8
	≥55	0	0	0
	Total	83	11	94
Black, Non-Hispanic	≤14	3	9	12
	15–19	89	164	253
	20–24	313	233	546
	25–29	322	163	485
	30–34	310	166	476
	35–39	385	183	568
	40–44	305	142	447
	45–54	370	112	482
	≥55	129	23	152
	Total	2,226	1,195	3,421
Hispanic	≤14	1	1	2
	15–19	37	25	62
	20–24	117	29	146
	25–29	139	26	165
	30–34	172	20	192
	35–39	178	22	200
	40–44	93	9	102
	45–54	69	14	83
	≥55	18	1	19
	Total	824	147	971
White, Non-Hispanic	≤14	3	1	4
	15–19	9	24	33
	20–24	89	40	129
	25–29	188	36	224
	30–34	373	31	404
	35–39	541	35	576
	40–44	429	23	452
	45–54	370	23	393
	≥55	106	4	110
	Total	2,108	217	2,325

Data Source: Centers for Disease Control and Prevention. Sexually Transmitted Disease Surveillance 2002. Atlanta: U.S. Department of Health and Human Services; 2003. p. 118.

Exercise 4.1

The data in Table 4.6 describe characteristics of the 38 persons who ate food at or from a church supper in Texas in August 2001. Fifteen of these persons later developed botulism[5]

1. Construct a table of the illness (botulism) by age group. Use botulism status (yes/no) as the column labels and age groups as the row labels.

2. Construct a two-by-two table of the illness (botulism) by exposure to chicken.

3. Construct a two-by-two table of the illness (botulism) by exposure to chili.

4. Construct a three-way table of illness (botulism) by exposure to chili and chili leftovers.

 Check your answers on page 4-73

Table 4.6 Line Listing for Exercise 4.1

ID	Age	Attended Supper	Case	Date of Onset	Case Status	Ate Any Food	Ate Chili	Ate Chicken	Ate Chili Leftovers
1	1	Y	N	-		Y	Y	Y	N
2	3	Y	Y	8/27	Lab-confirmed	Y	Y	N	N
3	7	Y	Y	8/31	Lab-confirmed	Y	Y	N	N
4	7	Y	N	-		Y	Y	Y	N
5	10	Y	N	-		Y	Y	N	Y
6	17	Y	Y	8/28	Lab-confirmed	Y	Y	Y	N
7	21	Y	N	-		N	N	N	N
8	23	Y	N	-		Y	Y	N	N
9	25	Y	Y	8/26	Epi-linked	Y	Y	N	N
10	29	N	Y	8/28	Lab-confirmed	Y	Unk	Unk	Y
11	38	Y	N	-		N	N	N	N
12	39	Y	N	-		N	N	N	N
13	41	Y	N	-		Y	Y	Y	N
14	41	Y	N	-		N	N	N	N
15	42	Y	Y	8/26	Lab-confirmed	Y	Y	Unk	N
16	45	Y	Y	8/26	Lab-confirmed	Y	Y	Y	Y
17	45	Y	Y	8/27	Epi-linked	Y	Y	Y	N
18	46	Y	N	-		Y	N	Y	N
19	47	Y	N	-		Y	N	Y	N
20	48	Y	Y	9/1	Lab-confirmed	Y	Y	Unk	N
21	50	Y	Y	8/29	Epi-linked	Y	Y	N	N
22	50	Y	N	-		Y	N	Y	N
23	50	Y	N	-		Y	N	N	Y
24	52	Y	Y	8/28	Lab-confirmed	Y	Y	Y	N
25	52	Y	N	-		N	N	N	N
26	53	Y	Y	8/27	Epi-linked	Y	Y	Y	N
27	53	Y	N	-		Y	Y	Y	N
28	62	Y	Y	8/27	Epi-linked	Y	Y	Y	N
29	62	Y	N	-		Y	N	Y	N
30	63	Y	N	-		N	N	N	N
31	67	Y	N	-		N	N	N	N
32	68	Y	N	-		N	N	N	N
33	69	Y	N	-		Y	Y	Y	N
34	71	Y	N	-		Y	N	Y	N
35	72	Y	Y	8/27	Lab-confirmed	Y	Y	Y	N
36	74	Y	N	-		Y	Y	N	N
37	74	Y	N	-		Y	N	Y	N
38	78	Y	Y	8/25	Epi-linked	Y	Y	Y	N

Data Source: Kalluri P, Crowe C, Reller M, Gaul L, Hayslett J, Barth S, Eliasberg S, Ferreira J, Holt K, Bengston S, Hendricks K, Sobel J. An outbreak of foodborne botulism associated with food sold at a salvage store in Texas. Clin Infect Dis 2003;37:1490–5.

Tables of statistical measures other than frequency

Tables 4.1–4.5 show case counts (frequency). The cells of a table could also display averages, rates, relative risks, or other epidemiological measures. As with any table, the title and/or headings must clearly identify what data are presented. For example, the title of Table 4.7 indicates that the data for reported cases of primary and secondary syphilis are rates rather than numbers.

Table 4.7 Rate per 100,000 Population for Reported Cases of Primary and Secondary Syphilis, by Age and Race — United States, 2002

Age Group (years)	Am. Indian/ Alaska Native	Asian/ Pacific Is.	Black, Non-Hispanic	Hispanic	White, Non-Hispanic	Total
10–14	0.0	0.1	0.3	0.1	0.0	0.1
15–19	0.5	0.2	8.6	1.9	0.3	1.7
20–24	5.0	1.5	20.7	4.3	1.1	4.4
25–29	2.7	1.6	19.1	4.9	1.8	4.6
30–34	2.0	2.2	18.2	6.1	3.0	5.4
35–39	4.8	1.6	20.1	7.1	3.6	6.0
40–44	4.5	1.6	16.6	4.4	2.8	4.6
45–54	6.1	0.6	11.8	2.7	1.4	2.6
55–64	1.4	0.0	4.6	0.6	0.5	0.9
65+	0.8	0.0	1.5	0.5	0.1	0.2
Totals	2.4	0.9	9.8	2.7	1.2	2.4

Data Source: Centers for Disease Control and Prevention. Sexually Transmitted Disease Surveillance 2002. Atlanta: U.S. Department of Health and Human Services; 2003.

Composite tables

To conserve space in a report or manuscript, several tables are sometimes combined into one. For example, epidemiologists often create simple frequency distributions by age, sex, and other demographic variables as separate tables, but editors may combine them into one large composite table for publication. Table 4.8 is an example of a composite table from the investigation of carbon monoxide poisoning following the power failure in Maine.[4]

It is important to realize that this type of table should not be interpreted as for a three-way table. The data in Table 4.8 have not been arrayed to indicate the interrelationship of sex, age, smoking, and disposition from medical care. Merely, several one variable tables (independently assessing the number of cases by each of these variables) have been concatenated for space conservation. So this table would not help in assessing the modification that smoking has on the risk of illness by age, for example. This difference also explains why portraying total values would be inappropriate and meaningless for Table 4.8.

Table 4.8 Number and Percentage of Confirmed Cases of Carbon Monoxide Poisoning Identified from Four Hospitals, by Selected Characteristics — Maine, January 1998

| | CASES | |
Characteristic	Number	Percent
Total cases	100	100
Sex (female)	59	59
Age (years)		
0–3	5	5
4–12	17	17
13–18	9	9
19–64	52	52
≥65	17	17
Smokers	20	20
Disposition		
Released from ED*	83	83
Admitted to hospital	11	11
Transferred	5	5
Died	1	1

* ED = Emergency department

Data Source: Daley RW, Smith A, Paz-Argandona E, Mallilay J, McGeehin M. An outbreak of carbon monoxide poisoning after a major ice storm in Maine. J Emerg Med 2000;18:87–93.

Table shells

Although you cannot analyze data before you have collected them, epidemiologists anticipate and design their analyses in advance to delineate what the study is going to convey, and to expedite the analysis once the data are collected. In fact, most protocols, which are written before a study can be conducted, require a description of how the data will be analyzed. As part of the analysis plan, you can develop table shells that show how the data will be organized and displayed. Table shells are tables that are complete except for the data. They show titles, headings, and categories. In developing table shells that include continuous variables such as age, we create more categories than we may later use, in order to disclose any interesting patterns and quirks in the data.

The following table shells were designed before conducting a case-control study of fractures related to falls in community-dwelling elderly persons. The researchers were particularly interested in assessing whether vigorous and/or mild physical activity was associated with a lower risk of fall-related fractures.

Table shells of epidemiologic studies usually follow a standard sequence from descriptive to analytic. The first and second tables in the sequence usually cover clinical features of the health event and demographic characteristics of the subjects. Next, the analyst portrays the association of most interest to the researchers, in this case, the association between physical activity and fracture. Subsequent tables may present stratified or adjusted analyses, refinements, and subset analyses. Of course, once the data are available and used for these tables, additional analyses will come to mind and should be pursued.

This sequence of table shells provides a systematic and logical approach to the analysis. The first two tables (Table shells 4.9a and 4.9b), describing the health problem of interest and the population studied, provide the background a reader would need to put the analytic results in perspective.

Table Shell 4.9a Anatomic Site of Fall-related Fractures Sustained by Participants, SAFE Study — Miami, 1987-1989

Fracture Site	Number	(Percent)
Skull	____	( )
Spine	____	( )
Clavicle (collarbone)	____	( )
Scapula (shoulderblade)	____	( )
Humerus (upper arm)	____	( )
Radius / ulna (lower arm)	____	( )
Bones of the hand	____	( )
Ribs, sternum	____	( )
Pelvis	____	( )
Neck of femur (hip)	____	( )
Other parts of femur (upper leg)	____	( )
Patella (knee)	____	( )
Tibia / fibula (lower leg)	____	( )
Ankle	____	( )
Bones of the foot	____	( )

Adapted from: Stevens, JA, Powell KE, Smith SM, Wingo PA, Sattin RW. Physical activity, functional limitations, and the risk of fall-related fractures in community-dwelling elderly. Annals of Epidemiology 1997;7:54–61.

Table Shell 4.9b Selected Characteristics of Case and Control Participants, SAFE Study — Miami, 1987–1989

		CASES		CONTROLS	
		Number	(Percent)	Number	(Percent)
Age	65–74	____	( )	____	( )
	75–84	____	( )	____	( )
	≥85	____	( )	____	( )
Sex	Male	____	( )	____	( )
	Female	____	( )	____	( )
Race	White	____	( )	____	( )
	Black	____	( )	____	( )
	Other	____	( )	____	( )
	Unknown	____	( )	____	( )
Ethnicity	Hispanic	____	( )	____	( )
	Non-Hispanic	____	( )	____	( )
	Unknown	____	( )	____	( )
Hours/day spent on feet					
	≤1	____	( )	____	( )
	2–4	____	( )	____	( )
	5–7	____	( )	____	( )
	≥8	____	( )	____	( )
Smoking status					
	Never smoked	____	( )	____	( )
	Former smoker	____	( )	____	( )
	Current smoker	____	( )	____	( )
	Unknown	____	( )	____	( )
Alcohol use (drinks / week)					
	None	____	( )	____	( )
	<1	____	( )	____	( )
	1–3	____	( )	____	( )
	≥4	____	( )	____	( )
	Unknown	____	( )	____	( )

Adapted from: Stevens, JA, Powell KE, Smith SM, Wingo PA, Sattin RW. Physical activity, functional limitations, and the risk of fall-related fractures in community-dwelling elderly. Annals of Epidemiology 1997;7:54–61.

Now that the data in Table shells 4.9a and 4.9b have illustrated descriptive characteristics of cases and controls in this study, we are ready to refine the analysis by demonstrating the variability of the data as assessed by statistical confidence intervals. Because of the study design in this example, we have chosen the odds ratio to assess statistical differences (see Lesson 3). Table shell 4.9c illustrates a useful display for this information.

Table Shell 4.9c Relationship Between Physical Activity (Vigorous and Mild) and Fracture, SAFE Study — Miami, 1987–1989

		CASES		CONTROLS		Odds Ratio (95% Confidence Interval)
		Number	(Percent)	Number	(Percent)	
Vigorous Activity	Yes	___	( )	___	( )	___ (___ – ___)
	No	___	( )	___	( )	
Vigorous Activity	Yes	___	( )	___	( )	___ (___ – ___)
	No	___	( )	___	( )	

Adapted from: Stevens, JA, Powell KE, Smith SM, Wingo PA, Sattin RW. Physical activity, functional limitations, and the risk of fall-related fractures in community-dwelling elderly. Annals of Epidemiology 1997;7:54–61.

Creating class intervals

If the epidemiologic hypothesis for the investigation involves variables such as "gender" or "exposure to a risk factor (yes/no)," the construction of tables as described thus far in this chapter should be straightforward. Often, however, the presumed risk factor may not be so conveniently packaged. We may need to investigate an infection acquired as a result of hospitalization and "days of hospitalization" may be relevant; for many chronic conditions, blood pressure is an important factor; if we are interested in the effect of alcohol consumption on health risk, number of drinks per week may be an important measurement. These examples illustrate relevant variables that have a broader range of possible responses than are easily handled by the methods described earlier in this chapter. One solution in this case is to create **class intervals** for your data, keeping the following guidelines in mind:

- Class intervals should be mutually exclusive and exhaustive. In plain language, that means that each individual in your data set should fit uniquely into one class interval, and all persons should fit into some class interval. So, for example, age ranges should not overlap. Most measures follow conventional rounding rules (see sidebar).

  A general tip is to use a large number of class intervals for the initial analysis to gain an appreciation for the variability of your data. You can combine your categories later.

- Use principles of biologic plausibility when constructing categories. For example, when analyzing infant and childhood mortality, we might use categories of 0–12 months (since neonatal problems are different epidemiologically from those of other childhood problems), 1–5 years (since these result

Conventional Rounding Rules

If a fraction is **greater than .5**, round it up (e.g., round 6.6 to 7).

If a fraction is **less than .5**, round it down (e.g., round 6.4 to 6).

If a fraction is **exactly .5**, it is recommended that you round it to the even value (e.g., round both 5.5 and 6.5 to 6). More common and also acceptable is to round it up (e.g., round 6.5 to 7) from causes of death primarily outside of institutions), and 5–10 years (since these may result from risks in school settings). Table 4.10 illustrates age groups that are sensible for the study of various health conditions that are behaviorally-related.

- A natural baseline group should be kept as a distinct category. Often the baseline group will include those who have not had an exposure, e.g., non-smokers (0 cigarettes per day).

- If you wish to calculate rates to illustrate the relative risk of adverse health events by these categories of risk factors, be sure that the intervals you choose for the classes of your data are the same as the intervals for the denominators that you will find for readily available data. For example, to compute rates of infant mortality by maternal age, you must find data on the number of live-born infants to women; in determining age groupings, consider what categories are used by the United States Census Bureau.

- Always consider a category for "unknown" or "not stated."

Table 4.10 Age Groupings Used for Different Conditions, as Reported in Surveillance Summaries, CDC, 2003

Overweight In Adults[7]	Traumatic Brain Injury[8]	Pregnancy-Related Mortality[9]	HIV/AIDS[10]	Vaccine Adverse Events[11]
18–24 years	<4 years	≤19 years	<13 years	<1 year
25–34	5–14	20–24	13–14	1–6
35–44	15–19	25–29	15–24	7–17
45–54	20–24	30–34	25–34	18–64
55–64	25–34	35–39	35–44	≥65
65–74	35–44	≥40	45–54	
≥75	45–64		55–64	
	≥65		≥65	
Total	Total	Total	Total	Total

In addition to these guidelines for creating class intervals, the analyst must decide how many intervals to portray. If no natural or standard class intervals are apparent, the strategies below may be helpful.

Strategy 1: Divide the data into groups of similar size

A particularly appropriate approach if you plan to create area maps (see later section on Maps) is to create a number of class intervals, each with the same number of observations. For example, to portray the rates of incidence of lung cancer by state (for men, 2001), one might group the rates into four class intervals, each with 10–12 observations:

Table 4.11 Rates of Lung Cancer in Men, 2001 by State (and the District of Columbia)

Rate	Number of States in the US	Cumulative Frequency
22.1–48.3	11	11
48.4–53.3	11	22
53.4–58.7	12	34
58.8–73.3	10	44
Missing data	7	51

Data Source: U.S. Cancer Statistics Working Group. United States Cancer Statistics: 2002 Incidence and Mortality. Atlanta: U.S. Department of Health and Human Services, Centers for Disease Control and Prevention and National Cancer Institute; 2005.

Strategy 2: Base intervals on mean and standard deviation

With this strategy, you can create three, four, or six class intervals. First, calculate the mean and standard deviation of the distribution of data. (Lesson 2 covers the calculation of these measures.) Then use the mean plus or minus different multiples of the standard deviation to establish the upper limits for the intervals. This strategy is most appropriate for large data sets. For example, let's suppose you are investigating a scoring system for preparedness of health departments to respond to emerging and urgent threats. You have devised a series of evaluation questions ranging from 0 to 100, with 100 being highest. You conduct a survey and find that the scores for health departments in your jurisdiction range from 19 to 82; the mean of the scores is 50, and the standard deviation is 10. Here, the strategy for establishing six intervals for these data specifies:

Upper limit of interval 6 = maximum value = 82
Upper limit of interval 5 = 50 + 20 = 70
Upper limit of interval 4 = 50 + 10 = 60
Upper limit of interval 3 = 50
Upper limit of interval 2 = 50 − 10 = 40
Upper limit of interval 1 = 50 − 20 = 30
Lower limit of interval 1 = 19

If you then select the obvious lower limit for each upper limit, you have the six intervals:

Interval 6 = 71–82   Interval 3 = 41–50
Interval 5 = 61–70   Interval 2 = 31–40
Interval 4 = 51–60   Interval 1 = 19–30

You can create three or four intervals by combining some of the adjacent six-interval limits.

Strategy 3: Divide the range into equal class intervals

This method is the simplest and most commonly used, and is most readily adapted to graphs. The selection of groups or categories is often arbitrary, but must be consistent (for example, age groups by

5 or 10 years throughout the data set). To use equal class intervals, do the following:

Find the range of the values in your data set. That is, find the difference between the maximum value (or some slightly larger convenient value) and zero (or the minimum value).

Decide how many class intervals (groups or categories) you want to have. For tables, choose between four and eight class intervals. For graphs and maps, choose between three and six class intervals. The number will depend on what aspects of the data you want to highlight.

Find what size of class interval to use by dividing the range by the number of class intervals you have decided on.

Begin with the minimum value as the lower limit of your first interval and specify class intervals of whatever size you calculated until you reach the maximum value in your data.

For example, to display 52 observations, say the percentage of men over age 40 screened for prostate cancer within the past two years in 2004 by state (including Puerto Rico and the District of Columbia), you could create five categories, each containing the number of states with percentages of screened men in the given range.

Table 4.12 Percentage of Men Over Age 40 Screened for Prostate Cancer, by State (including Puerto Rico and the District of Columbia), 2004

Percentage	Number of States	Cumulative Frequency
40.0–44.9	3	3
45.0–49.9	18	21
50.0–54.9	25	46
55.0–59.9	5	51
60.0–64.9	1	52

Data Source: Behavioral Risk Factor Surveillance System [Internet]. Atlanta: Centers for Disease Control and Prevention. Available from: http://www.cdc.gov/brfss.

EXAMPLE: Creating Class Interval Categories

Use each strategy to create four class interval categories by using the lung cancer mortality rates shown in Table 4.13.

Table 4.13 Age-adjusted Lung Cancer Death Rates per 100,000 population, in Rank Order by State — United States, 2000

Rank	State	Rate per 100,000	Rank	State	Rate per 100,000
1	Kentucky	116.1	26	Florida	75.3
2	Mississippi	111.7	27	Kansas	74.5
3	West Virginia	104.1	28	Massachusetts	73.6
4	Tennessee	103.4	29	Alaska	72.9
5	Alabama	100.8	30	Oregon	72.7
6	Louisiana	99.2	31	New Hampshire	71.2
7	Arkansas	99.1	32	New Jersey	71.2
8	North Carolina	94.6	33	Washington	71.2
9	Georgia	93.2	34	Vermont	70.2
10	South Carolina	92.4	35	South Dakota	68.1
11	Indiana	91.6	36	Wisconsin	67.0
12	Oklahoma	89.4	37	Montana	66.5
13	Missouri	88.5	38	Connecticut	66.4
14	Ohio	85.6	39	New York	66.2
15	Virginia	83.0	40	Nebraska	65.6
16	Maine	80.2	41	North Dakota	64.9
17	Illinois	80.0	42	Wyoming	64.4
18	Texas	79.3	43	Arizona	62.0
19	Maryland	79.2	44	Minnesota	60.7
20	Nevada	78.7	45	California	60.1
21	Delaware	78.2	46	Idaho	59.7
22	Rhode Island	77.9	47	New Mexico	52.3
23	Iowa	77.0	48	Colorado	52.1
24	Michigan	76.7	49	Hawaii	49.8
25	Pennsylvania	76.5	50	Utah	39.7
			Total	**United States**	**76.9**

Data Source: Stewart SL, King JB, Thompson TD, Friedman C, Wingo PA. Cancer Mortality–United States, 1990-2000. In: Surveillance Summaries, June 4, 2004. MMWR 2004;53 (No. SS-3):23–30.

Strategy 1: Divide the data into groups of similar size

(Note: If the states in Table 4.13 had been listed alphabetically rather than in rank order, the first step would have been to sort the data into rank order by rate. Fortunately, this has already been done.)

1. Divide the list into four equal sized groups of places:

   50 states / 4 = 12.5 states per group. Because states can't be cut in half, use two groups of 12 states and two groups of 13 states. Missouri (#13) could go into either the first or second group and Connecticut (#38) could go into either third or fourth group. Arbitrarily putting Missouri in the second category and Connecticut into the third results in the following groups:
   a. Kentucky through Oklahoma (States 1–12)
   b. Missouri through Pennsylvania (States 13–25)
   c. Florida through Connecticut (States 26–38)
   d. New York through Utah (States 39–50)

2. Identify the rate for the first and last state in each group:
   a. Oklahoma through Kentucky   89.4–116.1
   b. Pennsylvania through Missouri   76.5–88.5
   c. Connecticut through Florida   66.4–75.3
   d. Utah through New York   39.7–66.2

EXAMPLE: Creating Class Interval Categories (Continued)

3. Adjust the limits of each interval so no gap exists between the end of one class interval and beginning of the next. Deciding how to adjust the limits is somewhat arbitrary — you could split the difference, or use a convenient round number.
   a. Oklahoma through Kentucky   89.0–116.1
   b. Pennsylvania through Missouri   76.0–88.9
   c. Connecticut through Florida   66.3–75.9
   d. Utah through New York   39.7–66.2

Strategy 2: Base intervals on mean and standard deviation

1. Calculate the mean and standard deviation (see Lesson 2 for instructions in calculating these measures.):
   Mean = 77.1
   Standard deviation = 16.1

2. Find the upper limits of four intervals
   a. Upper limit of interval 4 = maximum value   = 116.1
   b. Upper limit of interval 3 = mean + 1 standard deviation   = 77.1 + 16.1   =   93.2
   c. Upper limit of interval 2 = mean   = 77.1
   d. Upper limit of interval 1 = mean − 1 standard deviation   = 77.1 − 16.1   =   61.0
   e. Lower limit of interval 1 = minimum value   = 39.7

3. Select the lower limit for each upper limit to define four full intervals. Specify the states that fall into each interval. (Note: To place the states with the highest rates first, reverse the order of the intervals):
   a. North Carolina through Kentucky (8 states)   93.3–116.1
   b. Rhode Island through Georgia (14 states)   77.1–93.2
   c. Arizona through Iowa (21 states)   61.1–77.1
   d. Utah through Minnesota (7 states)   39.7–61.0

Strategy 3: Divide the range into equal class intervals

1. Divide the range from zero (or the minimum value) to the maximum by 4:
   (116.1 − 39.7) / 4 = 76.4 / 4 = 19.1

2. Use multiples of 19.1 to create four categories, starting with 39.7:
   39.7 through (39.7 + 19.1) = 39.7 through 58.8
   58.9 through (39.7 + [2 x 19.1]) = 58.9 through 77.9
   78.0 through (39.7 + [3 x 19.1]) = 78.0 through 97.0
   97.1 through (39.7 + [4 x 19.1]) = 97.1 through 116.1

3. Final categories:
   a. Arkansas through Kentucky (7 states)   97.1–116.1
   b. Delaware through North Carolina (14 states)   78.0–97.0
   c. Idaho through Rhode Island (25 states)   58.9–77.9
   d. Utah through New Mexico (4 states)   39.7–58.8

4. Alternatively, since 19.1 is close to 20, multiples of 20 might be used to create the four categories that might look cleaner. For example, the final categories could look like:
   a. Arkansas through Kentucky (7 states)   97.0–116.9
   b. Iowa through North Carolina (16 states)   77.0–96.9
   c. Idaho through Michigan (23 states)   57.0–76.9
   d. Utah through New Mexico (4 states)   37.0–56.9
        OR
   a. Alabama through Kentucky (5 states)   100.0–119.9
   b. Illinois through Louisiana (12 states)   80.0–99.9
   c. California through Texas (28 states)   60.0–79.9
   d. Utah through Idaho (5 states)   39.7–59.9

Exercise 4.2

With the data on lung cancer mortality rates presented in Table 4.13, use each strategy to create three class intervals for the rates.

 Check your answers on page 4-74

Graphs

A graph (used here interchangeably with chart) displays numeric data in visual form. It can display patterns, trends, aberrations, similarities, and differences in the data that may not be evident in tables. As such, a graph can be an essential tool for analyzing and trying to make sense of data. In addition, a graph is often an effective way to present data to others less familiar with the data.

When designing graphs, the guidelines for categorizing data for tables also apply. In addition, some best practices for graphics include:

- Ensure that a graphic can stand alone by clear labeling of title, source, axes, scales, and legends;
- Clearly identify variables portrayed (legends or keys), including units of measure;
- Minimize number of lines on a graph;
- Generally, portray frequency on the vertical scale, starting at zero, and classification variable on horizontal scale;
- Ensure that scales for each axis are appropriate for data presented;
- Define any abbreviations or symbols; and
- Specify any data excluded.

In epidemiology, most graphs have two scales or axes, one horizontal and one vertical, that intersect at a right angle. The horizontal axis is known as the x-axis and generally shows values of the independent (or x) variable, such as time or age group. The vertical axis is the y-axis and shows the dependent (or y) variable, which, in epidemiology, is usually a frequency measure such as number of cases or rate of disease. Each axis should be labeled to show what it represents (both the name of the variable and the units in which it is measured) and marked by a scale of measurement along the line.

In constructing a useful graph, the guidelines for categorizing data for tables by types of data also apply. For example, the number of reported measles cases by year of report is technically a nominal variable, but because of the large number of cases when aggregated over the United States, we can treat this variable as a continuous one. As such, a line graph is appropriate to display these data.

"Charts...should fulfill certain basic objectives: they should be: (1) accurate representations of the facts, (2) clear, easily read, and understood, and (3) so designed and constructed as to attract and hold attention."[12]
- CF Schmid and SE Schmid

"Make the data stand out. Avoid superfluity."[13]
- WS Cleveland

Try It: Plotting a Graph

Scenario: Table 4.14 shows the number of measles cases by year of report from 1950 to 2003. The number of measles cases in years 1950 through 1954 has been plotted in Figure 4.1, below. The independent variable, years, is shown on the horizontal axis. The dependent variable, number of cases, is shown on the vertical axis. A grid is included in Figure 4.1 to illustrate how points are plotted. For example, to plot the point on the graph for the number of cases in 1953, draw a line up from 1953, and then draw a line from 449 cases to the right. The point where these lines intersect is the point for 1953 on the graph.

Your Turn: Use the data in Table 4.14 to plot the points for 1955 to 1959 and complete the graph in Figure 4.1.

Figure 4.1 Partial Graph of Measles by Year of Report — United States, 1950–1959

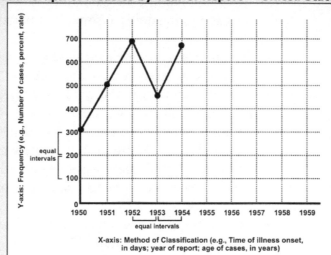

Table 4.14 Number of Reported Measles Cases, by Year of Report — United States, 1950–2003

Year	Cases	Year	Cases	Year	Cases
1950	319,000	1970	47,351	1990	27,786
1951	530,000	1971	75,290	1991	9,643
1952	683,000	1972	32,275	1992	2,237
1953	449,000	1973	26,690	1993	312
1954	683,000	1974	22,094	1994	963
1955	555,000	1975	24,374	1995	309
1956	612,000	1976	41,126	1996	508
1957	487,000	1977	57,345	1997	138
1958	763,000	1978	26,871	1998	100
1959	406,000	1979	13,597	1999	100
1960	442,000	1980	13,506	2000	86
1961	424,000	1981	3,124	2001	116
1962	482,000	1982	1,714	2002	44
1963	385,000	1983	1,497	2003	56
1964	458,000	1984	2,587		
1965	262,000	1985	2,822		
1966	204,000	1986	6,282		
1967	62,705	1987	3,655		
1968	22,231	1988	3,396		
1969	25,826	1989	18,193		

Data Sources: Centers for Disease Control and Prevention. Summary of notifiable diseases–United States, 1989. MMWR 1989;38(No. 54).
Centers for Disease Control and Prevention. Summary of notifiable diseases–United States, 2002. MMWR 2002;51(No. 53)
Centers for Disease Control and Prevention. Summary of notifiable diseases–United States, 2003. MMWR 2005;52(No. 54)

Arithmetic-scale line graphs

An arithmetic-scale line graph (such as Figure 4.1) shows patterns or trends over some variable, often time. In epidemiology, this type of graph is used to show long series of data and to compare several series. It is the method of choice for plotting rates over time.

In an arithmetic-scale line graph, a set distance along any axis represents the same quantity anywhere on that axis. In Figure 4.2, for example, the space between tick marks along the y-axis (vertical axis) represents an increase of 10,000 (10 x 1,000) cases anywhere along the axis — a continuous variable.

Furthermore, the distance between any two tick marks on the x-axis (horizontal axis) represents a period of time of one year. This represents an example of a discrete variable. Thus an arithmetic-scale line graph is one in which equal distances along either the x- or y- axis portray equal values.

Arithmetic-scale line graphs can display numbers, rates, proportions, or other quantitative measures on the y-axis. Generally, the x-axis for these graphs is used to portray the time period of data occurrence, collection, or reporting (e.g., days, weeks, months, or years). Thus, these graphs are primarily used to portray an overall trend over time, rather than an analysis of particular observations (single data points). For example, Figure 4.2 shows prevalence (of neural tube defects) per 100,000 births.

Figure 4.2 Trends in Neural Tube Defects (Anencephaly and Spina Bifida) Among All Births, 45 States and District of Columbia, 1990–1999

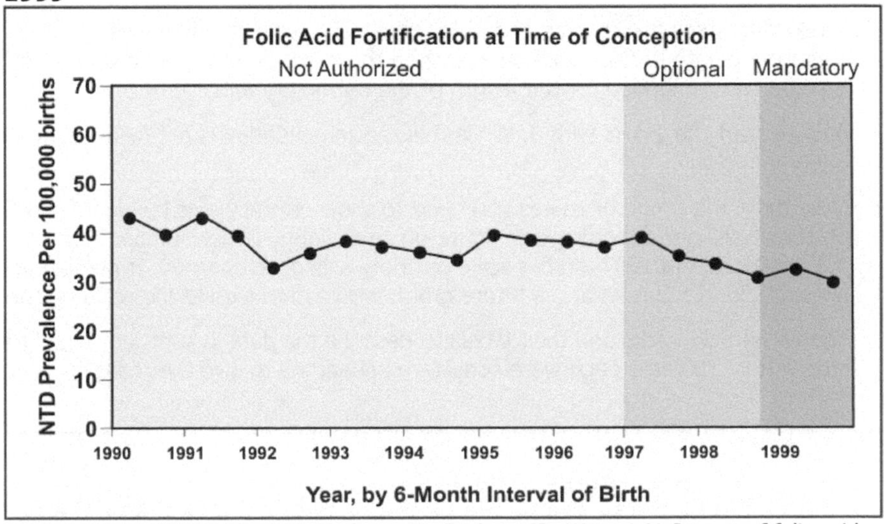

Source: Honein MA, Paulozzi LJ, Mathews TJ, Erickson JD, Wong L-Y. Impact of folic acid fortification of the US food supply on the occurrence of neural tube defects. JAMA 2001;285:2981–6.

Figure 4.3 shows another example of an arithmetic-scale line graph. Here the y-axis is a calculated variable, median age at death of people born with Down's syndrome from 1983–1997. Here also, we see the value of showing two data series on one graph; we can compare the mortality risk for males and females.

Figure 4.3 Median Age at Death of People with Down's Syndrome by Sex — United States, 1983–1997

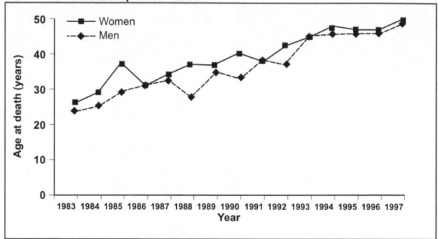

Source: Yang Q, Rasmussen A, Friedman JM. Mortality associated with Down's syndrome in the USA from 1983 to 1997: a population-based study. Lancet 2002;359:1019–25.

More About the X-axis and the Y-axis

When you create an arithmetic-scale line graph, you need to select a scale for the x- and y-axes. The scale should reflect both the data and the point of the graph. For example, if you use the data in Table 4.14 to graph the number of cases of measles cases by year from 1990 to 2002, then the scale of the x-axis will most likely be year of report, because that is how the data are available. Consider, however, if you had line-listed data with the actual dates of onset or report that spanned several years. You might prefer to plot these data by week, month, quarter, or even year, depending on the point you wish to make.

The following steps are recommended for creating a scale for the y-axis.
- Make the length of the y-axis shorter than the x-axis so that your graph is horizontal or "landscape." A 5:3 ratio is often recommended for the length of the x-axis to y-axis.

- Always start the y-axis with 0. While this recommendation is not followed in all fields, it is the standard practice in epidemiology.

- Determine the range of values you need to show on the y-axis by identifying the largest value you need to graph on the y-axis and rounding that figure off to a slightly larger number. For example, the largest y-value in Figure 4.3 is 49 years in 1997, so the scale on the y-axis goes up to 50. If median age continues to increase and exceeds 50 in future years, a future graph will have to extend the scale on the y-axis to 60 years.

- Space the tick marks and their labels to describe the data in sufficient detail for your purposes. In Figure 4.3, five intervals of 10 years each were considered adequate to give the reader a good sense of the data points and pattern.

Exercise 4.3

Using the data on measles rates (per 100,000) from 1955 to 2002 in Table 4.15:

1. *Construct an arithmetic-scale line graph of rate by year. Use intervals on the y-axis that are appropriate for the range of data you are graphing.*

2. *Construct a separate arithmetic-scale line graph of the measles rates from 1985 to 2002. Use intervals on the y-axis that are appropriate for the range of data you are graphing.*

Graph paper is provided at the end of this lesson.

Table 4.15 Rate (per 100,000 Population) of Reported Measles Cases by Year of Report — United States, 1955–2002

Year	Rate per 100,000	Year	Rate per 100,000	Year	Rate per 100,000
1955	336.3	1971	36.5	1987	1.5
1956	364.1	1972	15.5	1988	1.4
1957	283.4	1973	12.7	1989	7.3
1958	438.2	1974	10.5	1990	11.2
1959	229.3	1975	11.4	1991	3.8
1960	246.3	1976	19.2	1992	0.9
1961	231.6	1977	26.5	1993	0.1
1962	259.0	1978	12.3	1994	0.4
1963	204.2	1979	6.2	1995	0.1
1964	239.4	1980	6.0	1996	0.2
1965	135.1	1981	1.4	1997	0.06
1966	104.2	1982	0.7	1998	0.04
1967	31.7	1983	0.6	1999	0.04
1968	11.1	1984	1.1	2000	0.03
1969	12.8	1985	1.2	2001	0.04
1970	23.2	1986	2.6	2002	0.02

Data Sources: Centers for Disease Control. Summary of notifiable diseases–United States, 1989. MMWR 1989;38(No. 54). Centers for Disease Control and Prevention. Summary of notifiable diseases–United States, 2002. Published April 30, 2004 for MMWR 2002;51(No. 53).

 Check your answers on page 4-76

Semilogarithmic-scale line graphs

In some cases, the range of data observed may be so large that proper construction of an arithmetic-scale graph is problematic. For example, in the United States, vaccination policies have greatly reduced the incidence of mumps; however, outbreaks can still occur in unvaccinated populations. To portray these competing forces, an arithmetic graph is insufficient without an inset amplifying the problem years (Figure 4.4).

Figure 4.4 Mumps by Year — United States, 1978–2003

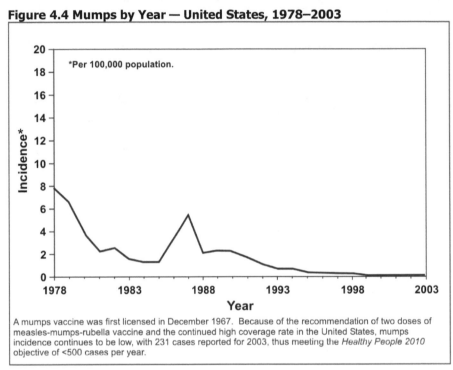

A mumps vaccine was first licensed in December 1967. Because of the recommendation of two doses of measles-mumps-rubella vaccine and the continued high coverage rate in the United States, mumps incidence continues to be low, with 231 cases reported for 2003, thus meeting the *Healthy People 2010* objective of <500 cases per year.

Source: Centers for Disease Control and Prevention. Summary of notifiable diseases–United States, 2003. Published April 22, 2005, for MMWR 2003;52(No. 54):54.

An alternative approach to this problem of incompatible scales is to use a **logarithmic transformation** for the y-axis. Termed a **"semi-log" graph**, this technique is useful for displaying a variable with a wide range of values (as illustrated in Figure 4.5). The x-axis uses the usual arithmetic-scale, but the y-axis is measured on a logarithmic rather than an arithmetic scale. As a result, the distance from 1 to 10 on the y- axis is the same as the distance from 10 to 100 or 100 to 1,000.

Another use for the semi-log graph is when you are interested in portraying the relative **rate of change** of several series, rather than the absolute value. Figure 4.5 shows this application. Note several aspects of this graph:

Cycle = order of magnitude

That is, from 1 to 10 is one cycle; from 10 to 100 is another cycle.

- The y-axis includes four cycles of the **order of magnitude**, each a multiple of ten (e.g., 0.1 to 1, 1 to 10, etc.) — each a constant multiple.

- Within a cycle, the ten tick-marks are spaced so that spaces become smaller as the value increases. Notice that the absolute distance from 1.0 to 2.0 is wider than the distance from 2.0 to 3.0, which is, in turn, wider than the distance from 8.0 to 9.0. This results from the fact that we are graphing the logarithmic transformation of numbers, which, in fact, shrinks them as they become larger. We can still compare series, however, since the shrinking process preserves the relative change between series.

Figure 4.5 Age-adjusted Death Rates for 5 of the 15 Leading Causes of Death — United States, 1958–2002

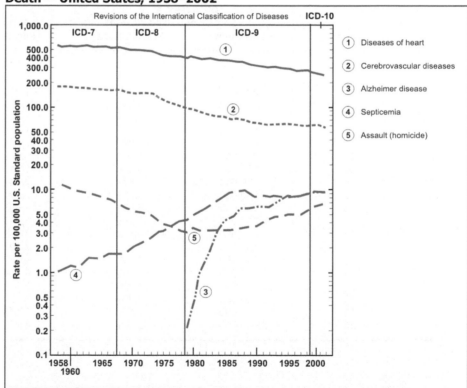

Adapted from: Kochanek KD, Murphy SL, Anderson RN, Scott C. Deaths: final data for 2002. National vital statistics report; vol 53, no 5. Hyattsville, Maryland: National Center for Health Statistics, 2004. p. 9.

Consider the data shown in Table 4.16. Two hypothetical countries begin with a population of 1,000,000. The population of Country A grows by 100,000 persons each year. The population of Country B grows by 10% each year. Figure 4.6 displays data from Country A on the left, and Country B on the right. Arithmetic-scale line graphs are above semilog-scale line graphs of the same data. Look at the left side of the figure. Because the population of Country A grows by a constant number of persons each year, the data on the arithmetic-scale line graph fall on a straight line. However, because the percentage growth in Country A declines each year, the curve on the semilog-scale line graph flattens. On the right side of the figure the population of Country B curves upward on the arithmetic-scale line graph but is a straight line on the semilog graph. In summary, a straight line on an arithmetic-scale line graph represents a constant change in the number or amount. A straight line on a semilog-scale line graph represents a constant percent change from a constant rate.

Table 4.16 Hypothetical Population Growth in Two Countries

Year	COUNTRY A (Constant Growth by 100,000)		COUNTRY B (Constant Growth by 10%)	
	Population	Growth Rate	Population	Growth Rate
0	1,000,000		1,000,000	
1	1,100,000	10.0%	1,100,000	10.0%
2	1,200,000	9.1%	1,210,000	10.0%
3	1,300,000	8.3%	1,331,000	10.0%
4	1,400,000	7.7%	1,464,100	10.0%
5	1,500,000	7.1%	1,610,510	10.0%
6	1,600,000	6.7%	1,771,561	10.0%
7	1,700,000	6.3%	1,948,717	10.0%
8	1,800,000	5.9%	2,143,589	10.0%
9	1,900,000	5.6%	2,357,948	10.0%
10	2,000,000	5.3%	2,593,742	10.0%
11	2,100,000	5.0%	2,853,117	10.0%
12	2,200,000	4.8%	3,138,428	10.0%
13	2,300,000	4.4%	3,452,271	10.0%
14	2,400,000	4.3%	3,797,498	10.0%
15	2,500,000	4.2%	4,177,248	10.0%
16	2,600,000	4.0%	4,594,973	10.0%
17	2,700,000	3.8%	5,054,470	10.0%
18	2,800,000	3.7%	5,559,917	10.0%
19	2,900,000	3.6%	6,115,909	10.0%
20	3,000,000	3.4%	6,727,500	10.0%

Figure 4.6 Comparison of Arithmetic-scale Line Graph and Semilogarithmic-scale Line Graph for Hypothetical Country A (Constant Increase in Number of People) and Country B (Constant Increase in Rate of Growth)

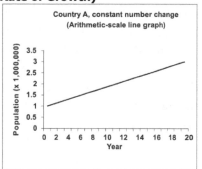

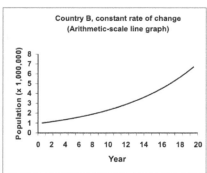

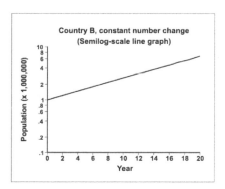

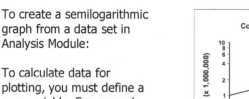

To create a semilogarithmic graph from a data set in Analysis Module:

To calculate data for plotting, you must define a new variable. For example, if you want a semilog plot for annual measles surveillance data in a variable called MEASLES, under the VARIABLES section of the Analysis commands:

- Select **Define**.
- Type **logmeasles** into the **Variable Name** box.
- Since your new variable is not used by other programs, the **Scope** should be **Standard**.
- Click on **OK** to define the new variable. Note that **logmeasles** now appears in the pull-down list of **Variables**.
- Under the **Variables** section of the Analysis commands, select **Assign**.

Types of variables and class intervals are discussed in Lesson 2.

Consequently, a semilog-scale line graph has the following features:

- The slope of the line indicates the rate of increase or decrease.
- A straight line indicates a constant rate (not amount) of increase or decrease in the values.
- A horizontal line indicates no change.
- Two or more lines following parallel paths show identical rates of change.

Semilog graph paper is available commercially, and most include at least three cycles.

Histograms

A histogram is a graph of the frequency distribution of a continuous variable, based on class intervals. It uses adjoining columns to represent the number of observations for each class interval in the distribution. The area of each column is proportional to the number of observations in that interval. Figures 4.7a and 4.7b show two versions of a histogram of frequency distributions with equal class intervals. Since all class intervals are equal in this histogram, the height of each column is in proportion to the number of observations it depicts.

Figures 4.7a, 4.7b, and 4.7c are examples of a particular type of histogram that is commonly used in field epidemiology — the epidemic curve. An epidemic curve is a histogram that displays the number of cases of disease during an outbreak or epidemic by times of onset. The y-axis represents the number of cases; the x-axis represents date and/or time of onset of illness. Figure 4.7a is a perfectly acceptable epidemic curve, but some epidemiologists prefer drawing the histogram as stacks of squares, with each square representing one case (Figure 4.7b). Additional information may be added to the histogram. The rendition of the epidemic curve shown in Figure 4.7c shades the individual boxes in each time period to denote which cases have been confirmed with culture results. Other information such as gender or presence of a related risk factor could be portrayed in this fashion.

Conventionally, the numbers on the x-axis are centered between the tick marks of the appropriate interval. The interval of time should be appropriate for the disease in question, the duration of the outbreak, and the purpose of the graph. If the purpose is to show the temporal relationship between time of exposure and onset of disease, then a widely accepted rule of thumb is to use intervals approximately one-fourth (or between one-eighth and one-third) of the incubation period of the disease shown. The incubation period for salmonellosis is usually 12–36 hours, so the x-axis of this epidemic curve has 12-hour intervals.

Figure 4.7a Number of Cases of *Salmonella* Enteriditis Among Party Attendees by Date and Time of Onset — Chicago, Illinois, February 2000

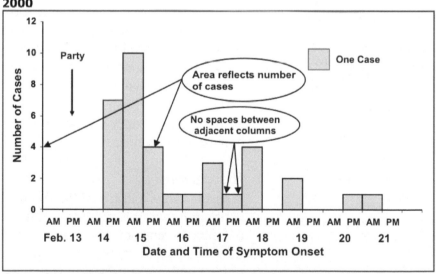

Source: Cortese M, Gerber S, Jones E, Fernandez J. A Salmonella Enteriditis outbreak in Chicago. Presented at the Eastern Regional Epidemic Intelligence Service Conference, March 23, 2000, Boston, Massachusetts.

Figure 4.7b Number of Cases of *Salmonella* Enteriditis Among Party Attendees by Date and Time of Onset — Chicago, Illinois, February 2000

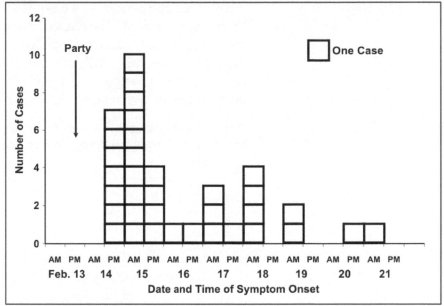

Source: Cortese M, Gerber S, Jones E, Fernandez J. A Salmonella Enteriditis outbreak in Chicago. Presented at the Eastern Regional Epidemic Intelligence Service Conference, March 23, 2000, Boston, Massachusetts.

The most common choice for the x-axis variable in field epidemiology is calendar time, as shown in Figures 4.7a–c. However, age, cholesterol level or another continuous-scale variable may be used on the x-axis of an epidemic curve.

Figure 4.7c Number of Cases of *Salmonella* Enteriditis Among Party Attendees by Date and Time of Onset — Chicago, Illinois, February 2000

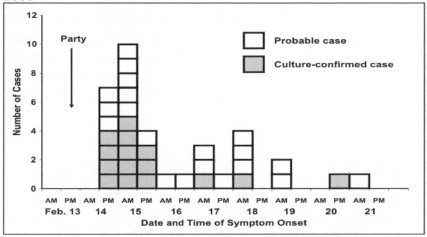

Source: Cortese M, Gerber S, Jones E, Fernandez J. A Salmonella Enteriditis outbreak in Chicago. Presented at the Eastern Regional Epidemic Intelligence Service Conference, March 23, 2000, Boston, Massachusetts.

In Figure 4.8, which shows a frequency distribution of adults with diagnosed diabetes in the United States, the x-axis displays a measure of body mass — weight (in kilograms) divided by height (in meters) squared. The choice of variable for the x-axis of an epidemic curve is clearly dependent on the point of the display. Figures 4.7a, 4.7b, or 4.7c are constructed to show the natural course of the epidemic over time; Figure 4.8 conveys the burden of the problem of overweight and obesity.

Figure 4.8 Distribution of Body Mass Index Among Adults with Diagnosed Diabetes — United States, 1999–2002

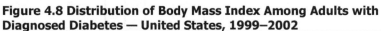
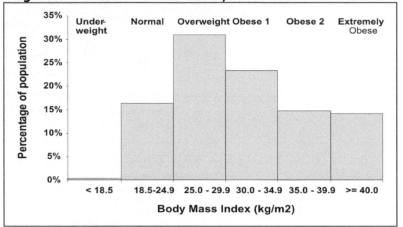

Data Source: Centers for Disease Control and Prevention. Prevalence of overweight and obesity among adults with diagnosed diabetes–United States, 1988-1994 and 1999-2002. MMWR 2004;53:1066–8.

The component of most interest should always be put at the bottom because the upper component usually has a jagged baseline that may make comparison difficult. Consider the data on pneumoconiosis in Figure 4.9a. The graph clearly displays a gradual decline in deaths from all pneumoconiosis between 1972 and 1999. It appears that deaths from asbestosis (top subgroup in Figure 4.9a) went against the overall trend, by increasing over the same period. However, Figure 4.9b makes this point more clearly by placing asbestosis along the baseline.

Figure 4.9a Number of Deaths with Any Death Certificate Mention of Asbestosis, Coal Worker's Pneumoconiosis (CWP), Silicosis, and Unspecified/Other Pneumoconiosis Among Persons Aged ≥ 15 Years, by Year — United States, 1968–2000

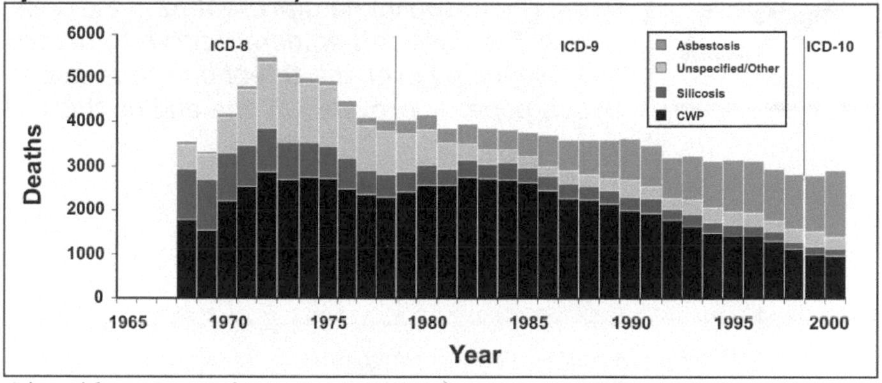

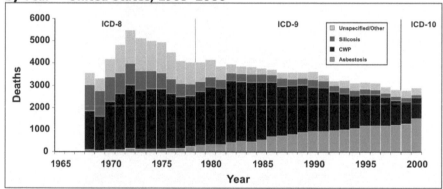

Adapted from: Centers for Disease Control and Prevention. Changing patterns of pneumoconiosis mortality–United States, 1968-2000. MMWR 2004;53:627–31.

Figure 4.9b Number of Deaths with Any Death Certificate Mention of Asbestosis, Coal Worker's Pneumoconiosis (CWP), Silicosis, and Unspecified/Other Pneumoconiosis Among Persons Aged ≥ 15 Years, by Year — United States, 1968–2000

Data Source: Centers for Disease Control and Prevention. Changing patterns of pneumoconiosis mortality–United States, 1968-2000. MMWR 2004;53:627–31.

Epidemic curves are discussed in more detail in Lesson 6.

Some histograms, particularly those that are drawn as stacks of squares, include a box that indicates how many cases are represented by each square. While a square usually represents one case in a relatively small outbreak, a square may represent five or ten cases in a relatively large outbreak.

Exercise 4.4

Using the botulism data presented in Exercise 4.1, draw an epidemic curve. Then use this epidemic curve to describe this outbreak as if you were speaking over the telephone to someone who cannot see the graph. Graph paper is provided at the end of this lesson.

 Check your answers on page 4-77

Population pyramid

A population pyramid displays the count or percentage of a population by age and sex. It does so by using two histograms — most often one for females and one for males, each by age group — turned sideways so the bars are horizontal, and placed base to base (Figures 4.10 and 4.11). Notice the overall pyramidal shape of the population distribution of a developing country with many births, relatively high infant mortality, and relatively low life expectancy (Figure 4.10). Compare that with the shape of the population distribution of a more developed country with fewer births, lower infant mortality, and higher life expectancy (Figure 4.11).

Figure 4.10 Population Distribution of Zambia by Age and Sex, 2000

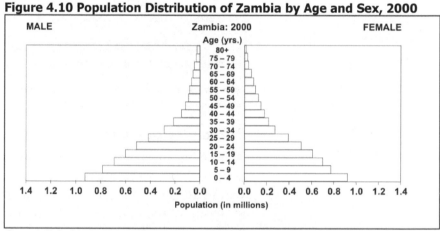

Source: U.S. Census Bureau [Internet]. Washington, DC: IDB Population Pyramids [cited 2004 Sep 10]. Available from: http://www.census.gov/ipc/www/idbpyr.html.

Figure 4.11 Population Distribution of Sweden by Age and Sex, 1997

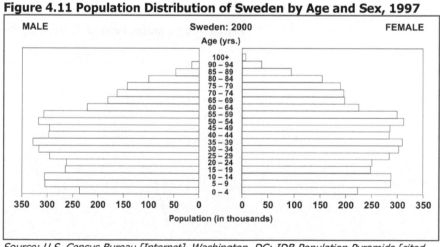

Source: U.S. Census Bureau [Internet]. Washington, DC: IDB Population Pyramids [cited 2004 Sep 10]. Available from: http://www.census.gov/ipc/www/idbpyr.html.

While population pyramids are used most often to display the distribution of a national population, they can also be used to display other data such as disease or a health characteristic by age and sex. For example, smoking prevalence by age and sex is shown in Figure 4.12. This pyramid clearly shows that, at every age, females are less likely to be current smokers than males.

Figure 4.12 Percentage of Persons ≥18 Years Who Were Current Smokers,* by Age and Sex — United States, 2002

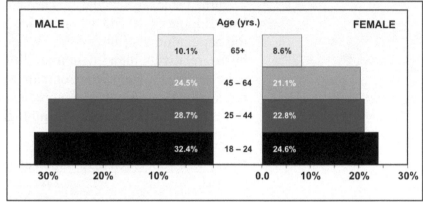

Answer "yes" to both questions: "Do you now smoke cigarettes everyday or some days?" and "Have you smoked at least 100 cigarettes in your entire life?"

Data Source: Centers for Disease Control and Prevention. Cigarette smoking among adults–United States, 2002. MMWR 2004;53:427–31.

Frequency polygons

A frequency polygon, like a histogram, is the graph of a frequency distribution. In a frequency polygon, the number of observations within an interval is marked with a single point placed at the midpoint of the interval. Each point is then connected to the next with a straight line. Figure 4.13 shows an example of a frequency polygon over the outline of a histogram for the same data. This graph makes it easy to identify the peak of the epidemic (4 weeks).

Figure 4.13 Comparison of Frequency Polygon and Histogram

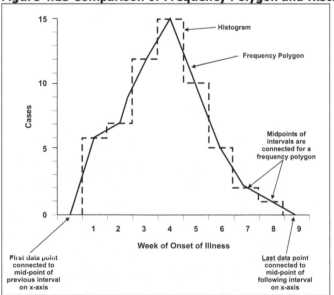

A frequency polygon contains the same area under the line as does a histogram of the same data. Indeed, the data that were displayed as a histogram in Figure 4.9a are displayed as a frequency polygon in Figure 4.14.

Figure 4.14 Number of Deaths with Any Death Certificate Mention of Asbestosis, Coal Worker's Pneumoconiosis (CWP), Silicosis, and Unspecified/Other Pneumoconiosis Among Persons Aged ≥ 15 Years, by Year — United States, 1968–2000

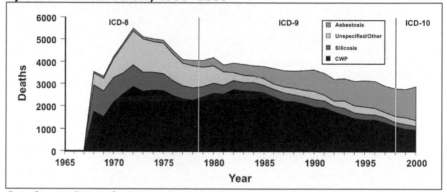

Data Source: Centers for Disease Control and Prevention. Changing patterns of pneumoconiosis mortality–United States, 1968-2000. MMWR 2004;53:627–31.

A frequency polygon differs from an arithmetic-scale line graph in several ways. A frequency polygon (or histogram) is used to display the entire frequency distribution (counts) of a continuous variable. An arithmetic-scale line graph is used to plot a series of observed data points (counts or rates), usually over time. A frequency polygon must be closed at both ends because the area under the curve is representative of the data; an arithmetic-scale line graph simply plots the data points. Compare the pneumoconiosis mortality data displayed as a frequency polygon in Figure 4.14 and as a line graph in Figure 4.15.

Figure 4.15 Number of Deaths with Any Death Certificate Mention of Asbestosis, Coal Worker's Pneumoconiosis (CWP), Silicosis, and Unspecified/Other Pneumoconiosis Among Persons Aged ≥ 15 Years, by Year — United States, 1968–2000

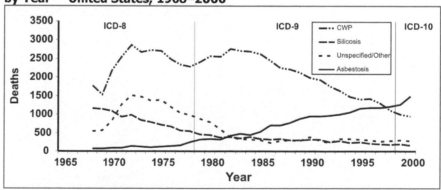

Data Source: Centers for Disease Control and Prevention. Changing patterns of pneumoconiosis mortality–United States, 1968-2000. MMWR 2004;53:627–31.

Exercise 4.5

Consider the epidemic curve constructed for Exercise 4.4. Prepare a frequency polygon for these same data. Compare the interpretations of the two graphs.

 Check your answers on page 4-77

Cumulative frequency and survival curves

As its name implies, a cumulative frequency curve plots the cumulative frequency rather than the actual frequency distribution of a variable. This type of graph is useful for identifying medians, quartiles, and other percentiles. The x-axis records the class intervals, while the y-axis shows the cumulative frequency either on an absolute scale (e.g., number of cases) or, more commonly, as percentages from 0% to 100%. The median (50% or half-way point) can be found by drawing a horizontal line from the 50% tick mark on the y-axis to the cumulative frequency curve, then drawing a vertical line from that spot down to the x-axis. Figure 4.16 is a cumulative frequency graph showing the number of days until smallpox vaccination scab separation among persons who had never received smallpox vaccination previously (primary vaccinees) and among persons who had been previously vaccinated (revaccinees). The median number of days until scab separation was 19 days among revaccinees, and 22 days among primary vaccinees.

Ogive (pronounced O'-jive) is another name for a cumulative frequency curve. Ogive also means the diagonal rib of a Gothic vault, a pointed arc, or the curved area making up the nose of a projectile.

Figure 4.16 Days to Smallpox Vaccination Scab Separation Among Primary Vaccinees (n=29) and Revaccinees (n=328) — West Virginia, 2003

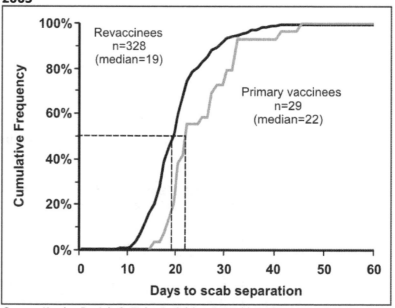

Source: Kaydos-Daniels S, Bixler D, Colsher P, Haddy L. Symptoms following smallpox vaccination–West Virginia, 2003. Presented at 53rd Annual Epidemic Intelligence Service Conference, April 19-23, 2004, Atlanta, Georgia.

A survival curve can be used with follow-up studies to display the proportion of one or more groups still alive at different time periods. Similar to the axes of the cumulative frequency curve, the x-axis records the time periods, and the y-axis shows percentages, from 0% to 100%, still alive.

The most striking difference is in the plotted curves themselves. While a cumulative frequency starts at zero in the lower left corner of the graph and approaches 100% in the upper right corner, a survival curve begins at 100% in the upper left corner and proceeds toward the lower right corner as members of the group die. The survival curve in Figure 4.17 shows the difference in survival in the early 1900s, mid-1900s, and late 1900s. The survival curve for 1900–1902 shows a rapid decline in survival during the first few years of life, followed by a relatively steady decline. In contrast, the curve for 1949–1951 is shifted right, showing substantially better survival among the young. The curve for 1997 shows improved survival among the older population.

Figure 4.17 Percent Surviving by Age in Death-registration States, 1900–1902 and United States, 1949–1951 and 1997

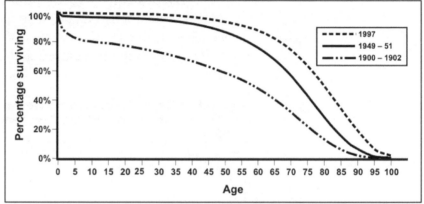

Source: Anderson RN. United States life tables, 1997. National vital statistics reports; vol 47, no. 28. Hyattsville, Maryland: National Center for Health Statistics, 1999.

Note that the smallpox scab separation data plotted as a cumulative frequency graph in Figure 4.16 can be plotted as a smallpox scab survival curve, as shown in Figure 4.18.

Figure 4.18 "Survival" of Smallpox Vaccination Scabs Among Primary Vaccines (n=29) and Revaccinees (n=328) — West Virginia, 2003

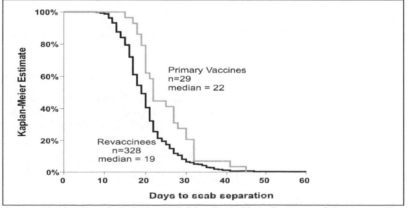

Source: Kaydos-Daniels S, Bixler D, Colsher P, Haddy L. Symptoms following smallpox vaccination–West Virginia, 2003. Presented at 53rd Annual Epidemic Intelligence Service Conference, April 19-23, 2004, Atlanta, Georgia.

Other Data Displays

Thus far in this lesson, we have covered the most common ways that epidemiologists and other public health analysts display data in tables and graphs. We now cover some additional graphical techniques that are useful in specific situations. While you may not find yourself constructing these figures often, our objective is to equip you to properly interpret these displays when you encounter them.

Scatter diagrams

A scatter diagram (or "scattergram") is a graph that portrays the relationship between two continuous variables, with the x-axis representing one variable and the y-axis representing the other.[15] To create a scatter diagram you must have a pair of values (one for each variable) for each person, group, country, or other entity in the data set, one value for each variable. A point is placed on the graph where the two values intersect. For example, demographers may be interested in the relationship between infant mortality and total fertility in various nations. Figure 4.19 plots the total fertility rate (estimated average number of children per woman) by the infant mortality rate in 194 countries, so this scatter diagram has 194 data points.

To interpret a scatter diagram, look at the overall pattern made by the plotted points. A fairly compact pattern of points from the lower left to the upper right indicates a positive correlation, in which one variable increases as the other increases. A compact pattern from the upper left to lower right indicates a negative or inverse correlation, in which one variable decreases as the other increases. Widely scattered points or a relatively flat pattern indicates little correlation. The data in Figure 4.19 seem to show a positive correlation between infant mortality and total fertility, that is, countries with high infant mortality seem to have high total fertility as well. Statistical tools such as linear regression can be applied to such data to quantify the correlation between variables in a scatter diagram. Similarly, scatter diagrams often display correlations that may provoke intriguing hypotheses about causal relationships, but additional investigation is almost always needed before any causal hypotheses should be accepted.

Figure 4.19 Correlation of Infant Mortality Rate and Total Fertility Rate Among 194 Nations, 1997

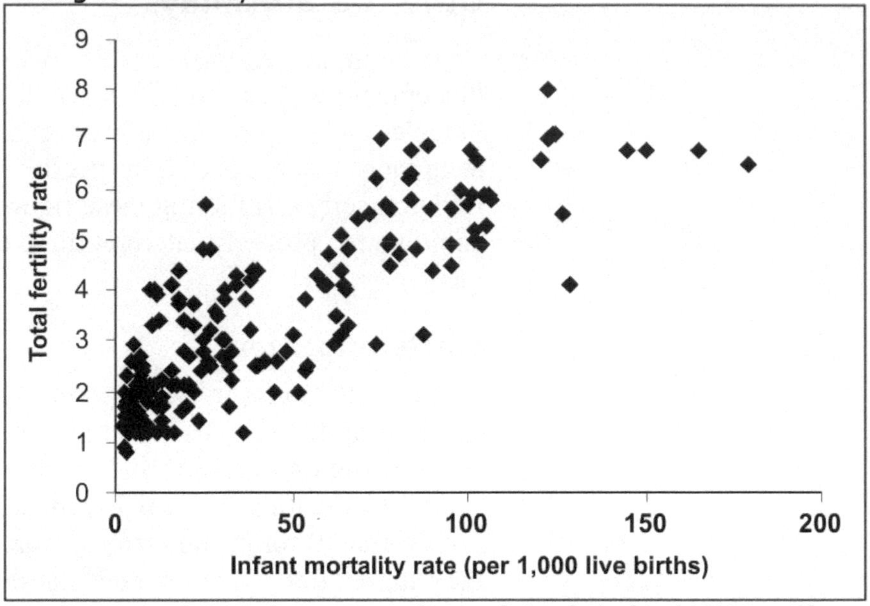

Data Source: Population Reference Bureau [Internet]. Datafinder [cited 2004 Dec 13]. Available from: http://www.prb.org/datafind/datafinder7.htm.

Bar charts

A bar chart uses bars of equal width to display comparative data. Comparison of categories is based on the fact that the length of the bar is proportional to the frequency of the event in that category. Therefore, breaks in the scale could cause the data to be misinterpreted and should not be used in bar charts. Bars for different categories are separated by spaces (unlike the bars in a histogram). The bar chart can be portrayed with the bars either vertical or horizontal. (This choice is usually made based on the length of text labels — long labels fit better on a horizontal chart than a vertical one) The bars are usually arranged in ascending or descending length, or in some other systematic order dictated by any intrinsic order of the categories. Appropriate data for bar charts include discrete data (e.g., race or cause of death) or variables treated as though they were discrete (age groups). (Recall that a histogram shows frequency of a continuous variable, such as dates of onset of symptoms).

The simplest bar chart is used to display the data from a one-variable table (see page 4-4). Figure 4.20 shows the number of deaths among persons ages 25–34 years for the six most common causes, plus all other causes grouped together, in the United States in 2003. Note that this bar chart is aligned horizontally to allow for long labels.

Figure 4.20 Number of Deaths by Cause Among 25–34 Year Olds — United States, 2003

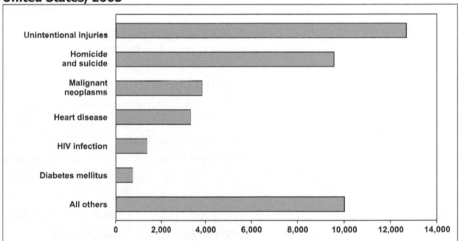

Data Source: Web-based Injury Statistics Query and Reporting System (WISQARS) [online database] Atlanta; National Center for Injury Prevention and Control. [cited 2006 Feb 15]. Available from: http://www.cdc.gov/ncipc/wisqars.

Grouped bar charts

A grouped bar chart is used to illustrate data from two-variable or three-variable tables. A grouped bar chart is particularly useful when you want to compare the subgroups within a group. Bars within a group are adjoining. The bars should be illustrated distinctively and described in a legend. For example, consider the data for Figure 4.12 — current smokers by age and sex. In Figure

4.21, each bar grouping represents an age group. Within the group, separate bars are used to represent data for males and females. This shows graphically that regardless of age, men are more likely to be current smokers than are women, but that difference declines with age.

Figure 4.21 Percentage of Persons Aged ≥18 Years Who Were Current Smokers, by Age and Sex — United States, 2002

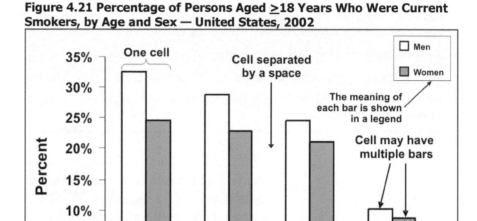

Data Source: Centers for Disease Control and Prevention. Cigarette smoking among adults–United States, 2002. MMWR 2004;53:427–31.

The bar chart in Figure 4.22a shows the leading causes of death in 1997 and 2003 among persons ages 25–34 years. The graph is more effective at showing the differences in causes of death during the same year than in showing differences in a single cause between years. While the decline in deaths due to HIV infection between 1997 and 2003 is quite apparent, the smaller drop in heart disease is more difficult to see. If the goal of the figure is to compare specific causes between the two years, the bar chart in Figure 4.22b is a better choice.

Figure 4.22a Number of Deaths by Cause Among 25–34 Year Olds — United States, 1997 and 2003

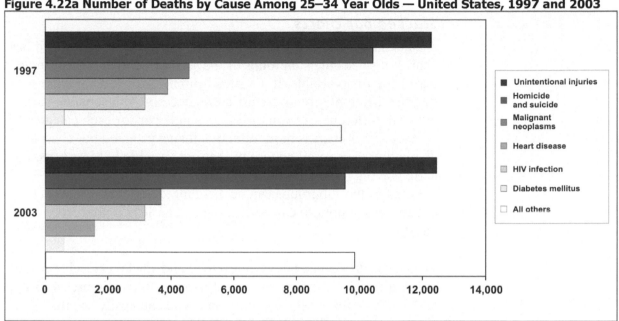

Data Source: Web-based Injury Statistics Query and Reporting System (WISQARS) [online database] Atlanta; National Center for Injury Prevention and Control. [cited 2006 Feb 15]. Available from: http://www.cdc.gov/ncipc/wisqars.

Figure 4.22b Number of Deaths by Cause Among 25–34 Year Olds — United States, 1997 and 2003

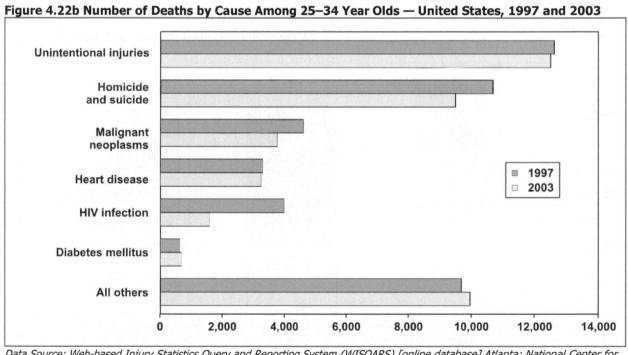

Data Source: Web-based Injury Statistics Query and Reporting System (WISQARS) [online database] Atlanta; National Center for Injury Prevention and Control. [cited 2006 Feb 15]. Available from: http://www.cdc.gov/ncipc/wisqars.

Stacked bar charts

A stacked bar chart is used to show the same data as a grouped bar chart but stacks the subgroups of the second variable into a single bar of the first variable. It deviates from the grouped bar chart in that the different groups are differentiated not with separate bars, but with different segments within a single bar for each category. A stacked bar chart is more effective than a grouped bar chart at displaying the overall pattern of the first variable but less effective at displaying the relative size of each subgroup. The trends or patterns of the subgroups can be difficult to decipher because, except for the bottom categories, the categories do not rest on a flat baseline.

To see the difference between grouped and stacked bar charts, look at Figure 4.23. This figure shows the same data as Figures 4.22a and 4.22b. With the stacked bar chart, you can easily see the change in the total number of deaths between the two years; however, it is difficult to see the values of each cause of death. On the other hand, with the grouped bar chart, you can more easily see the changes by cause of death.

Figure 4.23 Number of Deaths by Cause Among 25–44 Year Olds — United States, 1997 and 2003

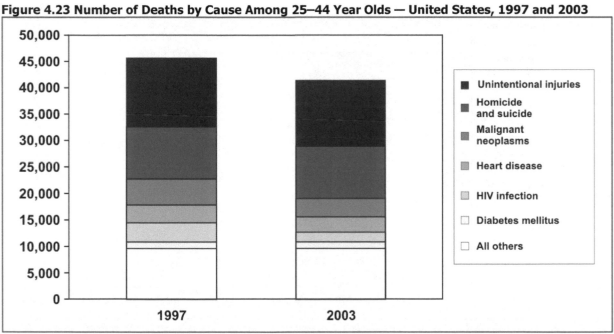

Data Source: Web-based Injury Statistics Query and Reporting System (WISQARS) [online database] Atlanta; National Center for Injury Prevention and Control. [cited 2006 Feb 15]. Available from: http://www.cdc.gov/ncipc/wisqars.

100% component bar charts

A 100% component bar chart is a variant of a stacked bar chart, in which all of the bars are pulled to the same height (100%) and show the components as percentages of the total rather than as actual values. This type of chart is useful for comparing the contribution of different subgroups within the categories of the main variable. Figure 4.24 shows a 100% component bar chart that compares lengths of hospital stay by age group. The figure clearly shows that the percentage of people who stay in the hospital for 1 day or less (bottom component) is greatest for children ages 0–4 years, and declines with increasing age. Concomitantly, lengths of stay of 7 or more days increase with age. However, because the columns are the same height, you cannot tell from the columns how many people in each age group were hospitalized for traumatic brain injury — putting numbers above the bars to indicate the totals in each age group would solve that problem.

Figure 4.24 Length of Hospital Stay for Traumatic Brain Injury-related Discharges — 14 States*, 1997

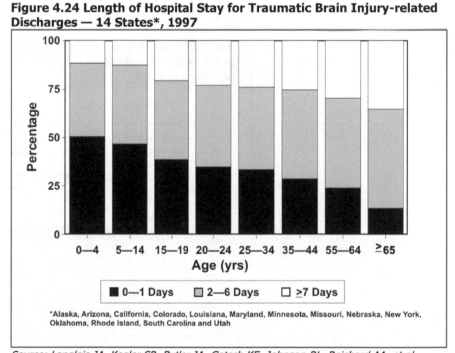

*Alaska, Arizona, California, Colorado, Louisiana, Maryland, Minnesota, Missouri, Nebraska, New York, Oklahoma, Rhode Island, South Carolina and Utah

Source: Langlois JA, Kegler SR, Butler JA, Gotsch KE, Johnson RL, Reichard AA, et al. Traumatic brain injury-related hospital discharges: results from a 14-state surveillance system. In: Surveillance Summaries, June 27, 2003. MMWR 2003;52(No. SS-04):1–18.

Deviation bar charts

While many bar charts show only positive values, a deviation bar chart displays both positive and negative changes from a baseline. (Imagine profit/loss data at different times.) Figure 4.25 shows such a deviation bar chart of selected reportable diseases in the United States. A similar chart appears in each issue of CDC's Morbidity and Mortality Weekly Report. In this chart, the number of cases reported during the past 4 weeks is compared to the average number reported during comparable periods of the past few years. The deviations to the right for hepatitis B and pertussis indicate increases over historical levels. The deviations to the left for measles, rubella, and most of the other diseases indicate declines in reported cases compared to past levels. In this particular chart, the x-axis is on a logarithmic scale, so that a 50% reduction (one-half of the cases) and a doubling (50% increase) of cases are represented by bars of the same length, though in opposite directions. Values beyond historical limits (comparable to 95% confidence limits) are highlighted for special attention.

Figure 4.25 Comparison of Current Four-week Totals with Historical Data for Selected Notifiable Diseases — United States, 4-weeks Ending December 11, 2004

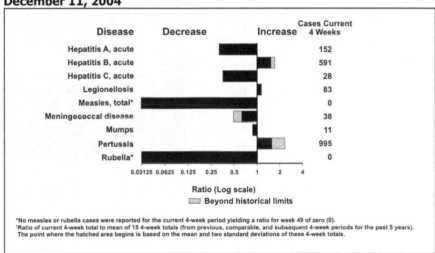

*No measles or rubella cases were reported for the current 4-week period yielding a ratio for week 49 of zero (0).
†Ratio of current 4-week total to mean of 15 4-week totals (from previous, comparable, and subsequent 4-week periods for the past 5 years). The point where the hatched area begins is based on the mean and two standard deviations of these 4-week totals.

Source: Centers for Disease Control and Prevention. Figure 1. Selected notifiable disease reports, United States, comparison of provisional 4-week totals ending December 11, 2004, with historical data. MMWR 2004;53:1161.

Exercise 4.6

Use the data in Table 4.17 to draw a stacked bar chart, a grouped bar chart, and a 100% component bar chart to illustrate the differences in the age distribution of syphilis cases among white males, white females, black males, and black females. What information is best conveyed by each chart? Graph paper is provided at the end of this lesson.

Table 4.17 Number of Reported Cases of Primary and Secondary Syphilis, by Age Group, Among Non-Hispanic Black and White Men and Women — United States, 2002

Age Group (Years)	Black Men	White Men	Black Women	White Women
≥40	804	905	277	50
30-39	695	914	349	66
20-29	635	277	396	76
<20	92	12	173	25

Data Source: Centers for Disease Control and Prevention. Sexually Transmitted Disease Surveillance 2002. Atlanta: U.S. Department of Health and Human Services; 2003.

 Check your answers on page 4-78

Pie charts

A pie chart is a simple, easily understood chart in which the size of the "slices" or wedges shows the proportional contribution of each component part.[16] Pie charts are useful for showing the proportions of a single variable's frequency distribution. Figure 4.26 shows a simple pie chart of the leading causes of death in 2003 among persons aged 25–34 years.

Figure 4.26 Number of Deaths by Cause Among 25–34 Year Olds — United States, 2003

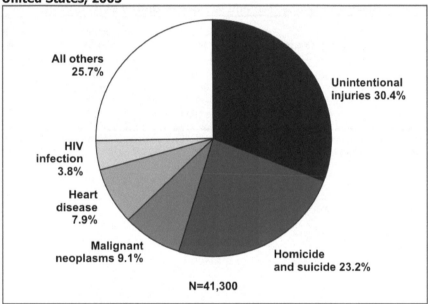

Data Source: Web-based Injury Statistics Query and Reporting System (WISQARS) [online database] Atlanta; National Center for Injury Prevention and Control. [cited 2006 Feb 15]. Available from: http://www.cdc.gov/ncipc/wisqars.

More About Constructing Pie Charts

- Conventionally, pie charts begin at 12 o'clock.

- The wedges should be labeled and arranged from largest to smallest, proceeding clockwise, although the "other" or "unknown" may be last.

- Shading may be used to distinguish between slices but is not always necessary.

- Because the eye cannot accurately gauge the area of the slices, the chart should indicate what percentage each slice represents either inside or near each slice.

Given current technology, pie charts are almost always generated by computer rather than drawn by hand. But the default settings of many computer programs differ from recommended epidemiologic practice. Many computer programs allow one or more slices to "explode" or be pulled out of the pie. In general, this technique should be limited to situations when you want to place special emphasis on one wedge, particularly when additional detail is provided about that wedge (Figure 4.27).

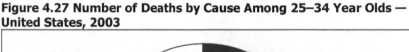
Figure 4.27 Number of Deaths by Cause Among 25–34 Year Olds — United States, 2003

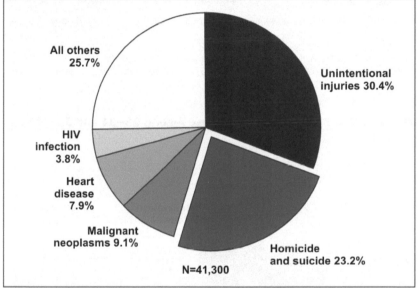

Data Source: Web-based Injury Statistics Query and Reporting System (WISQARS) [online database] Atlanta; National Center for Injury Prevention and Control. [cited 2006 Feb 15]. Available from: http://www.cdc.gov/ncipc/wisqars.

Multiple pie charts are occasionally used in place of a 100% component bar chart, that is, to display differences in proportional distributions. In some figures the size of each pie is proportional to the number of observations, but in others the pies are the same size despite representing different numbers of observations (Figure 4.28a and 4.28b).

Figure 4.28a Number of Deaths by Cause Among 25–34 and 35-44 Year Olds — United States, 2003

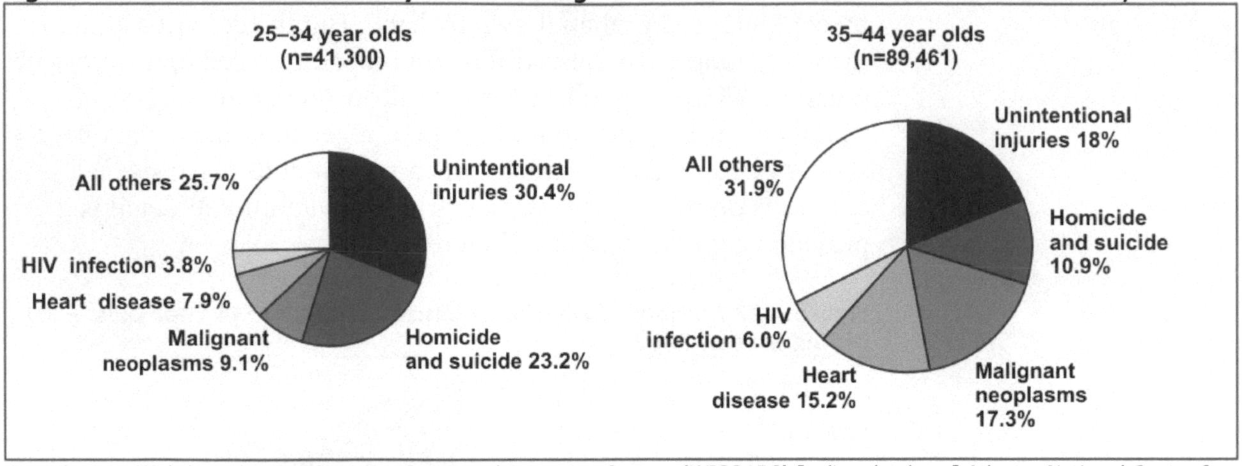

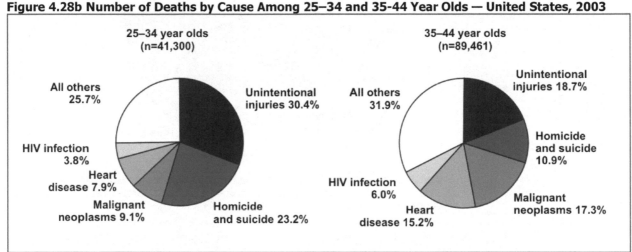

Data Source: Web-based Injury Statistics Query and Reporting System (WISQARS) [online database] Atlanta; National Center for Injury Prevention and Control. [cited 2006 Feb 15]. Available from: http://www.cdc.gov/ncipc/wisqars.

Figure 4.28b Number of Deaths by Cause Among 25–34 and 35-44 Year Olds — United States, 2003

Data Source: Web-based Injury Statistics Query and Reporting System (WISQARS) [online database] Atlanta; National Center for Injury Prevention and Control. [cited 2006 Feb 15]. Available from: http://www.cdc.gov/ncipc/wisqars.

Dot plots and box plots

A dot plot uses dots to show the relationship between a categorical variable on the x-axis and a continuous variable on the y-axis. A dot is positioned at the appropriate place for each observation. The dot plot displays not only the clustering and spread of observations for each category of the x-axis variable but also differences in the patterns between categories. In Figure 4.29 the villages using either antibacterial soap or plain soap have lower incidence rates of diarrhea than do the control (no soap) villages.[17]

Figure 4.29 Incidence of Childhood Diarrhea in Each Neighborhood by Hygiene Intervention Group — Pakistan, 2002–2003

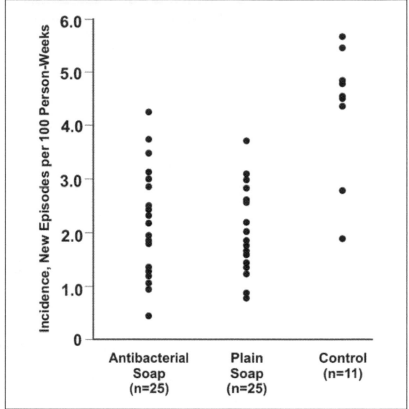

Source: Luby SP, Agboatwalla M, Painter J, Altaf A, Billhimer WL, Hoekstra RM. Effect of intensive handwashing promotion on childhood diarrhea in high-risk communities in Pakistan: a randomized controlled trial. JAMA 2004;291:2547–54.

A dot plot shows the relationship between a continuous and a categorical variable. The same data could also be displayed in a box plot, in which the data are summarized by using "box-and-whiskers." Figure 4.30 is an example of a box plot. The "box" represents values of the middle 50% (or interquartile range) of the data points, and the "whiskers" extend to the minimum and maximum values that the data assume. The median is usually marked with a horizontal line inside the box. As a result, you can use a box plot to show and compare the central location (median), dispersion (interquartile range and range), and skewness (indicated by a median line not centered in the box, such as for the cases in Figure 4.30).[18]

Figure 4.30 Risk Score for Alveolar Echinococcosis Among Cases and Controls — Germany, 1999–2000

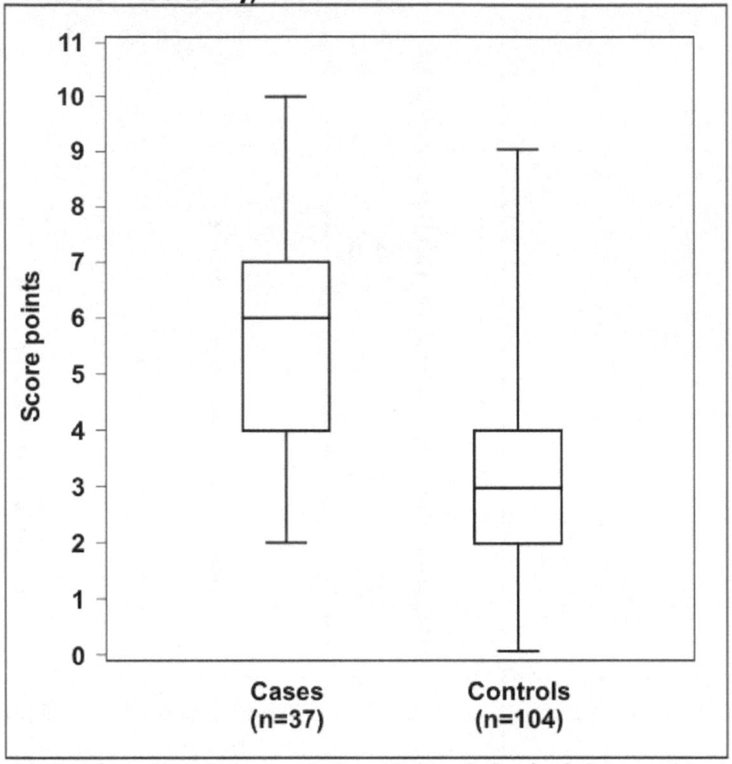

Adapted from: Kern P, Ammon A, Kron M, Sinn G, Sander S, Petersen LR, et al. Risk factors for alveolar echinococcosis in humans. Emerg Infect Dis 2004;10:2089-93.

Forest plots

A forest plot, also called a confidence interval plot, is used to display the point estimates and confidence intervals of individual studies assembled for a meta-analysis or systematic review.[19] In the forest plot, the variable on the x-axis is the primary outcome measure from each study (relative risk, treatment effects, etc.). If risk ratio, odds ratio, or another ratio measure is used, the x-axis uses a logarithmic-scale. This is because the logarithmic transformation of these risk estimates has a more symmetric distribution than do the risk estimates themselves (since the risk estimates can vary from zero to an arbitrarily large number). Each study is represented by a horizontal line — reflecting the confidence interval — and a dot or square — reflecting the point estimate — usually due to study size or some other aspect of study design (Figure 4.31). The shorter the horizontal line, the more precise the study's estimate. Point estimates (dots or squares) that line up reasonably well indicate that the studies show a relatively consistent effect. A vertical line indicates where no effect (relative risk = 1 or treatment effect = 0) falls on the x-axis. If a study's horizontal line does not cross the vertical line, that study's result is statistically significant. From a forest plot, one can easily ascertain patterns among studies as well as outliers.

Figure 4.31 Net Change in Glycohemoglobin (GHb) Following Self-management Education Intervention for Adults with Type 2 Diabetes, by Different Studies and Follow-up Intervals, 1980–1999

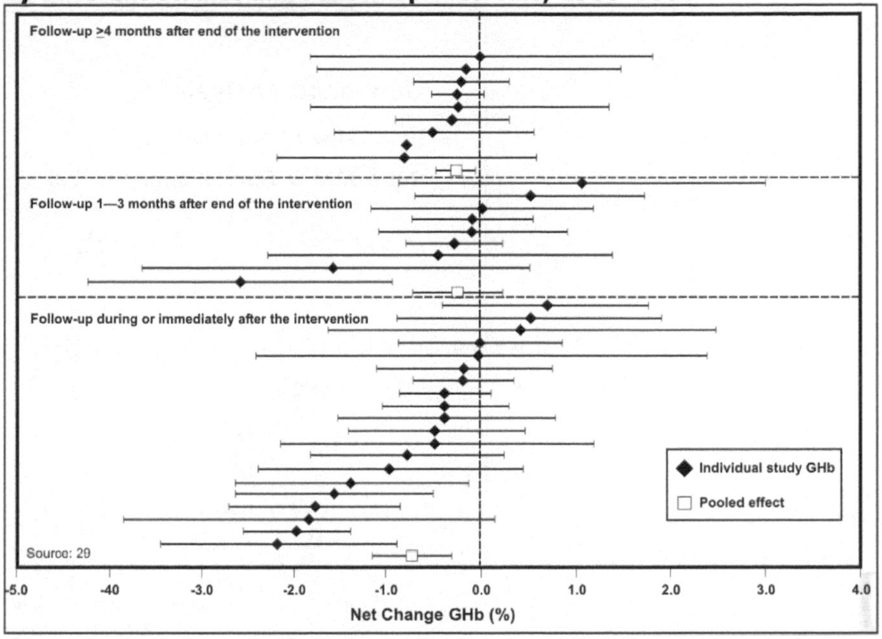

Source: Norris SL, Lau J, Smith SJ, Schmid CH, Engelgau MM. *Self-management education for adults with type 2 diabetes. Diabetes Care 2002;25:1159–71.*

Phylogenetic trees

A phylogenetic tree, a type of dendrogram, is a branching chart that indicates the evolutionary lineage or genetic relatedness of organisms involved in outbreaks of illness. Distance on the tree reflects genetic differences, so organisms that are close to one another on the tree are more related than organisms that are further apart. The phylogenetic tree in Figure 4.32 shows that the organisms isolated from patients with restaurant-associated hepatitis A in Georgia and North Carolina were identical and closely related to those from patients in Tennessee.[20] Furthermore, these organisms were similar to those typically seen in patients from Mexico. These microbiologic data supported epidemiologic data which implicated green onions from Mexico.

Figure 4.32 Comparison of Genetic Sequences of Hepatitis A Virus Isolates from Outbreaks in Georgia, North Carolina, and Tennessee in 2003 with Isolates from National Surveillance

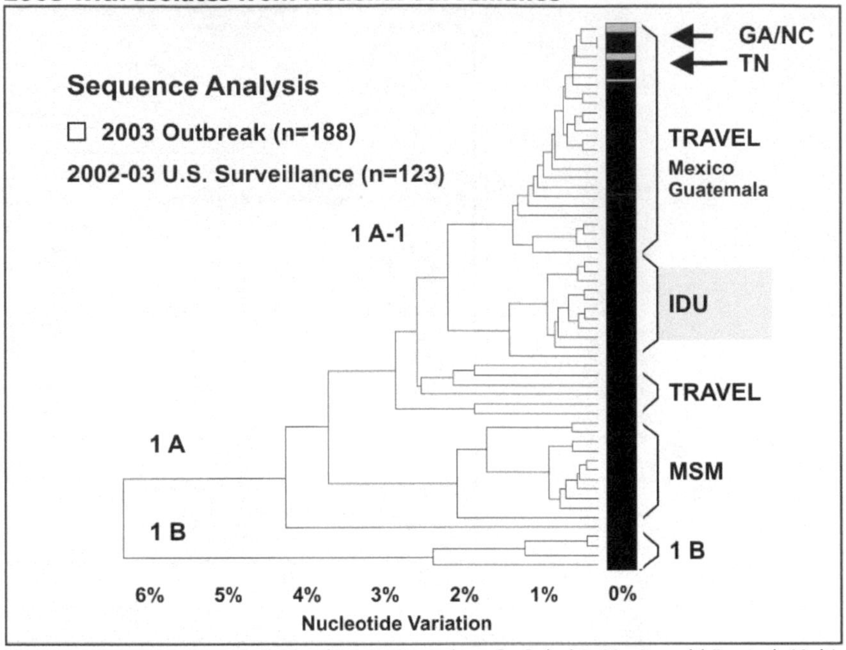

Source: Amon JJ, Devasia R, Guoliang X, Vaughan G, Gabel J, MacDonald P, et al. Multiple hepatitis A outbreaks associated with green onions among restaurant patrons–Tennessee, Georgia, and North Carolina, 2003. Presented at 53rd Annual Epidemic Intelligence Service Conference, April 19-23, 2004, Atlanta, Georgia.

Decision trees

A decision tree is a branching chart that represents the logical sequence or pathway of a clinical or public health decision.[21] **Decision analysis** is a systematic method for making decisions when outcomes are uncertain. The basic building blocks of a decision analysis are (1) decisions, (2) outcomes, and (3) probabilities.

A **decision** is a choice made by a person, group, or organization to select a course of action from among a set of mutually exclusive alternatives. The decision maker compares expected outcomes of available alternatives and chooses the best among them. This choice is represented by a **decision node**, a square, with branches representing the choices in the decision-tree diagram (for example, see Figure 4.33). For example, after receiving information that a person has a family history of a disease (colorectal cancer for this example), that person may decide (choose) to seek medical advice or choose not to do so.

Outcomes are the chance events that occur in response to a decision. Outcomes can be intermediate or final. Intermediate outcomes are followed by more decisions or chance events. For example, if a person decides to seek medical care for colorectal cancer screening, depending on the findings (outcomes) of the screening, his or her physician may advise diet or more frequent screenings; some combination of these two; or treatment. From the person's perspective, this is a chance outcome; from a health-care provider's perspective, it is a decision. Whether an outcome is intermediate or final may depend on the context of the decision problem. For example, colorectal cancer screening may be the final outcome in a decision analysis focusing on colorectal cancer as the health condition of interest, but it may be an intermediate outcome in a decision analysis focusing on more invasive cancer treatment. In a decision tree, outcomes follow a **chance node**, a circle, with branches representing different outcomes that occur by chance, one and only one of which occurs.

Each chance outcome has a probability by which it can occur written below the branch in a decision-tree diagram. The sum of probabilities for all outcomes that can occur at a chance node is one. The building blocks of decision analysis — decisions, outcomes, and probabilities — can be used to represent and examine complex decision problems.

Figure 4.33 Decision Tree Comparing Colorectal Screening Current Practice with a Targeted Family History Strategy

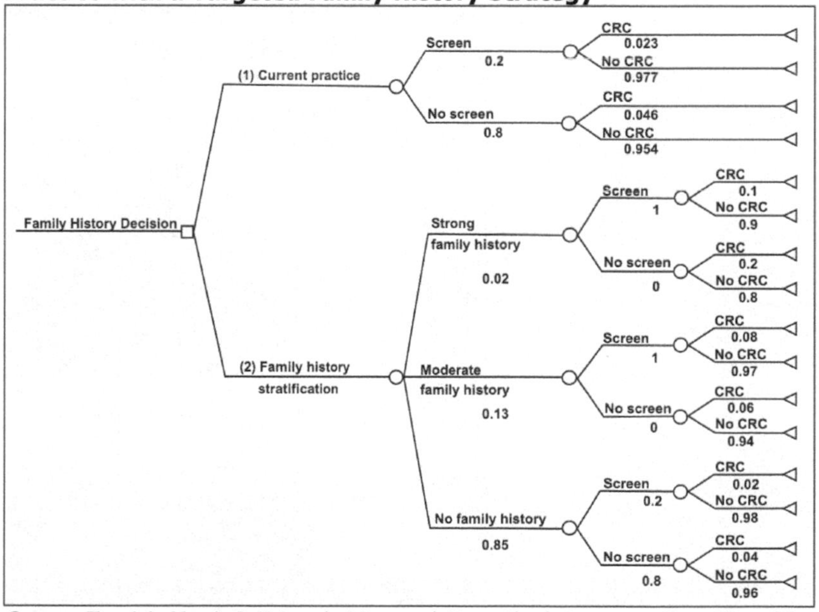

Source: Tyagi A, Morris J. Using decision analytic methods to assess the utility of family history tools. Am J Prev Med 2003;24:199–207.

Maps

Maps are used to show the geographic location of events or attributes. Two types of maps commonly used in field epidemiology are spot maps and area maps. Spot maps use dots or other symbols to show where each case-patient lived or was

EpiMap is an application of Epi Info for creating maps and overlaying survey data, and is available for download.

exposed. Figure 4.34 is a spot map of the residences of persons with West Nile Virus encephalitis during the outbreak in the New York City area in 1999. A spot map is useful for showing the geographic distribution of cases, but because it does not take the size of the population at risk into account a spot map does not show risk of disease. Even when a spot map shows a large number of dots in the same area, the risk of acquiring disease may not be particularly high if that area is densely populated.

More About Constructing Maps

- Excellent examples of the use of maps to display public health data are available in these selected publications:

- Atlas of United States Mortality, U. S. Department of Health and Human Services, Centers for Disease Control and Prevention, Hyattsville, MD, 1996 (DHHS Publication No. (PHS) 97-1015)

- Atlas of AIDS. Matthew Smallman-Raynor, Andrew Cliff, and Peter Haggett. Blackwell Publishers, Oxford, UK, 1992

- An Historical Geography of a Major Human Viral Disease: From Global Expansion to Local Retreat, 1840-1990. Andrew Cliff, Peter Haggett, Matthew Smallman-Raynor. Blackwell Publishers, Oxford, UK, 1988

Figure 4.34 Laboratory-confirmed Cases of West Nile Virus Disease — New York City, August–September 1999

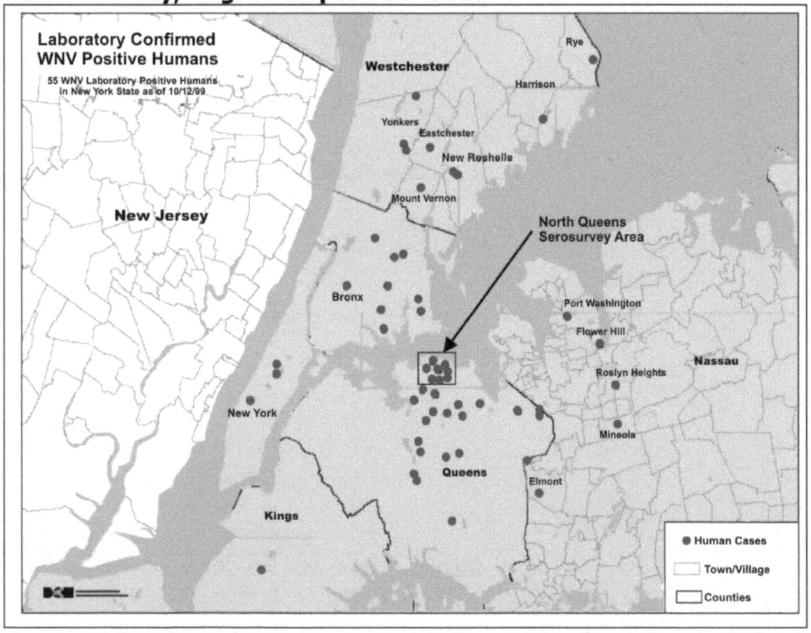

Source: Nash D, Mostashari F, Murray K, et al. Recognition of an outbreak of West Nile Virus disease. Presented at 49th Annual Epidemic Intelligence Service Conference, April 10–14, 2000, Atlanta, Georgia.

An area map, also called a chloropleth map, can be used to show rates of disease or other health conditions in different areas by using different shades or colors (Figure 4.35). When choosing shades or colors for each category, ensure that the intensity of shade or color reflects increasing disease burden. In Figure 4.35, as mortality rates increase, the shading becomes darker.

Figure 4.35 Mortality Rates (per 100,000) for Asbestosis by State — United States, 1982–2000

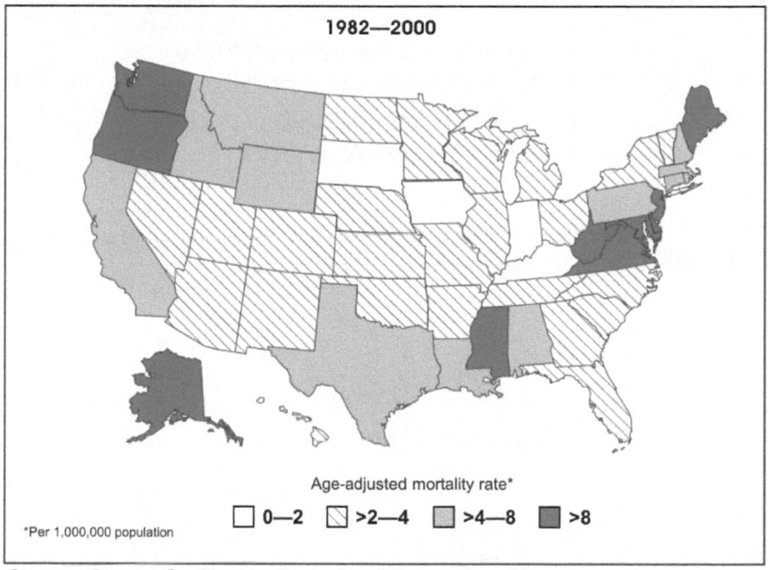

Source: Centers for Disease Control and Prevention. Changing patterns of pneumoconiosis mortality–United States, 1968-2000. MMWR 2004;53:627–31.

Exercise 4.7

Using the cancer mortality data in Table 4.13, construct an area map based on dividing the states into four quartiles as follows:

1. Oklahoma through Kentucky
2. Pennsylvania through Missouri
3. Connecticut through Florida
4. Utah through New York

A map of the United States is provided below for your use.

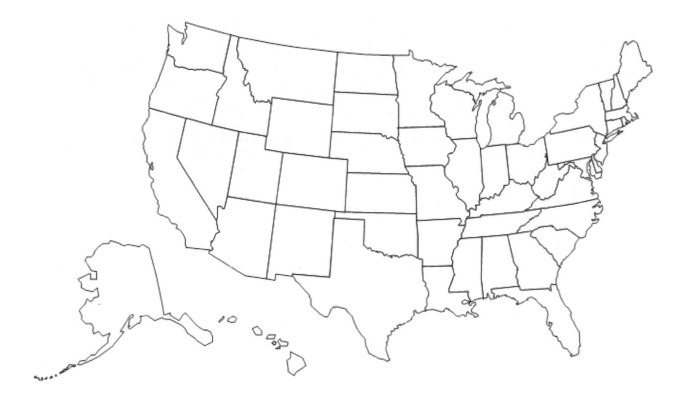

✓ **Check your answers on page 4-79**

More About Geographic Information Systems (GIS)

A geographic information system is a computer system for the input, editing, storage, retrieval, analysis, synthesis, and output of location-based information.22 In public health, GIS may use geographic distribution of cases or risk factors, health service availability or utilization, presence of insect vectors, environmental factors, and other location-based variables. GIS can be particularly effective when layers of information or different types of information about place are combined to identify or clarify geographic relationships. For example, in Figure 4.36, human cases of West Nile virus are shown as dots superimposed over areas of high crow mortality within the Chicago city limits.

Figure 4.36 High Crow-mortality Areas (HCMAs) and Reported Residences of A) West Nile Virus (WNV)-infected Case-patients, or B) WNV Meningoencephalitis Case-patients (WNV Fever Cases Excluded) — Chicago, Illinois, 2002

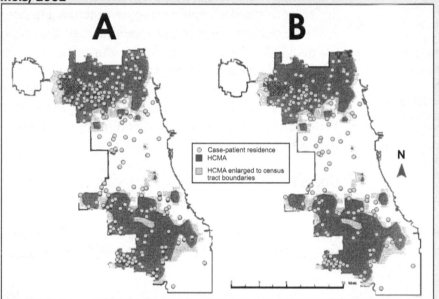

Source: Watson JT, Jones RC, Gibbs K, Paul W. Dead crow reports and location of human West Nile virus cases, Chicago, 2002. Emerg Infect Dis 2004;10:938–40.

Using Computer Technology

Many computer software packages are available to create tables and graphs. Most of these packages are quite useful, particularly in allowing the user to redraw a graph with only a few keystrokes. With these packages, you can now quickly and easily draw a number of graphs of different types and see for yourself which one best illustrates the point you wish to make when you present your data.[23-28]

On the other hand, these packages tend to have default values that differ from standard epidemiologic practice. Do not let the software package dictate the appearance of the graph. Remember the adage: let the computer do the work, but you still must do the thinking. Keep in mind the primary purpose of the graph — to communicate information to others. For example, many packages can draw bar charts and pie charts that appear three-dimensional. Will a three-dimensional chart communicate the information better than a two-dimensional one?

Compare and contrast the effectiveness of Figure 4.37a and 4.37b in communicating information.

Many software packages are available for producing all the tables and charts discussed in this chapter. One particularly helpful one is **R**,[29] used by universities and available for no charge around the world. In addition to graphical techniques, **R** provides a wide variety of statistical techniques (including linear and nonlinear modeling, classical statistical tests, time-series analysis, classification, and clustering).

Figure 4.37a Past Month Marijuana Use Among Youths Aged 12–17, by Geographic Region — United States, 2003 and 2004

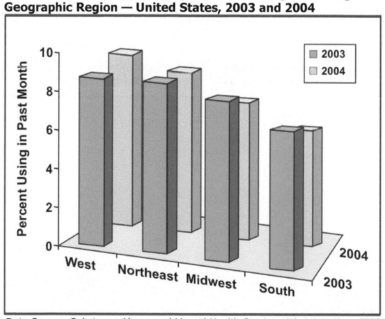

Data Source: Substance Abuse and Mental Health Services Administration. (2005). Results from the 2004 National Survey on Drug Use and Health: National Findings (Office of Applied Studies, NSDUH Series H-28, DHHS Publication No. SMA 05-4062). Rockville, MD.

Figure 4.37b Past Month Marijuana Use Among Youths Aged 12–17, by Geographic Region — United States, 2003 and 2004

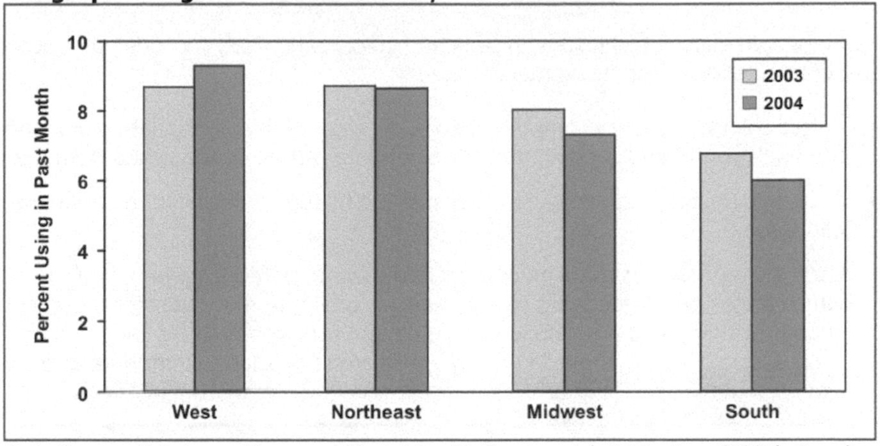

Data Source: Substance Abuse and Mental Health Services Administration. (2005). Results from the 2004 National Survey on Drug Use and Health: National Findings (Office of Applied Studies, NSDUH Series H-28, DHHS Publication No. SMA 05-4062). Rockville, MD.

"The problem with presenting information is simple – the world is high-dimensional, but our displays are not. To address this basic problem, answer 5 questions:
1. Quantitative thinking comes down to one question: Compared to what?
2. Try very hard to show cause and effect.
3. Don't break up evidence by accidents of means of production.
4. The world is multivariant, so the display should be high-dimensional.
5. The presentation stands and falls on the quality, relevance, and integrity of the content."[30]

  - ER Tufte

Most observers and analysts would agree that the three-dimensional graph does not communicate the information as effectively as the two-dimensional graph. For example, can you tell by a glance at the three-dimensional graph that marijuana use declined slightly in the Northeast in 2004? These differences are more distinct in the two-dimensional graph.

Similarly, does the three-dimensional pie chart in Figure 4.38a provide any more information than the two-dimensional chart in Figure 4.38b? The relative sizes of the components may be difficult to judge because of the tilting in the three-dimensional version. From Figure 4.38a, can you tell whether the wedge for heart disease is larger, smaller, or about the same as the wedge for malignant neoplasms? Now look at Figure 4.38b. The wedge for malignant neoplasms is larger.

Remember that communicating the names and relative sizes of the components (wedges) is the primary purpose of a pie chart. Keep the number of dimensions as small as possible to clearly convey the important points, and avoid using gimmicks that do not add information.

More About Using Color in Graphs

Many people misuse technology in selecting color, particularly for slides that accompany oral presentations.32 If you use colors, follow these recommendations.

- Select colors so that all components of the graph — title, axes, data plots, and legends — stand out clearly from the background and each plotted series of data can be distinguished from the others.

- Avoid contrasting red and green, because up to 10% of males in the audience may have some degree of color blindness.

- Use colors or shades to communicate information, particularly with area maps. For example, for an area map in which states are divided into four groups according to their rates for a particular disease, use a light color or shade for the states with the lowest rates and use progressively darker colors or shades for the groups with progressively higher rates. In this way, the colors or shades contribute directly to the impression you want the viewer to have about the data.

Figure 4.38a Leading Causes of Death in 25–34 Year Olds — United States, 2003

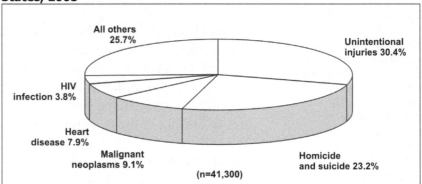

Data Source: Web-based Injury Statistics Query and Reporting System (WISQARS) [online database] Atlanta; National Center for Injury Prevention and Control. [cited 2006 Feb 15]. Available from: http://www.cdc.gov/ncipc/wisqars.

Figure 4.38b Leading Causes of Death in 25–34 Year Olds — United States, 2003

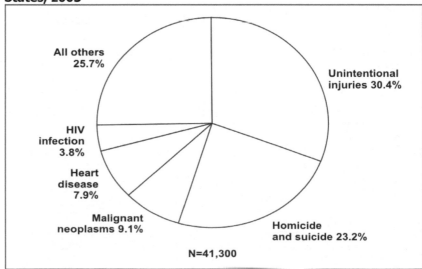

Data Source: Web-based Injury Statistics Query and Reporting System (WISQARS) [online database] Atlanta; National Center for Injury Prevention and Control. [cited 2006 Feb 15]. Available from: http://www.cdc.gov/ncipc/wisqars.

Summary

Much work has been done on other graphical methods of presentation.[33] One of the more creative is face plots.[34] Originally developed by Chernoff,[35] these give a way to display *n* variables on a two-dimensional surface. For instance, suppose you have several variables (x, y, z, etc.) that you have collected on each of *n* people, and for purposes of this illustration, suppose each variable can have one of 10 possible values. We can let *x* be eyebrow slant, *y* be eye size, *z* be nose length, etc. The figures below show faces produced using 10 characteristics — head eccentricity, eye size, eye spacing, eye eccentricity, pupil size, eyebrow slant, nose size, mouth shape, mouth size, and mouth opening) — each assigned one of 10 possible values.

Figure 4.39 Example of Face Plot Faces Produced Using 10 Characteristics

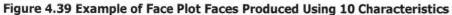
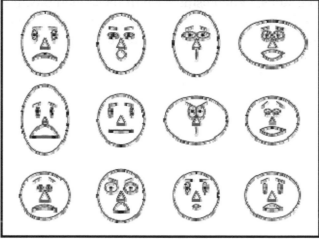

Source: Weisstein, Eric W. Chernoff Face. From MathWorld--A Wolfram Web Resource.
http://mathworld.wolfram.com/ChernoffFace.html.

To convey the messages of epidemiologic findings, you must first select the best illustration method. Tables are commonly used to display numbers, rates, proportions, and cumulative percents. Because tables are intended to communicate information, most tables should have no more than two variables and no more than eight categories (class intervals) for any variable. Printed tables should be properly titled, labeled, and referenced; that is, they should be able to stand alone if separated from the text.

Tables can be used with either nominal or continuous ordinal data. Nominal variables such as sex and state of residence have obvious categories. For continuous variables that do not have obvious categories, class intervals must be created. For some diseases, standard class intervals for age have been adopted. Otherwise a variety of methods are available for establishing reasonable class intervals. These include class intervals with an equal number of people or observations in each; class intervals with a constant width; and class intervals based on the mean and standard deviation.

Graphs can visually communicate data rapidly. Arithmetic-scale line graphs have traditionally been used to show trends in disease rates over time. Semilogarithmic-scale line graphs are preferred when the disease rates vary over two or more orders of magnitude. Histograms and frequency polygons are used to display frequency distributions. A special type of histogram known as an epidemic curve shows the number of cases by time of onset of illness or time of diagnosis during an epidemic period. The cases may be represented by squares that are stacked to form the columns of the histogram; the squares may be shaded to distinguish important characteristics of cases, such as fatal outcome.

Simple bar charts and pie charts are used to display the frequency distribution of a single variable. Grouped and stacked bar charts can display two or even three variables.

Spot maps pinpoint the location of each case or event. An area map uses shading or coloring to show different levels of disease numbers or rates in different areas.

The final pages of this lesson provide guidance in the selection of illustration methods and construction of tables and graphs. When using each of these methods, it is important to remember their purpose: to summarize and to communicate. Even the best method must be constructed properly or the message will be lost. Glitzy and colorful are not necessarily better; sometimes less is more!

Guide to Selecting a Graph or Chart to Illustrate Epidemiologic Data

Type of Graph or Chart	When to Use
Arithmetic scale line graph	Show trends in numbers or rates over time
Semilogarithmic scale line graph	Display rate of change over time; appropriate for values ranging over more than 2 orders of magnitude
Histogram	Show frequency distribution of continuous variable; for example, number of cases during epidemic (epidemic curve) or over longer period of time
Frequency polygon	Show frequency distribution of continuous variable, especially to show components
Cumulative frequency	Display cumulative frequency for continuous variables
Scatter diagram	Plot association between two variables
Simple bar chart	Compare size or frequency of different categories of a single variable
Grouped bar chart	Compare size or frequency of different categories of 2 4 series of data
Stacked bar chart	Compare totals and illustrate component parts of the total among different groups
Deviation bar chart	Illustrate differences, both positive and negative, from baseline
100% component bar chart	Compare how components contribute to the whole in different groups
Pie chart	Show components of a whole
Spot map	Show location of cases or events
Area map	Display events or rates geographically
Box plot	Visualize statistical characteristics (median, range, asymmetry) of a variable's distribution

Guide to Selecting a Method of Illustrating Epidemiologic Data

If data are:	And these conditions apply:		Then use:
Numbers or rates over time	Numbers	• 1 or 2 sets	Histogram
		• 2 or more sets	Frequency polygon
	Rates	• Range of values ≤ 2 orders of magnitude	Arithmetic-scale line graph
		• Range of values ≥ 2 orders of magnitude	Semilogarithmic-scale line graph
Continuous data other than time series	Frequency distribution		Histogram or frequency polygon
Data with discrete categories			Bar chart or pie chart
Place data Numbers	Not readily identifiable on map		Bar chart or pie chart
	Readily identifiable on map	• Specific site important	Spot map
		• Specific site unimportant	Area map
Rates			Area map

Checklist for Constructing Printed Tables

1. Title
- Does the table have a title?
- Does the title describe the objective of the data display and its content, including subject, person, place, and time?
- Is the title preceded by the designation "Table #"? ("Table" is used for typed text; "Figure" is used for graphs, maps, and illustrations. Separate numerical sequences are used for tables and figures in the same document (e.g., Table 4.1, Table 4.2; Figure 4.1, Figure 4.2).

2. Rows and Columns
- Is each row and column labeled clearly and concisely?
- Are the specific units of measurement shown? (e.g., years, mg/dl, rate per 100,000).
- Are the categories appropriate for the data?
- Are the row and column totals provided?

3. Footnotes
- Are all codes, abbreviations, or symbols explained?
- Are all exclusions noted?
- If the data are not original, is the source provided?
- If source is from website, is complete address specified; and is current, active, and reference date cited?

Checklist for Constructing Printed Graphs

1. Title
- Does the graph or chart have a title?
- Does the title describe the content, including subject, person, place, and time?
- Is the title preceded by the designation "Figure #"? ("Table" is used for typed text; "Figure" is used for graphs, charts, maps, and illustrations. Separate numerical sequences are used for tables and figures in the same document (e.g., Table 1, Table 2; Figure 1, Figure 2).

2. Axes
- Is each axis labeled clearly and concisely?
- Are the specific units of measurement included as part of the label? (e.g., years, mg/dl, rate per 100,000)
- Are the scale divisions on the axes clearly indicated?
- Are the scales for each axis appropriate for the data?
- Does the y axis start at zero?
- If a scale break is used with an arithmetic-scale line graph, is it clearly identified?
- Has a scale break been used with a histogram, frequency polygon, or bar chart? (Answer should be NO!)
- Are the axes drawn heavier than the other coordinate lines?
- If two or more graphs are to be compared directly, are the scales identical?

3. Grid Lines
- Does the figure include only as many grid lines as are necessary to guide the eye? (Often, these are unnecessary.)

4. Data plots
- Does the table have a title?
- Are the plots drawn clearly?
- Are the data lines drawn more heavily than the grid lines?
- If more than one series of data or components is shown, are they clearly distinguishable on the graph?
- Is each series or component labeled on the graph, or in a legend or key?
- If color or shading is used on an area map, does an increase in color or shading correspond to an increase in the variable being shown?
- Is the main point of the graph obvious, and is it the point you wish to make?

5. Footnotes
- Are all codes, abbreviations, or symbols explained?
- Are all exclusions noted?
- If the data are not original, is the source provided?

6. Visual Display
- Does the figure include any information that is not necessary?
- Is the figure positioned on the page for optimal readability?
- Do font sizes and colors improve readability?

Guide to Preparing Projected Slides

1. Legibility (make sure your audience can easily read your visuals)
- When projected, can your visuals be read from the farthest parts of the room?

2. Simplicity (keep the message simple)
- Have you used plain words?
- Is the information presented in the language of the audience?
- Have you used only key words?
- Have you omitted conjunctions, prepositions, etc.?
- Is each slide limited to only one major idea/concept/theme?
- Is the text on each slide limited to 2 or 3 colors (e.g., 1 color for title, another for text)?
- Are there no more than 6–8 lines of text and 6–8 words per line?

3. Color
- Colors have an impact on the effect of your visuals. Use warm/hot colors to emphasize, to highlight, to focus, or to reinforce key concepts. Use cool/cold colors for background or to separate items. The following table describes the effect of different colors.

	Hot	Warm	Cool	Cold
Colors:	Red	Light orange	Light blue	Dark blue
	Bright orange	Light yellow	Light green	Dark green
	Bright yellow	Light gold	Light purple	Dark purple
	Bright gold	Browns	Light gray	Dark gray
Effect:	Exciting	Mild	Subdued	Somber

- Are you using the best color combinations? The most important item should be in the text color that has the greatest contrast with its background. The most legible color combinations are:
  - Black on yellow
  - Black on white
  - Dark Green on white
  - Dark Blue on white
  - White on dark blue (yellow titles and white text on a dark blue background is a favorite choice among epidemiologists)
- Restrict use of red except as an accent.

4. Accuracy
- Slides are distracting when mistakes are spotted. Have someone who has not seen the slide before check for typos, inaccuracies, and errors in general.

Exercise Answers

Exercise 4.1

1.

Botulism Status by Age Group, Texas Church Supper Outbreak, 2001

Age Group (Years)	Botulism Status	
	Yes	No
≤9	2	2
10–19	1	1
20–29	2	2
30–39	0	2
40–49	4	4
50–59	3	4
60–69	1	5
70–79	2	3
≥80	0	0
Total	15	23

2.

Botulism Status by Exposure to Chicken,* Texas Church Supper Outbreak, 2001

Ate chicken?	Botulism?		Total
	Yes	No	
Yes	8	11	19
No	4	12	16
Total	12	23	35

* Excludes 3 botulism case-patients with unknown exposure to chicken

3.

Botulism Status by Exposure to Chili,* Texas Church Supper Outbreak, 2001

Ate chili?	Botulism?		Total
	Yes	No	
Yes	14	8	22
No	0	15	15
Total	14	23	37

* Excludes 1 botulism case-patient with unknown exposure to chili

4.

Number of Botulism Cases/Controls by Exposure to Chili and Leftover Chili

		Ate Leftover Chili		
		Yes	No	Total
Ate chili?	Yes	1 / 1	13 / 7	22
	No	0 / 1	0 / 14	15
	Total*	3	34	37*

* One case with unknown exposure to initial chili consumption

Exercise 4.2

Strategy 1: Divide the data into groups of similar size

1. Divide the list into three equal-sized groups of places:

    50 states ÷ 3 = 16.67 states per group. Because states can't be cut in thirds, two groups will contain 17 states and one group will contain 16 states.

    Illinois (#17) could go into either the first or second group, but its rate (80.0) is closer to #16 Maine's rate (80.2) than Texas' rate (79.3), so it makes sense to put Illinois in the first group. Similarly, #34 Vermont could go into either the second or third group.

    Arbitrarily putting Illinois into the first category and Vermont into the second results in the following groups:
    a. Kentucky through Illinois (States 1–17)
    b. Texas through Vermont (States 18–34)
    c. South Dakota through Utah (States 35–50)

2. Identify the rate for the first and last state in each group:
    a. Kentucky through Illinois   80.0–116.1
    b. Texas through Vermont   70.2–79.3
    c. South Dakota through Utah   39.7–68.1

3. Adjust the limits of each interval so no gap exists between the end of one class interval and beginning of the next. Deciding how to adjust the limits is somewhat arbitrary — you could split the difference, or use a convenient round number.

    a. Kentucky through Illinois   80.0–116.1
    b. Texas through Vermont   70.0–79.9
    c. South Dakota through Utah   39.7–69.9

Strategy 2: Base intervals on mean and standard deviation

1. Create three categories based on the mean (77.1) and standard deviation (16.1) by finding the upper limits of three intervals:
    a. Upper limit of interval 3 = maximum value = 116.1
    b. Upper limit of interval 2 = mean + 1 standard deviation = 77.1 + 16.1 = 93.2

c. Upper limit of interval 1 = mean − 1 standard deviation = 77.1 − 16.1 = 61.0

d. Lower limit of interval 1 = minimum value = 39.7

2. Select the lower limit for each upper limit to define three full intervals. Specify the states that fall into each interval. (Note: To place the states with the highest rates first, reverse the order of the intervals):

   a. North Carolina through Kentucky (8 states)   93.3–116.1
   b. Arizona through Georgia (35 states)   61.1–93.2
   c. Utah through Minnesota (7 states)   39.7–61.0

Strategy 3: Divide the range into equal class intervals

1. Divide the range from zero (or the minimum value) to the maximum by 3:
   (116.1 − 39.7) / 3 = 76.4 / 3 = 25.467

2. Use multiples of 25.467 to create three categories, starting with 39.7:
   39.7 through (39.7 + 1 x 25.467) = 39.7 through 65.2
   65.3 through (39.7 + 2 x 25.467) = 65.3 through 90.6
   90.7 through (39.7 + 3 x 25.467) = 90.7 through 116.1

3. Final categories:

   a. Indiana through Kentucky (11 states)   90.7–116.1
   b. Nebraska through Oklahoma (29 states)   65.3–90.6
   c. Utah through North Dakota (10 states)   39.7–65.2

4. Alternatively, since 90.6 is close to 90 and 65.2 is close to 65.0, the categories could be reconfigured with no change in state assignments. For example, the final categories could look like:

   Indiana through Kentucky (11 states)   90.1–116.1
   Nebraska through Oklahoma (29 states)   65.1–90.0
   Utah through North Dakota (10 states)   39.7–65.0

Exercise 4.3

1. Highest rate is 438.2 per 100,000 (in 1958), so maximum on y-axis should be 450 or 500 per 100,000.

Rate (per 100,000 Population) of Reported Measles Cases by Year of Report — United States, 1955–2002

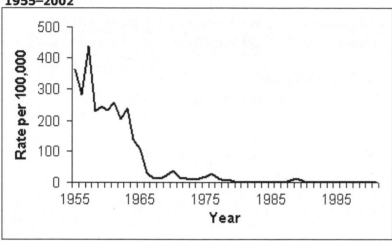

2. Highest rate between 1985 and 2002 was 11.2 per 100,000 in 1990), so maximum on y-axis should be 12 per 100,000.

Rate (per 100,000 Population) of Reported Measles Cases by Year of Report — United States, 1985–2002

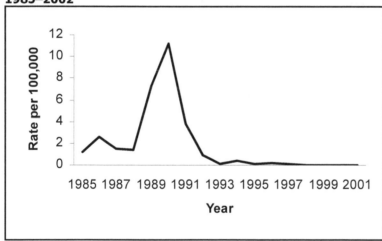

Exercise 4.4

Number of Cases of Botulism by Date of Onset of Symptoms, Texas Church Supper Outbreak, 2001

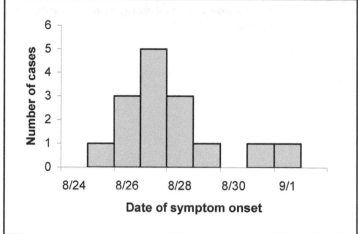

The first case occurs on August 25, rises to a peak two days later on August 27, then declines symmetrically to 1 case on August 29. A late case occurs on August 31 and September 1.

Exercise 4.5

Number of Cases of Botulism by Date of Onset of Symptoms, Texas Church Supper Outbreak, 2001

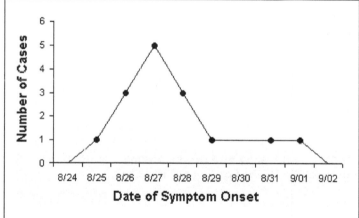

The area under the line in this frequency polygon is the same as the area in the answer to Exercise 4.4 The peak of the epidemic (8/27) is easier to identify.

Exercise 4.6

Number of Reported Cases of Primary and Secondary Syphilis, by Age Group, Among Non-Hispanic Black and White Men and Women — United States, 2002 (Stacked Bar Chart)

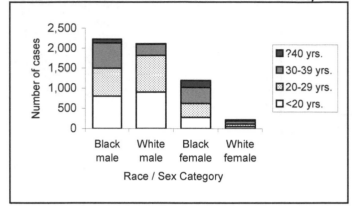

Number of Reported Cases of Primary and Secondary Syphilis, by Age Group, Among Non-Hispanic Black and White Men and Women — United States, 2002 (Grouped Bar Chart)

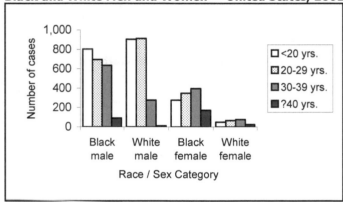

Percent of Reported Cases of Primary and Secondary Syphilis, by Age Group, Among Non-Hispanic Black and White Men and Women — United States, 2002 (100% Component Bar Chart)

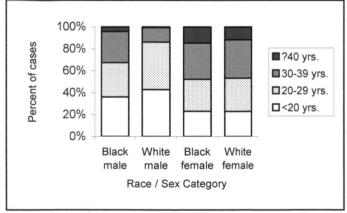

Source: Centers for Disease Control and Prevention. Sexually Transmitted Disease Surveillance 2002. Atlanta, Georgia. U.S. Department of Health and Human Services; 2003.

The stacked bar chart clearly displays the differences in total number of cases, as reflected by the overall height of each column. The number of cases in the lowest category (age <20 years) is also easy to compare across race-sex groups, because it rests on the x-axis. Other categories might be a little harder to compare because they do not have a consistent baseline. If the size of each category in a given column is different enough and the column is tall enough, the categories within a column can be compared.

The grouped bar chart clearly displays the size of each category within a given group. You can also discern different patterns across the groups. Comparing categories across groups takes work.

The 100% component bar chart is best for comparing the percent distribution of categories across groups. You must keep in mind that the distribution represents percentages, so while the 30-39 year category in white females appears larger than the 30-39 year category in the other race-sex groups, the actual numbers are much smaller.

Exercise 4.7

Age-adjusted Lung Cancer Death Rates per 100,000 Population, by State — United States, 2002

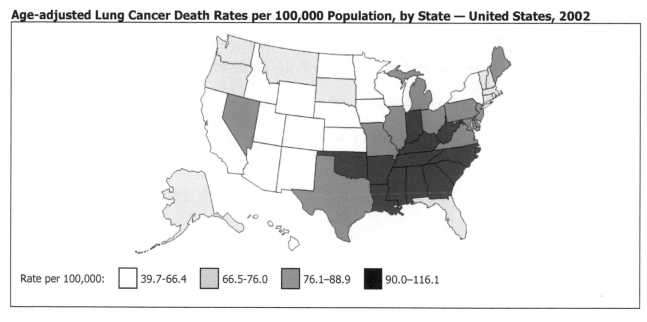

Rate per 100,000: ☐ 39.7-66.4   ◻ 66.5-76.0   ▨ 76.1–88.9   ■ 90.0–116.1

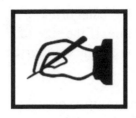

Self-Assessment Quiz

Now that you have read Lesson 4 and have completed the exercises, you should be ready to take the self-assessment quiz. This quiz is designed to help you assess how well you have learned the content of this lesson. You may refer to the lesson text whenever you are unsure of the answer.

Unless otherwise instructed, choose ALL correct choices for each question.

1. Tables and graphs are important tools for which tasks of an epidemiologist?
   A. Data collection
   B. Data summarization (descriptive epidemiology)
   C. Data analysis
   D. Data presentation

2. A table in a report or manuscript should include:
   A. Title
   B. Row and column labels
   C. Footnotes that explain abbreviations, symbols, exclusions
   D. Source of the data
   E. Explanation of the key findings

3. The following table is unacceptable because the percentages add up to 99.9% rather than 100.0%
   A. True
   B. False

Age group	No.	Percent
< 1 year	10	19.6%
1 – 4	9	17.6%
5 – 9	9	17.6%
10 – 14	17	33.3%
≥ 15	6	11.8%
Total	53	

4. In the following table, the total number of persons with the disease is:
   A. 3
   B. 22
   C. 25
   D. 34
   E. 50

	Cases	Controls	Total
Exposed	22	12	34
Unexposed	3	13	16
Total	25	25	50

5. A table shell is the:
   A. Box around the outside of a table
   B. Lines ("skeleton") of a table without the labels or title
   C. Table with data but without the title, labels or data
   D. Table with labels and title but without the data

6. The best time to create table shells is:
   A. Just before planning a study
   B. As part of planning the study
   C. Just after collecting the data
   D. Just before analyzing the data
   E. As part of analyzing the data

7. Recommended methods for creating categories for continuous variables include:
   A. Basing the categories on the mean and standard deviation
   B. Dividing the data into categories with similar numbers of observations in each
   C. Dividing the range into equal class intervals
   D. Using categories that have been used in national surveillance summary reports
   E. Using the same categories as your population data are grouped

8. In frequency distributions, observations with missing values should be excluded.
   A. True
   B. False

9. The following are reasonable categories for a disease that mostly affects people over age 65 years:
   A. True
   B. False

   Age Group
   < 65 years
   65 – 70
   70 – 75
   75 – 80
   80 – 85
   > 85

10. In general, before you create a graph to display data, you should put the data into a table.
    A. True
    B. False

11. On an arithmetic-scale line graph, the x-axis and y-axis each should:
    A. Begin at zero on each axis
    B. Have labels for the tick marks and each axis
    C. Use equal distances along the axis to represent equal quantities (although the quantities measured on each axis may differ)
    D. Use the same tick mark spacing on the two axes

12. Use the following choices for Questions 12a–d:
    A. Arithmetic-scale line graph
    B. Semilogarithmic-scale line graph
    C. Both
    D. Neither

    12a. _____ A wide range of values can be plotted and seen clearly, regardless of magnitude
    12b. _____ A constant rate of change would be represented by a curved line
    12c. _____ The y-axis tick labels could be 0.1, 1, 10, and 100
    12d. _____ Can plot numbers or rates

13. Use the following choices for Questions 13a–d:
    A. Histogram
    B. Bar chart
    C. Both
    D. Neither

    13a. _____ Used for categorical variables on the x-axis
    13b. _____ Columns can be subdivided with color or shading to show subgroups
    13c. _____ Displays continuous data
    13d. _____ Epidemic curve

14. Which of the following shapes of a population pyramid is most consistent with a young population?
    A. Tall, narrow rectangle
    B. Short, wide rectangle
    C. Triangle base down
    D. Triangle base up

15. A frequency polygon differs from a line graph because a frequency polygon:
    A. Displays a frequency distribution; a line graph plots data points
    B. Must be closed (plotted line much touch x-axis) at both ends
    C. Cannot be used to plot data over time
    D. Can show percentages on the y-axis; a line graph cannot

16. Use the following choices for Questions 16a–d:
    A. Cumulative frequency curve
    B. Survival curve
    C. Both
    D. Neither

    16a. _____ Y-axis shows percentages from 0% to 100%
    16b. _____ Plotted curve usually begins in the upper left corner
    16c. _____ Plotted curve usually begins in the lower left corner
    16d. _____ Horizontal line drawn from 50% tick mark to plotted curve intersects at median

17. A scatter diagram is the graph of choice for plotting:
    A. Anabolic steroid levels measured in both blood and urine among a group of athletes
    B. Mean cholesterol levels over time in a population
    C. Infant mortality rates by mean annual income among different countries
    D. Systolic blood pressure by eye color (brown, blue, green, other) measured in each person

18. Which of the following requires more than one variable?
    A. Frequency distribution
    B. One-variable table
    C. Pie chart
    D. Scatter diagram
    E. Simple bar chart

19. Compared with a scatter diagram, a dot plot:
    A. Is another name for the same type of graph
    B. Differ because a scatter diagram plots two continuous variables; a dot plot plots one continuous and one categorical variable
    C. Differ because a scatter diagram plots one continuous and one categorical variable; a dot plot plots two continuous variables
    D. Plots location of cases on a map

20. A spot map must reflect numbers; an area map must reflect rates.
    A. True
    B. False

21. To display different rates on an area map using different colors, select different colors that have the same intensity, so as not to bias the audience.
    A. True
    B. False

22. In an oral presentation, three-dimensional pie charts and three-dimensional columns in bar charts are desirable because they add visual interest to a slide.
    A. True
    B. False

23. A 100% component bar chart shows the same data as a stacked bar chart. The key difference is in the units on the x-axis.
    A. True
    B. False

24. When creating a bar chart, the decision to use vertical or horizontal bars is usually based on:
    A. The magnitude of the data being graphed and hence the scale of the axis
    B. Whether the data being graphed represent numbers or percentages
    C. Whether the creator is an epidemiologist (who almost always use vertical bars)
    D. Which looks better, such as whether the label fits below the bar

25. Use the following choices for Questions 25a-d (match all that apply):
    A. Grouped bar chart
    B. Histogram
    C. Line graph
    D. Pie chart

    25a. _____ Number of cases of dog bites over time
    25b. _____ Number of cases of dog bites by age group (adult or child) and sex of the victim
    25c. _____ Number of cases of dog bites by breed of the dog
    25d. _____ Number of cases of dog bites per 100,000 population over time

Answers to Self-Assessment Quiz

1. B, C, D. Tables and graphs are important tools for summarizing, analyzing, and presenting data. While data are occasionally collected using a table (for example, counting observations by putting tick marks into particular cells in table), this is not a common epidemiologic practice.

2. A, B, C, D. A table in a printed publication should be self-explanatory. If a table is taken out of its original context, it should still convey all the information necessary for the reader to understand the data. Therefore, a table should include, in addition to the data, a proper title, row and column labels, source of the data, and footnotes that explain abbreviations, symbols, and exclusions, if any. Tables generally present the data, while the accompanying text of the report may contain an explanation of key findings.

3. B (False). Rounding that results in totals of 99.9% or 100.1% is common in tables that show percentages. Nonetheless, the total percentage should be displayed as 100.0%, and a footnote explaining that the difference is due to rounding should be included.

4. C. In the two-by-two table presented in Question 4, the total number of cases is shown as the total of the left column (labeled "Cases"). That column total number is 25.

5. D. A table shell is the skeleton of a table, complete with titles and labels, but without the data. It is created when designing the analysis phase of an investigation. Table shells help guide what data to collect and how to analyze the data.

6. B. Creation of table shells should be part of the overall study plan or protocol. Creation of table shells requires the investigator to decide how to analyze the data, which dictates what questions should be asked on the questionnaire.

7. A, B, C, D, E. All of the methods listed are in Question 6 are appropriate and commonly used by epidemiologists

8. B (False). The number of observations with missing values is important when interpreting the data, particularly for making generalizations.

9. B (False). The limits of the class intervals must not overlap. For example, would a 70-year-old be counted in the 65-70 category or in the 70-75 category?

10. A (True). In general, before you create a graph, you should observe the data in a table. By reviewing the data in the table, you can anticipate the range of values that must be covered by the axes of a graph. You can also get a sense of the patterns in the data, so you can anticipate what the graph should look 1ike.

11. B, C. On an arithmetic-scale line graph, the axes and tick marks should be clearly labeled. For both the x- and y-axis, a particular distance anywhere along the axis should represent the same increase in quantity, although the x- and y-axis usually differ in what is measured. The y-axis, measuring frequency, should begin at zero. But the x-axis, which often measures time, need not start at zero.

12a. B. One of the key advantages of a semilogarithmic-scale line graph is that it can display a wide range of values clearly.

12b. A. A starting value of, say, 100,000 and a constant rate of change of, say, 10%, would result in observations of 100,000, 110,000, 121,000, 133,100, 146, 410, 161,051, etc. The resulting plotted line on an arithmetic-scale line graph would curve upwards. The resulting plotted line on a semilogarithmic-scale line graph would be a straight line.

12c. B. Values of 0.1, 1,10, and 100 represent orders of magnitude typical of the y-axis of a semilogarithmic-scale line graph.

12d. C. Both arithmetic-scale and semilogarithmic-scale line graphs can be used to plot numbers or rates.

13a. B. A bar chart is used to graph the frequency of events of a categorical variable such as sex, or geographic region.

13b. C. The columns of either a histogram or a bar chart can be shaded to distinguish subgroups. Note that a bar chart with shaded subgroups is called a stacked bar chart.

13c. A. A histogram is used to graph the frequency of events of a continuous variable such as time.

13d. A. An epidemic curve is a particular type of histogram in which the number of cases (on the y-axis) that occur during an outbreak or epidemic are graphed over time (on the x-axis).

14. C. A typical population pyramid usually displays the youngest age group at the bottom and the oldest age group at the top, with males on one side and females on the other side. A young population would therefore have a wide bar at the bottom with gradually narrowing bars above.

15. A, B. A frequency polygon differs from a line graph in that a frequency polygon represents a frequency distribution, with the area under the curve proportionate to the frequency. Because the total area must represent 100%, the ends of the frequency polygon must be closed. Although a line graph is commonly used to display frequencies over time, a frequency polygon can display the frequency distribution of a given period of time as well. Similarly, the y-axis of both types of graph can measure percentages.

16a. C. The y-axis of both cumulative frequency curves and survival curves typically display percentages from 0% at the bottom to 100% at the top. The main difference is that a cumulative frequency curve begins at 0% and increases, whereas a survival curve begins at 100% and decreases.

16b. B. Because a survival curve begins at 100%, the plotted curve begins at the top of the y-axis and at the beginning time interval (sometimes referred to as time-zero) of the x-axis, i.e., in the upper left corner.

16c. A. Because a cumulative frequency curve begins at 0%., the plotted curve begins at the base of the y-axis and at the beginning time interval (sometimes referred to as time-zero) of the x-axis, i.e., in the lower left corner.

16d. C. Because the y-axis represents proportions, a horizontal line drawn from the 50% tick mark to the plotted curve will indicate 50% survival or 50% cumulative frequency. The median is another name for the 50% mark of a distribution of data.

17. A, C. A scatter diagram graphs simultaneous data points of two continuous variables for individuals or communities. Drug levels, infant mortality, and mean annual income are all examples of continuous variables. Eye color, at least as presented in the question, is a categorical variable.

18. D. A frequency distribution, one-variable table, pie chart, and simple bar chart are all used to display the frequency of categories of a single variable. A scatter diagram requires two variables.

19. B. A scatter diagram graphs simultaneous data points of two continuous variables for individuals or communities; whereas a dot plot graphs data points of a continuous variable according to categories of a second, categorical variable.

20. B (False). The spots on a spot map usually reflect one or more cases, i.e., numbers. The shading on an area map may represent numbers, proportions, rates, or other measures.

21. B (False). Shading should be consistent with frequency. So rather than using different colors of the same intensity, increasing shades of the same color or family of colors should be used.

22. B (False). The primary purpose of any visual is to communicate information clearly. 3-D columns, bars, and pies may have pizzazz, but they rarely help communicate information, and sometimes they mislead.

23. A (False). The difference between a stacked bar chart and a 100% component bar chart is that the bars of a 100% component bar chart are all pulled to the top of the y-axis (100%). The units on the x-axis are the same.

24. D. Any bar chart can be oriented vertically or horizontally. The creator of the chart can choose, and often does so on the basis of consistency with other graphs in a series, opinion about which orientation looks better or fits better, and whether the labels fit adequately below vertical bars or need to placed beside horizontal bars.

25a. B, C. Both line graphs and histograms are commonly used to graph numbers of cases over time. Line graphs are commonly used to graph secular trends over longer time periods; histograms are often used to graph cases over a short period of observation, such as during an epidemic.

25b. A. A grouped bar chart (or a stacked bar chart) is ideal for graphing frequency over two categorical variables. A pie chart is used for a single variable.

25c. D. A pie chart (or a simple bar chart) is used for graphing the frequency of categories of a single categorical variable such as breed of dog.

25d. C. Rates over time are traditionally plotted by using a line graph.

References

1. Koschat MA. A case for simple tables. The American Statistician 2005;59:31–40.

2. Centers for Disease Control and Prevention. Sexually Transmitted Disease Surveillance, 2002. Atlanta, GA: U.S. Department of Health and Human Services, Centers for Disease Control and Prevention, September 2003.

3. Pierchala C. The choice of age groupings may affect the quality of tabular presentations. ASA Proceedings of the Joint Statistical Meetings; 2002; Alexandria, VA: American Statistical Association; 2002:2697–702.

4. Daley RW, Smith A, Paz-Argandona E, Mallilay J, McGeehin M. An outbreak of carbon monoxide poisoning after a major ice storm in Maine. J Emerg Med 2000;18:87–93.

5. Kalluri P, Crowe C, Reller M, Gaul L, Hayslett J, Barth S, Eliasberg S, Ferreira J, Holt K, Bengston S, Hendricks K, Sobel J. An outbreak of foodborne botulism associated with food sold at a salvage store in Texas. Clin Infect Dis 2003;37:1490–5.

6. Stevens JA, Powell KE, Smith SM, Wingo PA, Sattin RW. Physical activity, functional limitations, and the risk of fall-related fractures in community-dwelling elderly. Ann Epidemiol 1997;7:54–61.

7. Ahluwalia IB, Mack K, Murphy W, Mokdad AH, Bales VH. State-specific prevalence of selected chronic disease-related characteristics–Behavioral Risk Factor Surveillance System, 2001. In: Surveillance Summaries, August 22, 2003. MMWR 2003;52(No. SS-08):1–80.

8. Langlois JA, Kegler SR, Butler JA, Gotsch KE, Johnson RL, Reichard AA, et al. Traumatic brain injury-related hospital discharges: results from a 14-state surveillance system. In: Surveillance Summaries, June 27, 2003. MMWR 2003;52(No. SS-04):1–18.

9. Chang J, Elam-Evans LD, Berg CJ, Herndon J, Flowers L, Seed KA, Syverson CJ. Pregnancy-related mortality surveillance–United States, 1991-1999. In: Surveillance Summaries, February 22, 2003. MMWR 2003;52(No. SS-02):1–8.

10. Centers for Disease Control and Prevention. HIV/AIDS Surveillance Report, 2003 (Vol. 15). Atlanta, Georgia: US Department of Health and Human Services;2004:1–46.

11. Zhou W, Pool V, Iskander JK, English-Bullard R, Ball R, Wise RP, et al. Surveillance for safety after immunization: Vaccine Adverse Event Reporting System (VAERS)–1991-2001. In: Surveillance Summaries, January 24, 2003. MMWR 2003;52(No. SS-01):1–24.

12. Schmid CF, Schmid SE. Handbook of graphic presentation. New York: John Wiley & Sons, 1954.

13. Cleveland WS. The elements of graphing data. Summit, NJ: Hobart Press, 1994.

14. Brookmeyer R, Curriero FC. Survival curve estimation with partial non-random exposure information. Statistics in Medicine 2002;21:2671–83.

15. Korn EL, Graubard BI. Scatterplots with survey data. The American Statistician 1998;52,58–69.

16. Souvaine DL, Van Wyk CJ. How hard can it be to draw a pie chart? Mathematics Magazine 1990;63:165–72.

17. Luby SP, Agboatwalla M, Painter J, Altaf A, Billhimer WL, Hoekstra RM. Effect of intensive handwashing promotion on childhood diarrhea in high-risk communities in Pakistan: a randomized controlled trial. JAMA 2004; 291(21):2547–54.

18. Kafadar K. John Tkey and robustness. Statistical Science 2003:18:319–31.

19. Urbank S. Exploring statistical forests. ASA Proceedings of the Join Statistical Meetings; 2002; Alexandria, VA: American Statistical Association, 2002: 3535–40.

20. Amon J, Devasia R, Guoliang X, Vaughan G, Gabel J, MacDonald P, et al. Multiple hepatitis A outbreaks associated with green onions among restaurant patrons–Tennessee, Georgia, and North Carolina, 2003. Presented at 53rd Annual Epidemic Intelligence Service Conference, April 19-23, 2004, Atlanta, Georgia.

21. Haddix AC, Teutsch SM, Corso PS. Prevention effectiveness: a guide to decision analysis and economic evaluation. 2nd ed. New York, New York: Oxford University Press; October 2002.

22. Croner CM. Public health GIS and the internet. Annu Rev Public Health 2003;24:57–82.

23. Hilbe JM. Statistical computing software reviews. The American Statistician 2004;58:92.

24. Devlin SJ. Statistical graphs in customer survey research. ASA Proceedings of the Joint Statistical Meetings 2003:1212–16.

25. Taub GE. A review of {\it ActivStats for SPSS\/}: Integrating SPSS instruction and multimedia in an introductory statistics course. Journal of Educational and Behavioral Statistics 2003;28:291–3.

26. Hilbe J. Computing and software: editor's notes. Health Services & Outcomes Research Methodology 2000;1:75–9.

27. Oster RA. An examination of five statistical software packages for epidemiology. The American Statistician 1998;52:267–80.

28. Morgan WT. A review of eight statistics software packages for general use. The American Statistician 1998;52:70–82.

29. Anderson-Cook CM. Data analysis and graphics using R: an example-based approach. Journal of the American Statistical Association 2004;99:901–2.

30. Tufte ER. The visual display of quantitative information. Cheshire CT: Graphics Press, LLC; 2002.

31. Tufte ER. The visual display of quantitative information. Cheshire, CT: Graphics Press; 1983.

32. Olsen J. 2002. Using color in statistical graphs and maps. ASA Proceedings of the Joint Statistical Meetings; 2002; Alexandria, VA: American Statistical Association; 2002: 2524-9.

33. Wainer H, Velleman PF. Statistical Graphics: mapping the pathways of science. Annual Review of Psychology 2001;52:305–35.

34. Benedetto DD. Faces and the others: interactive expressions for observations. ASA Proceedings of the Joint Statistical Meetings; 2003; Alexandria, VA: American Statistical Association; 2003:520–7.

35. Weisstein EW. [Internet] MathWorld–A Wolfram Web Resource [updated 2006]. Chernoff Face. Available from: http://mathworld.wolfram.com/ChernoffFace.html.

Websites

For more information on:	Visit the following websites:
Age categorization used by CDC's National Center for Health Statistics	http://www.cdc.gov/nchs
Age groupings used by the United States Census Bureau	http://www.census.gov
CDC's Morbidity and Mortality Weekly Report	http://www.cdc.gov/mmwr
Epi Info and EpiMap	http://www.cdc.gov/epiinfo
GIS	http://wwww.atsdr.cdc.gov/GIS
R	http://www.r-project.org
Selecting color schemes for graphics	http://www.colorbrewer.org

Instructions for Epi Info 6 (DOS)

To create a frequency distribution from a data set in Analysis Module:
  EpiInfo6: >freq *variable.* Output provides columns for number, percentage, and cumulative percentage.

To create a two-variable table from a data set in Analysis Module:
  EpiInfo6: >Tables exposure_variable outcome_variable. Output shows table plus chi-square and p-value. For a two-by-two table, output also provides risk ratio, odds ratio, and confidence intervals.

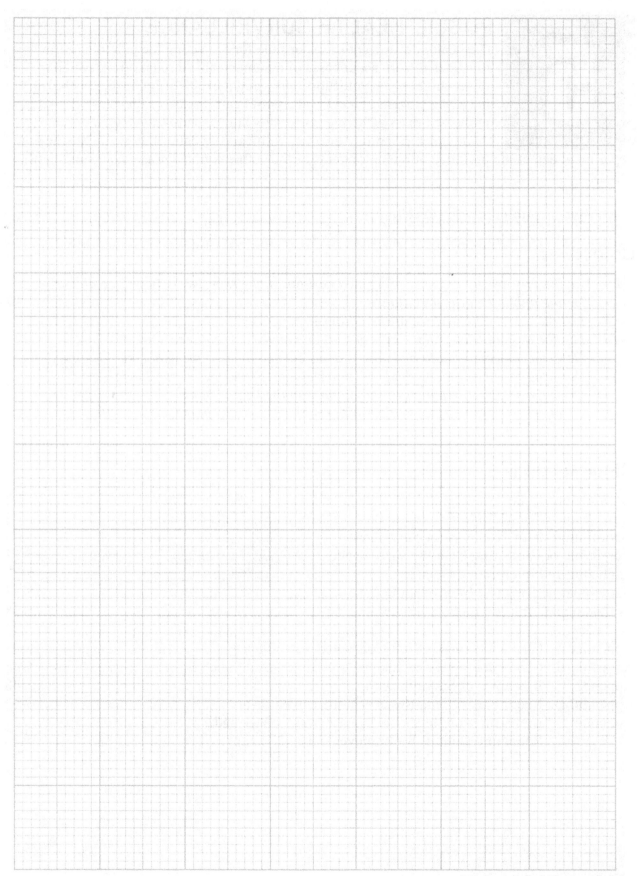

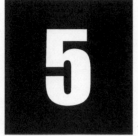

PUBLIC HEALTH SURVEILLANCE

The health department is responsible for protecting the public's health, but how does it learn about cases of communicable diseases from which the public might need protection? How might health officials track behaviors that place citizens at increased risk of heart disease or diabetes? If a highly publicized mass gathering potentially attracts terrorists (e.g., a championship sporting event or political convention), how might a health department detect the presence of biologic agents or the outbreak of a disease the agent might cause?

The answer is **public health surveillance**.

Objectives

After studying this lesson and answering the questions in the exercises, you will be able to:
- *Define public health surveillance*
- *List the essential activities of surveillance*
- *List the desirable characteristics of well-conducted surveillance activities*
- *Describe sources of data and data systems commonly used for public health surveillance*
- *Describe the principal methods of analyzing and presenting surveillance data*
- *Describe selected examples of surveillance in the United States*
- *Given a scenario and a specific health problem, design a plan for conducting surveillance of the problem*

Major Sections

Introduction

Surveillance — from the French **sur** (over) and **veiller** (to watch) — is the "close and continuous observation of one or more persons for the purpose of direction, supervision, or control."[1] In his classic 1963 paper, Alexander Langmuir applied **surveillance** for a disease to mean "the continued watchfulness over the distribution and trends of incidence [of a disease] through the systematic collection, consolidation, and evaluation of morbidity and mortality reports and other relevant data." He illustrated this application with four communicable diseases: malaria, poliomyelitis, influenza, and hepatitis.[2] Since then, surveillance has been extended to non-communicable diseases and injuries (and to their risk factors), and we now use the term **public health surveillance** to describe the general application of surveillance to public health problems.[3]

Evolution of Surveillance

The term **surveillance** was used initially in public health to describe the close monitoring of persons who, because of an exposure, were at risk for developing highly contagious and virulent infectious diseases that had been controlled or eradicated in a geographic area or among a certain population (e.g., cholera, plague, and yellow fever in the United States in the latter 1800s). These persons were monitored so that, if they exhibited evidence of disease, they could be quarantined to prevent spreading the disease to others.

In 1952, the U.S. Communicable Disease Center described its effort to redirect large-scale control programs for multiple infectious diseases, which had achieved their purpose, "toward the establishment of a continuing surveillance program. The objective of this redirected program is to maintain constant vigilance to detect the presence of serious infectious diseases anywhere in the country, and when necessary, to mobilize all available forces to control them."[4]

In 1968 at the 21st World Health Assembly, surveillance was defined as "the systematic collection and use of epidemiologic information for the planning, implementation, and assessment of disease control."[5] In the 1980s and 1990s, Thacker[3] and others[6-8] expanded the term to encompass not just disease, but any outcome, hazard, or exposure. In fact, the term **surveillance** is often applied to almost any effort to monitor, observe, or determine health status, diseases, or risk factors within a population. Care should be taken, however, in applying the term **surveillance** to virtually any program for or method of gathering information about a population's health, because this might lead to disagreement and confusion among public health policymakers and practitioners. Other terms (e.g., survey, health statistics, and health information system) might be more appropriate for describing specific information-gathering activities or programs.[9]

The essence of public health surveillance is the use of data to monitor health problems to facilitate their prevention or control. Data, and interpretations derived from the evaluation of surveillance data, can be useful in setting priorities, planning, and conducting disease control programs, and in assessing the effectiveness of control efforts. For example, identifying geographic areas or populations with higher rates of disease can be helpful in planning control programs and targeting interventions, and monitoring the temporal trend of the rate of disease after implementation of control efforts.

Those persons conducting surveillance should: (1) identify, define, and measure the health problem of interest; (2) collect and compile data about the problem (and if possible, factors that influence it); (3) analyze and interpret these data; (4) provide these data and their interpretation to those responsible for controlling the health problem; and (5) monitor and periodically evaluate the usefulness and quality of surveillance to improve it for future use. Note that surveillance of a problem does **not** include actions to control the problem.[2]

In this lesson, we describe these five essential activities of surveillance, enumerate the desirable characteristics of surveillance, and provide examples of surveillance for multiple health problems.

Purpose and Characteristics of Public Health Surveillance

Public health surveillance provides and interprets data to facilitate the prevention and control of disease. To achieve this purpose, surveillance for a disease or other health problem should have clear objectives. These objectives should include a clear description of how data that are collected, consolidated, and analyzed for surveillance will be used to prevent or control the disease. For example, the objective of surveillance for tuberculosis might be to identify persons with active disease to ensure that their disease is adequately treated. For such an objective, data collection should be sufficiently frequent, timely, and complete to allow effective treatment. Alternatively, the objective might be to determine whether control measures for tuberculosis are effective. To meet this objective, one might track the temporal trend of tuberculosis, and data might not need to be collected as quickly or as frequently. Surveillance for a health problem can have more than one objective.

After the objectives for surveillance have been determined, critical characteristics of surveillance are usually apparent, including:

- **Timeliness**, to implement effective control measures;
- **Representation**, to provide an accurate picture of the temporal trend of the disease;
- **Sensitivity**, to allow identification of individual persons with disease to facilitate treatment; quarantine, or other appropriate control measures; and
- **Specificity**, to exclude persons not having disease.

Other characteristics of well-conducted surveillance are described in Appendix A. The importance of each of these characteristics can vary according to the purpose of surveillance, the disease under surveillance, and the planned use of surveillance data (See Table 5.7 in Appendix A). To establish the objectives of surveillance for a particular disease in a specific setting and to select an appropriate method of conducting surveillance for that disease, asking and answering the following questions will be helpful.

- What is the **health-related event** under surveillance? What is its **case definition**?
- What is the **purpose** and what are the **objectives** of surveillance?
- What are the **planned uses** of the surveillance data?
- What is the **legal authority** for any data collection?
- Where is the **organizational home** of the surveillance?

- Is the system **integrated** with other surveillance and health information systems?
- What is the **population** under surveillance?
- What is the **frequency** of data collection (weekly, monthly, annually)?
- What **data** are collected and **how**? Would a **sentinel** approach or **sampling** be more effective?
- What are the **data sources**? What **approach** is used to obtain data?
- During what **period** should surveillance be conducted? Does it need to be continuous, or can it be intermittent or short-term?
- How are the data **processed** and **managed**? How are they routed, transferred, stored? Does the system comply with applicable standards for data formats and coding schemes? How is **confidentiality** maintained?
- How are the data **analyzed**? By whom? How often? How thoroughly?
- How is the information **disseminated**? How often are reports distributed? To whom? Does it get to all those who need to know, including the medical and public health communities and policymakers? [9,10]

Identifying Health Problems for Surveillance

Multiple health problems confront the populations of the world. Certain problems present an immediate threat to health, whereas others are persistent, long-term problems with relatively stable incidence and prevalence among the populations they affect. Examples of the former include influenza epidemics and hurricanes; the latter include atherosclerotic cardiovascular disease and colon cancer. Health problems also vary for different populations and settings, and an immediate threat among one population might be a chronic problem among another. For example, an outbreak of malaria in the United States in 2006 would be an immediate threat, but malaria in Africa is a chronic problem.

Selecting a Health Problem for Surveillance

Because conducting surveillance for a health problem consumes time and resources, taking care in selecting health problems for surveillance is critical. In certain countries, selection is based on criteria developed for prioritizing diseases, review of available morbidity and mortality data, knowledge of diseases and their geographic and temporal patterns, and impressions of public and political concerns, sometimes augmented with surveys of the general public or nonhealth-associated government officials. Criteria developed for selecting and prioritizing health problems for surveillance include the following: [9,10,11,12]

Public health importance of the problem:
- incidence, prevalence,
- severity, sequela, disabilities,
- mortality caused by the problem,
- socioeconomic impact,
- communicability,
- potential for an outbreak,
- public perception and concern, and
- international requirements.

Ability to prevent, control, or treat the health problem:
- preventability and
- control measures and treatment.

Capacity of health system to implement control measures for the health problem:
- speed of response,
- economics,
- availability of resources, and
- what surveillance of this event requires.

In the United States, the Centers for Disease Control and Prevention (CDC) and the Council of State and Territorial Epidemiologists (CSTE) periodically review communicable diseases and other health conditions to determine which ones should be reported to federal authorities by the states. Because of their greater likelihood of producing immediate, increased threats to public health, communicable diseases are the most common diseases under surveillance. Table 5.1 presents nationally notifiable infectious diseases for the United States for 2006. The Morbidity and Mortality Weekly Report (MMWR) presents a weekly and annual summary of nationally notifiable infectious diseases in the U.S. After priorities have been set, the extent to which a state or local health department can conduct surveillance for particular diseases is dependent on available resources.

Table 5.1 Nationally Notifiable Infectious Diseases — United States, 2006

Acquired immunodeficiency syndrome (AIDS)
Anthrax
Arboviral neuroinvasive and nonneuroinvasive diseases
- California serogroup virus disease
- Eastern equine encephalitis virus disease
- Powassan virus disease
- St. Louis encephalitis virus disease
- West Nile virus disease
- Western equine encephalitis virus disease
Botulism
- Botulism, foodborne
- Botulism, infant
- Botulism, other (wound and unspecified)
Brucellosis
Chancroid
Chlamydia trachomatis, genital infections
Cholera
Coccidioidomycosis
Cryptosporidiosis
Cyclosporiasis
Diphtheria
Ehrlichiosis
- Ehrlichiosis, human granulocytic
- Ehrlichiosis, human monocytic
- Ehrlichiosis, human, other or unspecified agent
Giardiasis
Gonorrhea
Haemophilus influenzae, invasive disease
Hansen disease (leprosy)

Hantavirus pulmonary syndrome
Hemolytic uremic syndrome, postdiarrheal
Hepatitis, viral, acute
- Hepatitis A, acute
- Hepatitis B, acute
- Hepatitis B virus, perinatal infection
- Hepatitis, C, acute
Hepatitis, viral, chronic
- Chronic Hepatitis B
- Hepatitis C Virus Infection (past or present)
HIV infection
- HIV infection, adult (aged ≥13 years)
- HIV infection, pediatric (aged <13 years)
Influenza-associated pediatric mortality
Legionellosis
Listeriosis
Lyme disease
Malaria
Measles
Meningococcal disease
Mumps
Pertussis
Plague
Poliomyelitis, paralytic
Psittacosis
Q Fever
Rabies
- Rabies, animal
- Rabies, human
Rocky Mountain spotted fever
Rubella
Rubella, congenital syndrome
Salmonellosis
Severe acute respiratory syndrome-associated coronavirus (SARS-CoV) disease

Shiga toxin-producing Escherichia coli (STEC)
Shigellosis
Smallpox
Streptococcal disease, invasive, Group A
Streptococcal toxic-shock syndrome
Streptococcus pneumoniae, drug resistant, invasive disease
Streptococcus pneumoniae, invasive in children aged <5 years
Syphilis
- Syphilis, primary
- Syphilis, secondary
- Syphilis, latent
- Syphilis, early latent
- Syphilis, late latent
- Syphilis, latent, unknown duration
- Neurosyphilis
- Syphilis, latent, nonneurological
Syphilis, congenital
- Syphilitic stillbirth
Tetanus
Toxic-shock syndrome (other than streptococcal)
Trichinellosis (trichinosis)
Tuberculosis
Tularemia
Typhoid fever
Vancomycin — intermediate Staphylococcus aureus (VISA)
Vancomycin-resistant Staphylococcus aureus (VRSA)
Varicella (morbidity)
Varicella (deaths only)
Yellow fever

Adapted from: National Notifiable Diseases Surveillance System [Internet]. Atlanta: CDC [updated 2006 Jan 13]. Nationally Notifiable Infectious Diseases United States 2006 . Available from: http://www.cdc.gov/epo/dphsi/phs/infdis2006.htm.

Exercise 5.1

A researcher at the state university's medical center is urging the state health department to add chlamydial infections to the state's list of diseases for which surveillance is required. On the basis of the information about chlamydial infections provided in Appendix B, draw conclusions on the table below and discuss the advantages and disadvantages of adding chlamydia infections to the state's list of notifiable diseases.

Public health importance of chlamydia	
Incidence	
Severity	
Mortality caused by chlamydia	
Socioeconomic impact	
Communicability	
Potential for an outbreak	
Public perception and concern	
International requirements	

Ability to prevent, control, or treat chlamydia	
Preventability	
Control measures and treatment	

Capacity of health system to implement control measures for chlamydia	
Speed of response	
Economics	
Availability of resources	
What surveillance of this event requires	

Advantages	Disadvantages

 Check your answers on page 5-57

Defining the health problem, identifying needed information, and establishing the scope for surveillance

After a decision has been made to undertake surveillance for a particular health problem, adopting — or, if necessary, developing — an operational definition of the health problem for surveillance is necessary for the health problem to be accurately and reliably recognized and counted. The operational definition consists of one or more criteria and is known as the **case definition for surveillance**. The case definition criteria might differ from the clinical criteria for diagnosing the disease and from the case definition of the disease used in outbreak investigations. For example, the case definition of listeriosis for surveillance is provided in the box below. (See Lesson 1 for further discussion of case definitions and for an example of a case definition of listeriosis for outbreak investigation). CDC and CSTE have developed case definitions for common communicable diseases,[13] certain chronic diseases, and selected injuries.

Case Definition of Listeriosis for Surveillance Purposes

Clinical description
Infection caused by *Listeria monocytogenes*, which can produce any of multiple clinical syndromes, including stillbirth, listeriosis of the newborn, meningitis, bacteremia, or localized infections.

Laboratory criteria for diagnosis
Isolation of *L. monocytogenes* from a normally sterile site (e.g., blood or cerebrospinal fluid or, less commonly, joint, pleural, or pericardial fluid).

Case classification
Confirmed: A clinically compatible case that is laboratory-confirmed.

Source: Centers for Disease Control and Prevention. Case definitions for infectious conditions under public health surveillance. MMWR 1997;46(No.RR-10):p. 43.

Situations might exist in which the criteria for identifying and counting occurrences of a disease consist of a constellation of signs and symptoms, chief complaints or presumptive diagnoses, or other characteristics of the disease, rather than specific clinical or laboratory diagnostic criteria. Surveillance using less specific criteria is sometimes referred as **syndromic surveillance**.

For example, a syndromic surveillance system was put in place in New York City after the World Trade Center (WTC) attacks in 2001. Here, the objectives were to detect illness related to either a bioterrorist event or an outbreak because of concern that the WTC attack could be followed by terrorists' use of biological or chemical agents in the city. One example of non-bioterrorist syndromic surveillance is surveillance for acute flaccid paralysis (syndrome) in order to capture possible cases of poliomyelitis. This is an example where the syndrome is monitored as a proxy for the disease, and the syndrome is infrequent and severe enough to warrant investigation of each identified case.

The goal of syndromic surveillance is to provide an earlier indication of an unusual increase in illnesses than traditional surveillance might, to facilitate early intervention (e.g., vaccination or chemoprophylaxis). For syndromic surveillance, a syndrome is a constellation of signs and symptoms. Signs and symptoms are grouped into syndrome categories (e.g., the category of "respiratory" includes cough, shortness of breath, difficulty breathing, and so forth).

The term, as used in the United States, often refers to observing emergency department visits for multiple syndromes (e.g., "respiratory disease with fever") as an early detection system for a biologic or chemical terrorism event. The advantage of syndromic surveillance is that persons can be identified when they seek medical attention, which is often 1–2 days before a diagnosis is made. In addition, syndromic surveillance does not rely on a clinician's ability to think of and test for a specific disease or on the availability of local laboratory or other diagnostic resources. Because syndromic surveillance focuses on syndromes instead of diagnoses and suspect diagnoses, it is less specific and more likely to identify multiple persons without the disease of interest. As a result, more data have to be handled, and the analyses tend to be more complex. Syndromic surveillance relies on computer methods to look for deviations above baseline (certain methods look for space-time clusters). Emergency department data are the most common data source for syndromic surveillance systems.

You might use syndromic surveillance when:
- Timeliness is key either for naturally occurring infectious diseases (e.g., severe acute respiratory syndrome [SARS]), or a terrorism event;
- Making a diagnosis is difficult or time-consuming (e.g., a new, emerging, or rare pathogen);
- Trying to detect outbreaks (e.g., when syndromic surveillance identified an increase in gastroenteritis after a widespread electrical blackout, probably from consuming spoiled food); or
- Defining the scope of an outbreak (e.g., investigators quickly having information on the age breakdown of patients or being able to determine geographic clustering).

Syndromic surveillance is a key adjunct reporting system that can detect terrorism events early. Syndromic surveillance is not intended to replace traditional surveillance, but rather to supplement it. However, evaluation of these approaches is needed because syndromic surveillance is largely untested (fortunately, no terrorism events have occurred that test the available models); its usefulness has not been proven, given the early stage of the science and the relative lack of specificity of the systems. Criticism and concern have arisen regarding the associated costs and the number of false alarms that will be fruitlessly pursued and whether syndromic surveillance will work to detect outbreaks (See below for a possible scenario).

Possible Scenario for Syndromic Surveillance

Consider the time sequence of an unsuspecting person exposed to an aerosolized agent (e.g., anthrax).

- Two days after exposure, the person experiences a prodrome of headache and fever and visits a local pharmacy to buy acetaminophen or another over-the-counter medicine.
- On day 3, he develops a cough and calls his health-care provider.
- On day 4, feeling worse, he visits his physician's office and receives a diagnosis of influenza.
- On day 5, he feels weaker, calls 9-1-1, and is taken by ambulance to his local hospital's emergency department, but is then sent home.
- By day 6, he is admitted to the hospital with a diagnosis of pneumonia.
- The following day, the radiologist identifies the characteristic feature of pulmonary anthrax on the chest radiograph and indicates a diagnosis. Laboratory tests are also positive. The infection-control practitioner, familiar with notifiable disease reporting, immediately calls the health department, which is on day 7 after exposure.

Thus, the health department learns about this case and perhaps others a full 7 days after exposure. However, if enough persons had been exposed on day 0, the health department might have detected an increase days earlier by using a syndromic surveillance system that tracks pharmacy over-the-counter medicine sales, nurses' hotlines, managed care office visits, school or work absenteeism, ambulance dispatches, emergency medical system or 9-1-1 calls, or emergency room visits.

After a case definition has been developed, the persons conducting surveillance should determine the specific information needed from surveillance to implement control measures. For example, the geographic distribution of a health problem at the county level might be sufficient to identify counties to be targeted for control measures, whereas the names and addresses of persons affected with sexually transmitted diseases are needed to identify contacts for follow-up investigation and treatment. How quickly this information must be available for effective control is also critical in planning surveillance. For example, knowing of new cases of hepatitis A within a week of diagnosis is helpful in preventing further spread, but knowing of new cases of colon cancer within a year might be sufficient for tracking its long-term trend and the effectiveness of prevention strategies and treatment regimens.

Another key component of establishing surveillance for a health problem is defining the scope of surveillance, including the geographic area and population to be covered by surveillance. Establishing a period during which surveillance initially will be conducted is also useful. At the end of this period, the results of surveillance can be reviewed to determine whether surveillance should be continued. This approach might prevent the continuation of surveillance when it is no longer needed.

Identifying or Collecting Data for Surveillance

After the problem for surveillance has been identified and defined and the needs and scope determined, available reports and other relevant data should be located that can be used to conduct surveillance. These reports and data are gathered for different purposes from multiple sources by using selected methods. Data might be collected initially to serve health-related purposes, whereas data might later serve administrative, legal, political, or economic purposes. Examples of the former include collecting data from death certificates regarding the cause and circumstances of death and collecting data from national health surveys regarding health-related behaviors; examples of the latter include collecting data on cigarette and alcohol sales and administrative data generated from the reimbursement of health-care providers.

Before describing available local and national data resources for surveillance, understanding the principal sources and methods of obtaining data about health problems is helpful. As you recall from Lesson 1, the majority of diseases have a characteristic natural history. An understanding of the natural history of a disease is critical to conducting surveillance for that disease because someone — either the patient or a health-care provider — must recognize, or diagnose, the disease and create a record of its existence for it to be identified and counted for surveillance. For diseases that cause severe illness or death (e.g., lung cancer or rabies), the likelihood that the disease will be diagnosed and recorded by a health-care provider is high. For diseases that produce limited or no symptoms in the majority of those affected, the likelihood that the disease will be recognized is low. Certain diseases fall between these extremes. The characteristics and natural history of a disease determine how best to conduct surveillance for that disease.

Sources and Methods for Gathering Data

Examples of documentation of financial, legal, and administrative activities that might be used for surveillance
- Receipts for cigarette and other tobacco product sales.
- Automated reports of pharmaceutical sales.
- Electronic records of billing and payment for health-care services.
- Laws and regulations related to drug use.

Data collected for health-related purposes typically come from three sources, individual persons, the environment, and health-care providers and facilities. Moreover, data collected for nonhealth–related purposes (e.g., taxes, sales, or administrative data) might also be used for surveillance of health-related problems. Because a researcher might wish to calculate rates of disease, information about the size of the population under surveillance and its geographic distribution are also helpful. Table 5.2 summarizes health and nonhealth-related sources of data, and the box to the left provides examples of nonhealth-related data that can be used for surveillance of specific health problems.

Table 5.2 Typical Sources of Data

Individual persons

Health-care providers, facilities, and records
- Physician offices
- Hospitals
- Outpatient departments
- Emergency departments
- Inpatient settings
- Laboratories

Environmental conditions
- Air
- Water
- Animal vectors

Administrative actions

Financial transactions
- Sales of goods and services
- Taxation

Legal actions

Laws and regulations

A limited number of methods are used to collect the majority of health-related data, including environmental monitoring, surveys, notifications, and registries. These methods can be further characterized by the approach used to obtain information from the sources described previously. For example, the method of collecting information might be an annual population survey that uses an in-person interview and a standardized questionnaire for obtaining data from women aged 18–45 years; or the method might be a notification that requires completion and submission of a form by health-care providers about occurrences of specific diseases that they see in their practices.

Depending on the situation, these methods might be used to obtain information about a sample of a population or events or about all members of the population or all occurrences of a specific event (e.g., birth or death). Information might be collected continuously, periodically, or for a defined period, depending on the need. Careful consideration of the objectives of surveillance for a particular disease and a thorough understanding of the advantages and disadvantages of different sources and methods for gathering data are critical in deciding what data are needed for surveillance and the most appropriate sources and methods for obtaining it.[9,14] We now discuss each of these four methods.

Environmental Monitoring

Monitoring the environment is critical for ensuring that it is healthy and safe (see Examples of Environmental Monitoring). Multiple qualitative and quantitative approaches are used to monitor the environment, depending on the problem, setting, and planned use of the monitoring data.

Survey

A survey is an investigation that uses a "structured and systematic gathering of information" from a sample of "a population of interest to describe the population in quantitative terms."[15] The majority of surveys gather information from a representative sample of a population so that the results of the survey can be generalized to the entire population. Surveys are probably the most common method used for gathering information about populations. The subjects of a survey can be members of the general public, patients, health-care providers, or organizations. Although their topics might vary widely, surveys are typically designed to obtain specific information about a population and can be conducted once or on a periodic basis.

Notification

A notification is the reporting of certain diseases or other health-related conditions by a specific group, as specified by law, regulation, or agreement. Notifications are typically made to the state or local health agency. Notifications are often used for surveillance, and they aid in the timely control of specific health problems or hazardous conditions. When reporting is required by law, the diseases or conditions to be reported are known as **notifiable** diseases or conditions.

Individual notifiable disease case reports are considered confidential and are not available for public inspection. In most states, a case report from a physician or hospital is sent to the local health department, which has primary responsibility for taking appropriate action. The local health department then forwards a copy of the case report to the state health department. In states that have no local health departments or in which the state heath department has primary responsibility for collecting and investigating case reports, initial case reports go directly to the state health department. In some states all laboratory reports are sent to the state health department, which informs the local health department responsible for following up with the physician.

This form of data collection, in which health-care providers send reports to a health department on the basis of a known set of rules and regulations, is called **passive surveillance** (provider-initiated). Less commonly, health department staff may contact healthcare providers to solicit reports. This **active surveillance** (health department- initiated) is usually limited to specific diseases over a limited period of time, such as after a community exposure or during an outbreak.

Table 5.3 shows the types of notification and examples.

Table 5.3 Types of Notification and Examples

1. Disease or hazard-specific notifications
   a. Communicable diseases
      i. World Health Organization: International health regulations require reporting of cholera, plague, and yellow fever
      ii. National: United States and Canada specify diseases that require notification by all states and provinces, respectively
      iii. Provincial, state, or subnational: for example, coccidioidomycosis in California
   b. Chemical and physical hazards in the environment
      i. Childhood lead poisoning
      ii. Occupational hazards
      iii. Firearm-related injury
      iv. Consumer product-related injury
2. Notifications related to treatment administration
   a. Adverse effect of drugs or medical products
   b. Adverse effect from vaccines
3. Notifications related to persons at risk
   a. Elevated blood lead among adults
   b. Elevated blood lead among children

Adapted from: Koo D, Wingo P, Rothwell C. Health Statistics from Notifications, Registration Systems, and Registries. In: Friedman D, Parrish RG, Hunter E (editors). Health Statistics: Shaping Policy and Practice to Improve the Population's Health. New York: Oxford University Press; 2005, p. 82.

Use of sentinel sites has become the preferred approach for human immunodeficiency virus/acquired immunodeficiency syndrome (HIV/AIDS) surveillance for certain countries where national population-based surveillance for HIV infection is not feasible. This approach is based on periodic serologic surveys conducted at selected sites with well-defined population subgroups (e.g., prenatal clinics). Under this strategy, health officials define the population subgroups and the regions to study and then identify health-care facilities serving those populations that are capable and willing to participate. These facilities then conduct serologic surveys at least annually to provide statistically valid estimates of HIV prevalence.

Because underreporting is common for certain diseases, an alternative to traditional reporting is **sentinel** reporting, which relies on a prearranged sample of health-care providers who agree to report all cases of certain conditions. These sentinel providers are clinics, hospitals, or physicians who are likely to observe cases of the condition of interest. The network of physicians reporting influenza-like illness, as described in one of the examples in Appendix C, is an example of surveillance that uses sentinel providers. Although the sample used in sentinel surveillance might not be representative of the entire population, reporting is probably consistent over time because the sample is stable and the participants are committed to providing high-quality data.

Registries

Maintaining registries is a method for documenting or tracking events or persons over time (Table 5.4). Certain registries are required by law (e.g., registries of vital events). Although similar to notifications, registries are more specific because they are intended to be a permanent record of persons or events. For example, birth and death certificates are permanent legal records that also contain important health-related information. A disease registry (e.g., a cancer registry) tracks a person with disease over time and usually includes diagnostic, treatment, and outcome information. Although the majority of disease registries require health facilities to report information on patients with disease, an active component might exist in which the registry periodically updates patient information through review of health, vital, or other records.

Reanalysis or Secondary Use of Data

Surveillance for a health problem can use data originally collected for other purposes — a practice known as the reanalysis or secondary use of data. This approach is efficient but can suffer from a lack of timeliness, or it can lack sufficient detail to address the problem under surveillance. Because the primary collection of data for surveillance is time-consuming and resource-intensive if done well, it should be undertaken only if the health problem is of high priority and no other adequate source of data exists.

Table 5.4 Types of Registries and Examples of Selected Types

1. Vital event registration
   a. Birth registration
   b. Marriage and divorce registration
   c. Death registration
2. Registries used in preventive medicine
   a. Immunization registries
   b. Registries of persons at risk for selected conditions
   c. Registries of persons positive for genetic conditions
3. Disease-specific registries
   a. Blind registries
   b. Birth defects registries
   c. Cancer registries
   d. Psychiatric case registries
   e. Ischemic heart disease registries
4. Treatment registries
   a. Radiotherapy registries
   b. Follow-up registries for detection of iatrogenic thyroid disease
5. After-treatment registries
   a. Handicapped children
   b. Disabled persons
6. Registries of persons at risk or exposed
   a. Children at high risk for developing a health problem
   b. Occupational hazards registries
   c. Medical hazards registries
   d. Older persons or chronically ill registries
   e. Atomic bomb survivors (Japan)
   f. World Trade Center survivors (New York City)
7. Skills and resources registries
8. Prospective research studies
9. Specific information registries

Adapted from: Koo D, Wingo P, Rothwell C. Health Statistics from Notifications, Registration Systems, and Registries. In: Friedman D, Parrish RG, Hunter E (editors). Health Statistics: Shaping Policy and Practice to Improve the Population's Health. New York: Oxford University Press; 2005, p. 91.
Weddell JM. Registers and registries: a review. Int J Epid 1973;2:221–8.

Exercise 5.2

State funding for a childhood asthma program has just become available. To initiate surveillance for childhood asthma, the staff is reviewing different sources of data on asthma. Discuss the advantages and disadvantages of the following sources of data and methods for conducting surveillance for asthma. (Figure 5.12 in Appendix C indicates national data for these different sources.)

- Self-reported asthma prevalence and asthmatic attacks obtained by a telephone survey of the general population.
- Asthma-associated outpatient visits obtained from periodic surveys of local health-care providers, including emergency departments and hospital outpatient clinics.

 Check your answers on page 5-58

Major health data systems

Data regarding the characteristics of diseases and injuries are critical for guiding efforts for preventing and controlling those diseases. Multiple systems exist in the United States to gather such data, as well as other health-related data, at national, state, and local levels. These systems provide the "morbidity and mortality reports and other relevant data" for surveillance, as described by Langmuir, and examples of such systems are listed in Appendix E. Remember, however, that surveillance is an activity — the continued watchfulness over a disease by using data collected about it — and not the data about a disease or the different data systems used to collect or manage such data.

Surveillance for communicable diseases principally relies upon reports of notifiable diseases from health-care providers and laboratories and the registration of deaths. Because the most common use of surveillance for communicable diseases at the local level is to prevent or control cases of disease, local surveillance relies on finding individual cases of disease through notifications or, where more complete reporting is required, actively contacting health-care facilities or providers on a regular basis.[10] At the state and national level, the principal notification system in the United States is the National Notifiable Disease Surveillance System (NNDSS). State and local vital registration provides data for monitoring deaths from certain infectious diseases (e.g., influenza and AIDS).

More About the National Notifiable Disease Surveillance System

A notifiable disease is one for which regular, frequent, and timely information regarding individual cases is considered necessary for preventing and controlling the disease.

The list of nationally notifiable diseases is revised periodically. For example, a disease might be added to the list as a new pathogen emerges, and diseases are deleted as incidence declines. Public health officials at state health departments and CDC collaborate in determining which diseases should be nationally notifiable. The Council of State and Territorial Epidemiologists, with input from CDC, makes recommendations annually for additions and deletions. However, reporting of nationally notifiable diseases to CDC by the states is voluntary. Reporting is mandated (i.e., by legislation or regulation) only at the state and local levels. Thus, the list of diseases considered notifiable varies slightly by state. All states typically report diseases for which the patients must be quarantined (i.e., cholera, plague, and yellow fever) in compliance with the World Health Organization's International Health Regulations.

Data in the National Notifiable Disease Surveillance System (NNDSS) are derived primarily from reports transmitted to CDC by the 50 states, two cities, and five territorial health departments.

Source: National Notifiable Diseases Surveillance System [Internet]. Atlanta: CDC [updated 2006 Jan 13]. Available from: http://www.cdc.gov/epo/dphsi/nndsshis.htm

Surveillance for chronic diseases usually relies upon health-care–related data (e.g., hospital discharges, surveys of the public, and mortality data from the vital statistics system). Given the slow rate of change in the incidence and prevalence of these diseases, data for surveillance of chronic conditions need not be as timely as those for acute infectious diseases.

Surveillance for behaviors that influence health and for other markers for health (e.g., smoking, blood pressure, and serum cholesterol) is accomplished by population surveys, which might be supplemented with health-care related data. The Behavioral Risk Factor Surveillance System (BRFSS), the Youth Risk Behavior Surveillance System (YRBSS), the National Health Interview Survey (NHIS), and the National Household Survey on Drug Abuse are all surveys that gather data regarding behaviors that influence health. The National Health and Nutrition Examination Survey (NHANES), probably the most comprehensive survey in the United States of health and the factors that influence it, gathers extensive data on physiologic and biochemical measures of the population and on the presence of chemicals among the population resulting from environmental exposures (e.g., lead, pesticides, and cotinine from secondhand smoke). Data from NHANES have been used for approximately 40 years to monitor the lead burden among the general public, demonstrating its marked elevation and then substantial decline after the mandated removal of lead from gasoline and paint.

Exercise 5.3

Assume you work in a state in which none of the following conditions is on the state list of notifiable diseases. For each condition, list at least one existing source of data that you need for conducting surveillance on the condition. What factors make the selected source or data system more appropriate than another?

Listeriosis: A serious infection can result from eating food contaminated with the bacterium *Listeria monocytogenes*. The disease affects primarily pregnant women, newborns, and adults with weakened immune systems. A person with listeriosis has fever, muscle aches, and sometimes gastrointestinal symptoms (e.g., nausea or diarrhea). If infection spreads to the nervous system, such symptoms as headache, stiff neck, confusion, loss of balance, or convulsions can occur. Infected pregnant women might experience only a mild influenza-like illness; however, infections during pregnancy can lead to miscarriage or stillbirth, premature delivery, or infection of the newborn. In the United States, approximately 800 cases of listeriosis are reported each year. Of those with serious illness, 15% die; newborns and immunocompromised persons are at greatest risk for serious illness and death.

Spinal cord injury: Approximately 11,000 persons sustain a spinal cord injury (SCI) each year in the United States, and 200,000 persons in the United States live with a disability related to an SCI. More than half of the persons who sustain SCIs are aged 15-29 years. The leading cause of SCI varies by age. Motor vehicle crashes are the leading cause of SCIs among persons aged <65 years. Among persons aged ≥65 years, falls cause the majority of spinal cord injuries. Sports and recreation activities cause an estimated 18% of spinal cord injuries.

Lung cancer among nonsmokers: A usually fatal cancer of the lung can occur in a person who has never smoked. An estimated 10%-15% of lung cancer cases occur among nonsmokers, and this type of cancer appears to be more common among women and persons of East Asian ancestry.

 Check your answers on page 5-60

Analyzing and Interpreting Data

After morbidity, mortality, and other relevant data about a health problem have been gathered and compiled, the data should be analyzed by time, place, and person. Different types of data are used for surveillance, and different types of analyses might be needed for each. For example, data on individual cases of disease are analyzed differently than data aggregated from multiple records; data received as text must be sorted, categorized, and coded for statistical analysis; and data from surveys might need to be weighted to produce valid estimates for sampled populations.

For analysis of the majority of surveillance data, descriptive methods are usually appropriate. The display of frequencies (counts) or rates of the health problem in simple tables and graphs, as discussed in Lesson 4, is the most common method of analyzing data for surveillance. Rates are useful — and frequently preferred — for comparing occurrence of disease for different geographic areas or periods because they take into account the size of the population from which the cases arose. One critical step before calculating a rate is constructing a denominator from appropriate population data. For state- or countywide rates, general population data are used. These data are available from the U.S. Census Bureau or from a state planning agency. For other calculations, the population at risk can dictate an alternative denominator. For example, an infant mortality rate uses the number of live-born infants; rates of surgical wound infections in a hospital requires the number of such procedures performed. In addition to calculating frequencies and rates, more sophisticated methods (e.g., space-time cluster analysis, time series analysis, or computer mapping) can be applied.

To determine whether the incidence or prevalence of a health problem has increased, data must be compared either over time or across areas. The selection of data for comparison depends on the health problem under surveillance and what is known about its typical temporal and geographic patterns of occurrence.

For example, data for diseases that indicate a seasonal pattern (e.g., influenza and mosquito-borne diseases) are usually compared with data for the corresponding season from past years. Data for diseases without a seasonal pattern are commonly compared with data for previous weeks, months, or years, depending on the nature of the disease. Surveillance for chronic diseases typically requires data covering multiple years. Data for acute infectious diseases might only require data covering weeks or months, although data extending over multiple years can also be helpful in the analysis of the natural history of disease. Data from one geographic area are sometimes compared with data from another area. For example, data from a county might be compared with data from adjacent counties or with data from the state. We now describe common methods for, and provide examples of, the analysis of data by time, place, and person.

Analyzing by time

Basic analysis of surveillance data by time is usually conducted to characterize trends and detect changes in disease incidence. For notifiable diseases, the first analysis is usually a comparison of the number of case reports received for the current week with the number received in the preceding weeks. These data can be organized into a table, a graph, or both (Table 5.5 and Figures 5.2 and 5.3). An abrupt increase or a gradual buildup in the number of cases can be detected by looking at the table or graph. For example, health officials reviewing the data for Clark County in Table 5.5 and Figures 5.2 and 5.3 will have noticed that the number of cases of hepatitis A reported during week 4 exceeded the numbers in the previous weeks. This method works well when new cases are reported promptly.

Table 5.5 Reported Cases of Hepatitis A, by County and Week of Report, 1991

County	Week of report								
	1	2	3	4	5	6	7	8	9
Adams	—	—	—	1	—	—	1	—	—
Asotin	—	—	—	—	—	—	—	—	—
Benton	—	—	—	2	1	—	2	—	3
Chelen	—	—	1	3	1	1	—	—	1
Clallam	—	—	1	—	—	—	—	2	—
Clark	—	—	3	8	14	13	11	6	—
Columbia	—	—	—	—	—	—	—	—	—
Cowlitz	2	—	3	—	—	6	4	9	—
Douglas	—	—	—	—	—	—	—	—	—
Ferry	—	—	—	—	—	—	—	—	—
Franklin	—	—	3	2	3	—	5	—	4
Garfield	—	—	—	—	—	—	—	1	—
Etc.									

Another common analysis is a comparison of the number of cases during the current period to the number reported during the same period for the last 2–10 years (Table 5.6). For example, health officials will have noted that the 11 cases reported for Clark County during weeks 1–4 during 1991 exceeded the numbers reported during the same 4-week period during the previous 3 years. A related method involves comparing the cumulative number of cases reported to date during the current year (or during the previous 52 weeks) to the cumulative number reported to the same date during previous years.

Table 5.6 Reported Cases of Hepatitis A, by County for Weeks 1–4, 1988–1991

County	Year			
	1988	1989	1990	1991
Adams	—	—	—	1
Asotin	—	—	—	—
Benton	—	—	3	2
Chelen	—	1	2	4
Clallam	—	1	1	1
Clark	6	3	—	11
Columbia	—	—	—	—
Cowlitz	—	5	—	5
Douglas	—	—	2	—
Ferry	1	—	—	—
Franklin	—	2	3	5
Garfield	—	—	—	—
Etc.				

Analysis of long-term time trends, also known as *secular* trends, usually involves graphing occurrence of disease by year. Figure 5.1 illustrates the rate of reported cases of malaria for the United States during 1932–2003. Graphs can also indicate the occurrence of events thought to have an impact on the secular trend (e.g., implementation or cessation of a control program or a change in the method of conducting surveillance). Figure 5.2 illustrates reported morbidity from malaria for 1932–1962, along with events and control activities that influenced its incidence.[2]

Figure 5.1 Rate (per 100,000 Persons) of Reported Cases of Malaria, By Year — United States, 1932–2003

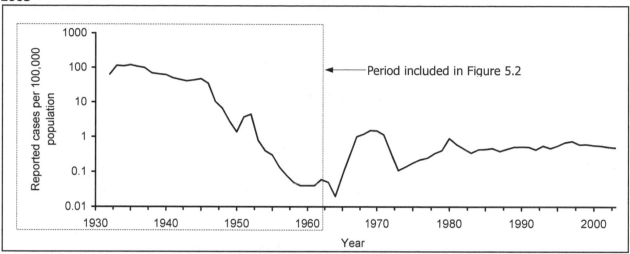

Adapted from: Centers for Disease Control and Prevention. Summary of notifiable diseases, United States, 1993b. MMWR 1993; 42(53):38, and Langmuir AD. The surveillance of communicable diseases of national importance. N Engl J Med 1963;268:182–92.

Figure 5.2 Reported Malaria Morbidity — United States, 1932–1962

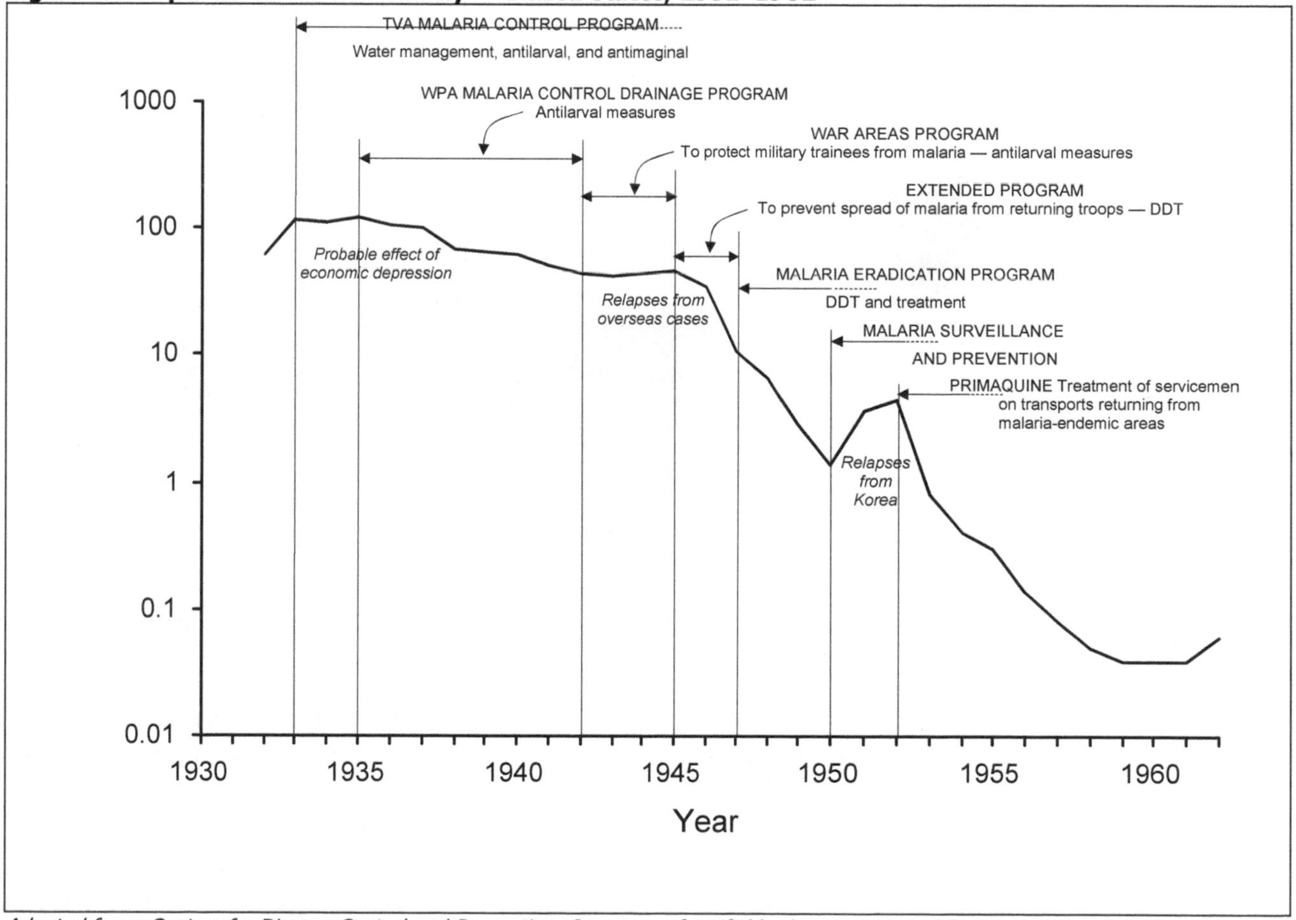

Adapted from: Centers for Disease Control and Prevention. Summary of notifiable diseases, United States, 1993b. MMWR 1993;42(53):38, and National Notifiable Diseases Surveillance System [Internet]. Atlanta: CDC [updated 2005 Oct 14; cited 2005 Nov 16]. Available from: http://www.cdc.gov/epo/dphsi/nndsshis.htm, Langmuir AD. The surveillance of communicable diseases of national importance. N Engl J Med 1963;268:184.

Statistical methods can be used to detect changes in disease occurrence. The Early Aberration Detection System (EARS) is a package of statistical analysis programs for detecting aberrations or deviations from the baseline, by using either long- (3–5 years) or short-term (as short as 1–6 days) baselines.[16]

Analyzing by place

The analysis of cases by place is usually displayed in a table or a map. State and local health departments usually analyze surveillance data by neighborhood or by county. CDC routinely analyzes surveillance data by state. Rates are often calculated by adjusting for differences in the size of the population of different counties, states, or other geographic areas. Figure 5.3 illustrates lung cancer mortality rates for white males for all U.S. counties for 1998–2002. To deal with county-to-county variations in population size and age distribution, age-adjusted rates are displayed.

Figure 5.3 Age-Adjusted Lung and Bronchus Cancer Mortality Rates (per 100,000 Population) By State — United States, 1998–2002

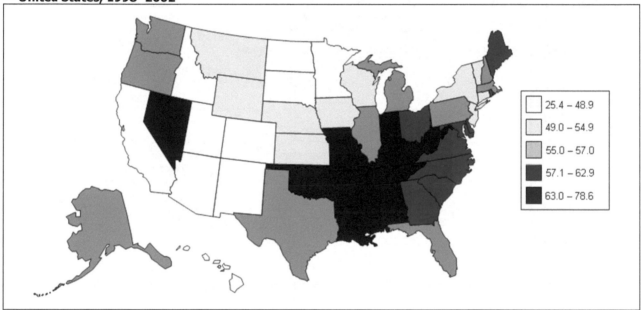

Data Source: National Cancer Institute [Internet] Bethesda: NCI [cited 2006 Mar 22] Surveillance Epidemiology and End Results (SEER). Available from: http://seer.cancer.gov/faststats/.

The advent of geographic information systems (GIS) allows more robust analysis of data by place and has moved spot and shaded, or **choropleth**, maps to much more sophisticated applications.[17] Using GIS is particularly effective when different types of information about place are combined to identify or clarify geographic relationships. For example, in Figure 5.4, the absence or presence of the tick that transmits Lyme disease, *Ixodes scapularis,* are illustrated superimposed over habitat suitability.[18] Such software packages as SatScan™ (Martin Kulldorff, Harvard

University and Information Management System, Inc., Silver Spring, Maryland), EpiInfo™ (CDC, Atlanta, Georgia), and Health Mapper (World Health Organization, Geneva, Switzerland) provide GIS functionality and can be useful when analyzing surveillance data.[19-21]

Figure 5.4 Predictive Risk Map of Habitat Suitability for *Ixodes scapularis* in Wisconsin and Illinois

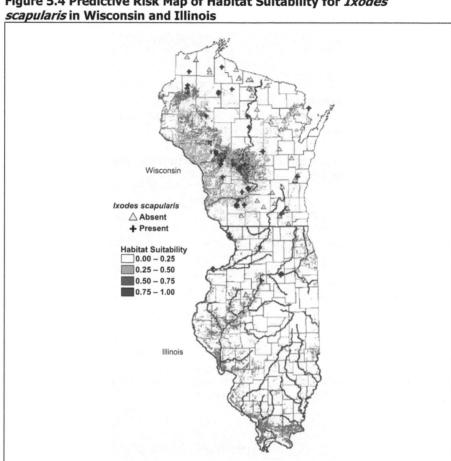

Source: Guerra M, Walker E, Jones C, Paskewitz S, Cortinas MR, Stancil A, Beck L, Bobo M, Kitron U. Predicting the risk of Lyme disease: habitat suitability for Ixodes scapularis in the north central United States. Emerg Infect Dis. 2002;8:289–97.

Analyzing by time and place

As a practical matter, disease occurrence is often analyzed by time and place simultaneously. An analysis by time and place can be organized and presented in a table or in a series of maps highlighting different periods or populations (Figures 5.5 and 5.6).

Figure 5.5 Age-Adjusted Colon Cancer Mortality Rates* for White Females by State — United States, 1950–1954, 1970–1974, and 1990–1994

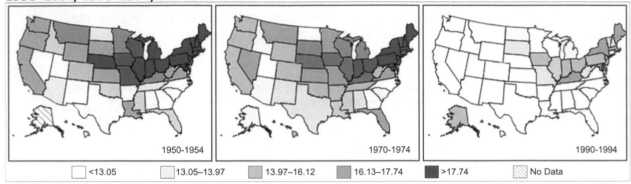

	<13.05		13.05–13.97		13.97–16.12		16.13–17.74		>17.74		No Data

Scale based on 1950–1994 rates (per 100,000 person years).
Data Source: Customizable Mortality Maps [Internet] Bethesda: National Cancer Institute [cited 2006 Mar 22]. Available from: http://cancercontrolplanet.cancer.gov/atlas/index.jsp.

Figure 5.6 Age-Adjusted Colon Cancer Mortality Rates* for White Males by State — United States, 1950–1954, 1970–1974, and 1990–1994

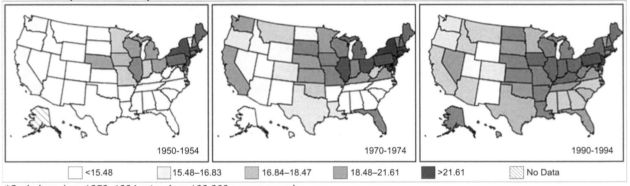

	<15.48		15.48–16.83		16.84–18.47		18.48–21.61		>21.61		No Data

Scale based on 1950–1994 rates (per 100,000 person years).
Data Source: Customizable Mortality Maps [Internet] Bethesda: National Cancer Institute [cited 2006 Mar 22]. Available from: http://cancercontrolplanet.cancer.gov/atlas/index.jsp.

Analyzing by person

The most commonly collected and analyzed person characteristics are age and sex. Data regarding race and ethnicity are less consistently available for analysis. Other characteristics (e.g., school or workplace, recent hospitalization, and the presence of such risk factors for specific diseases as recent travel or history of cigarette smoking) might also be available and useful for analysis, depending on the health problem.

Age

Meaningful age categories for analysis depend on the disease of interest. Categories should be mutually exclusive and all-inclusive. Mutually exclusive means the end of one category cannot overlap with the beginning of the next category (e.g., 1–4 years and 5–9 years rather than 1–5 and 5–9). All-inclusive means that the categories should include all possibilities, including the extremes of age (e.g., <1 year and ≥84 years) and unknowns.

Standard age categories for childhood illnesses are usually <1 year and ages 1–4, 5–9, 10–14, 15–19, and ≥20 years. For pneumonia and influenza mortality, which usually disproportionally affects older persons, the standard categories are <1 year and 1–24, 25–44, 45–64, and ≥65 years. Because two-thirds of all deaths in the United States occur among persons aged ≥65 years, researchers often divide the last category into ages 65–74, 75–84, and ≥85 years.

The characteristic age distribution of a disease should be used in deciding the age categories — multiple narrow categories for the peak ages, broader categories for the remainder. If the age distribution changes over time or differs geographically, the categories can be modified to accommodate those differences.

To use data in the calculation of rates, the age categories must be consistent with the age categories available for the population at risk. For example, census data are usually published as <5 years, 5–9, 10–14, and so on in 5-year age groups. These denominators could not be used if the surveillance data had been categorized in different 5-year age groups (e.g., 1–5 years, 6–10, 11–15, and so forth).

Other Person- or Disease-Related Risk Factor

For certain diseases, information on other specific risk factors (e.g., race, ethnicity, and occupation) are routinely collected and regularly analyzed. For example, have any of the reported cases of hepatitis A occurred among food-handlers who might expose (or might have exposed) unsuspecting patrons? For hepatitis B case reports, have two or more reports listed the same dentist as a potential source? For a varicella (chickenpox) case report, had the patient been vaccinated? Analysis of risk-factor data can provide information useful for disease control and prevention. Unfortunately, data regarding risk factors are often not available for analysis, particularly if a generic form (i.e., one report form for all diseases) or a secondary data source is used.

Interpreting results of analyses

When the incidence of a disease increases or its pattern among a specific population at a particular time and place varies from its expected pattern, further investigation or increased emphasis on prevention or control measures is usually indicated. The amount of increase or variation required for action is usually determined locally and reflects the priorities assigned to different diseases, the local health department's capabilities and resources, and sometimes, public, political, or media attention or pressure.

For certain diseases (e.g., botulism), a single case of an illness of public health importance or suspicion of a common source of infection for two or more cases is often sufficient reason for initiating an investigation. Suspicion might also be aroused from finding that patients have something in common (e.g., place of residence, school, occupation, racial/ethnic background, or time of onset of illness). Or a physician or other knowledgeable person might report that multiple current or recent cases of the same disease have been observed and are suspected of being related (e.g., a report of multiple cases of hepatitis A within the past 2 weeks from one county).

Observed increases or decreases in incidence or prevalence might, however, be the result of an aspect of the way in which surveillance was conducted rather than a true change in disease occurrence. Common causes of such artifactual changes are:
- Changes in local reporting procedures or policies (e.g., a change from passive to active surveillance).
- Changes in case definition (e.g., AIDS in 1993).
- Increased health-seeking behavior (e.g., media publicity prompts persons with symptoms to seek medical care).
- Increase in diagnosis.
- New laboratory test or diagnostic procedure.
- Increased physician awareness of the condition, or a new physician is in town.
- Increase in reporting (i.e., improved awareness of requirement to report).
- Outbreak of similar disease, misdiagnosed as disease of interest.
- Laboratory error.
- Batch reporting in which reports from previous periods are held and reported all at once during another reporting period (e.g., reporting all cases received during December and the first week of January during the second week of January).

Artifactual changes include an increase in population size, improved diagnostic procedures, enhanced reporting, and duplicate reporting. Compare the sharp increases in disease incidence illustrated in Figures 5.7 and 5.8. Although they appear similar, the increase displayed in Figure 5.7 represents a true increase in incidence, whereas the increase displayed in Figure 5.8 resulted from a change in the case definition.[22,23] Nonetheless, because a health department's primary responsibility is to protect the health of the public, public health officials usually consider an apparent increase real, and respond accordingly, until proven otherwise.

Figure 5.7 Reported Cases of Salmonellosis per 100,000 Population, By Year — United States, 1972–2002

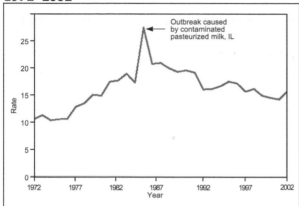

Source: Centers for Disease Control and Prevention. Summary of notifiable diseases–United States, 2002. Published April 30, 2004, for MMWR 2002;51(No. 53): p. 59.

Figure 5.8 Reported Cases of AIDS, by Year — United States* and U.S. Territories, 1982–2002

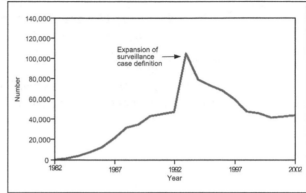

* Total number of AIDS cases includes all cases reported to CDC as of December 31, 2002. Total includes cases among residents in the U.S. territories and 94 cases among persons with unknown state of residence.

Source: Centers for Disease Control and Prevention. Summary of notifiable diseases–United States, 2002. Published April 30, 2004, for MMWR 2002;51(No. 53): p. 59.

Exercise 5.4

During the previous 6 years, one to three cases per year of tuberculosis had been reported to a state health department. During the past 3 months, 17 cases have been reported. All but two of these cases have been reported from one county. The local newspaper published an article about one of the first reported cases, which occurred in a girl aged 3 years. Describe the possible causes of the increase in reported cases.

 Check your answers on page 5-60

Disseminating Data and Interpretations

As Langmuir[2] emphasized, the timely, regular dissemination of basic data and their interpretations is a critical component of surveillance. Data and interpretations should be sent to those who provided reports or other data (e.g., health-care providers and laboratory directors). They should also be sent to those who use them for planning or managing control programs, administrative purposes, or other health-related decision-making.

Dissemination of surveillance information can take different forms. Perhaps the most common is a surveillance report or summary, which serves two purposes: to inform and to motivate. Information on the occurrence of health problems by time, place, and person informs local physicians about their risk for their encountering the problem among their patients. Other useful information accompanying surveillance data might include prevention and control strategies and summaries of investigations or other studies of the health problem. A report should be prepared on a regular basis and distributed by mail or e-mail and posted on the health department's Internet or intranet site, as appropriate. Increasingly, surveillance data are available in a form that can be queried by the general public on health departments' Internet sites.[24]

A surveillance report can also be a strong motivational factor in that it demonstrates that the health department actually looks at the case reports that are submitted and acts on those reports. Such efforts are important in maintaining a spirit of collaboration among the public health and medical communities, which in turn, improves the reporting of diseases to health authorities.

State and local health departments often publish a weekly or monthly newsletter that is distributed to the local medical and public health community. These newsletters usually provide tables of current surveillance data (e.g., the number of cases of disease identified since the last report for each disease and geographic area under surveillance), the number of cases previously identified (for comparison with current numbers), and other relevant information. They also usually contain information of current interest about the prevention, diagnosis, and treatment of selected diseases and summarize current or recently completed epidemiologic investigations.

At the national level, CDC provides similar information through the MMWR, MMWR Annual Summary of Notifiable Diseases, MMWR Surveillance Summaries, and individual surveillance

> "Development of a reasonably effective primary surveillance system took time. Usually, 2 full years were required. Experience showed that development was best achieved by establishing for each administrative unit of perhaps 2–5 million population, a surveillance team of perhaps two to four persons with transport. Each team, in addition to its other duties in outbreak containment, visited each reporting unit regularly to explain and discuss the program, to distribute forms (and often vaccine), and to check on those who were delinquent in reporting. Regularly distributed surveillance reports also helped to motivate these units. *Undoubtedly, the greatest stimulus to reporting was the prompt visit of the surveillance team for outbreak investigations and control whenever cases were reported. This simple, obvious, and direct indication that the routine weekly reports were actually seen and were a cause for public health action did more, I am sure, than the multitude of government directives which were issued.*" [Emphasis added][25]

reports published either by CDC or in peer-reviewed public health and medical journals.

When faced with a health problem of immediate public concern, whether it is a rapid increase in the number of heroin-related deaths in a city or the appearance of a new disease (e.g., AIDS in the early 1980s or West Nile Virus in the United States in 1999), a health department might need to disseminate information more quickly and to a wider audience than is possible with routine reports, summaries, or newsletters. Following the appearance of West Nile Virus in New York City in late August 1999, the following measures were taken:

> *"Emergency telephone hotlines were established in New York City on September 3 and in Westchester County on September 21 to address public inquiries about the encephalitis outbreak and pesticide application. As of September 28, approximately 130,000 calls [had] been received by the New York City hotline and 12,000 by the WCDH [Westchester County Health Department] hotline. Approximately 300,000 cans of DEET-based mosquito repellant were distributed citywide through local firehouses, and 750,000 public health leaflets were distributed with information about personal protection against mosquito bites. Recurring public messages were announced on radio, television, on the New York City and WCDH World-Wide Web sites, and in newspapers, urging personal protection against mosquito bites, including limiting outdoor activity during peak hours of mosquito activity, wearing long-sleeved shirts and long pants, using DEET-based insect repellents, and eliminating any potential mosquito breeding niches. Spraying schedules also were publicized with recommendations for persons to remain indoors while spraying occurred to reduce pesticide exposure."* [26]

Depending on the circumstances, reports of surveillance data and their interpretation might also be directed at the general public, particularly when a need exists for a public response to a particular problem.

Exercise 5.5

You have recently been hired by a state health department to direct surveillance activities for notifiable diseases, among other tasks. All notifiable disease surveillance data are entered and stored in computer files at the state and transmitted to CDC once each week. CDC publishes these data for all states in the MMWR each week, but health department staff do not routinely review these data in the MMWR. The state has never generated its own set of tables for analysis and dissemination, and you believe that it would be valuable to do so to educate and increase interest among health department staff.

1. What three tables might you want to generate by computer each week for use by health department staff?

2. You next decide that it would be a good idea to share these data with health-care providers, as well. What tables or figures might you generate for distribution to health-care providers, and how frequently would you distribute them?

 Check your answers on page 5-61

Exercise 5.6

Last week, the state public health laboratory diagnosed rabies among four raccoons that had been captured in a wooded residential neighborhood. This information will be duly reported in the tables of the monthly state health department newsletter. Who needs to know this information?

 Check your answers on page 5-62

Evaluating and Improving Surveillance

Surveillance for a disease or other health-related problem should be evaluated periodically to ensure that it is serving a useful public health function and is meeting its objectives. Such an evaluation: (1) identifies elements of surveillance that should be enhanced to improve its attributes, (2) assesses how surveillance findings affect control efforts, and (3) improves the quality of data and interpretations provided by surveillance.

Although the aspects of surveillance that are emphasized in an evaluation can differ, depending on the purpose and objectives of surveillance, the evaluation's overall scope and approach should be similar for any health-related problem. The evaluation usually begins by identifying and interviewing key stakeholders and by collecting background documents, forms, and reports. The evaluation should address the purpose of surveillance, objectives, and mechanics of conducting surveillance; the resources needed to conduct surveillance; the usefulness of surveillance; and the presence or absence of the characteristics or qualities of optimal surveillance. The outcome of the evaluation should provide recommendations for improvement.[9,27,28] We discuss these main components in the following sections.

Stakeholders

Stakeholders are the persons and organizations who contribute to, use, and benefit from surveillance. They typically include public health officials and staff, health-care providers, data providers and users, community representatives, government officials, and others interested in the health condition under surveillance. Stakeholders should be identified not only because they contribute to or use surveillance results, but also because they might be interested in, and can contribute to the evaluation. Stakeholders should be engaged early in the evaluation process because some might have a hand in implementing recommendations that emerge from the evaluation. Evaluations conducted without early buy-in from those responsible for conducting surveillance are often viewed as unwanted criticism and interference from outsiders and are usually ignored.

Purpose, objectives, and operations

The evaluation should start with a clear statement of the purpose of surveillance, which usually facilitates prevention or control of a health-related problem. The purpose should be followed by clearly stated objectives describing how surveillance data and their interpretations are used. Considering the information needed for effective prevention and control of the health problem is also helpful. For example, an objective of surveillance for gonorrhea might be to detect individual cases and their contacts so that both can be treated. To meet this objective, sufficient information will be needed to identify cases and contacts for follow-up. To characterize the purpose, objectives, and operations of surveillance, addressing the questions at the beginning of this lesson will be helpful.

Sketching a flow chart of the method of conducting surveillance is recommended. First, identify gaps in the evaluator's knowledge of how surveillance is being conducted. Second, provide a clear visual display of the activities of and flow of data for surveillance for those not familiar with it (Figure 5.9).

Usefulness

Usefulness refers to whether surveillance contributes to prevention and control of a health-related problem. Note that usefulness can include improved understanding of the public health implications of the health problem. Usefulness is typically assessed by determining whether surveillance meets its objectives. For example, if the primary objective of surveillance is to identify individual cases of disease to facilitate timely and effective control measures, does surveillance permit timely and accurate identification, diagnosis, treatment, or other handling of contacts when appropriate?

Usefulness of surveillance is influenced greatly by its operation, including its feedback mechanism to those who need to know, and by the presence or absence of the characteristics of optimal surveillance. Qualities or characteristics described previously in this lesson and in Appendix A affect the operation and usefulness of surveillance. Evaluation of surveillance requires assessment, either qualitatively or quantitatively, of each characteristic.

Figure 5.9 Simplified Diagram of Surveillance for a Health Problem

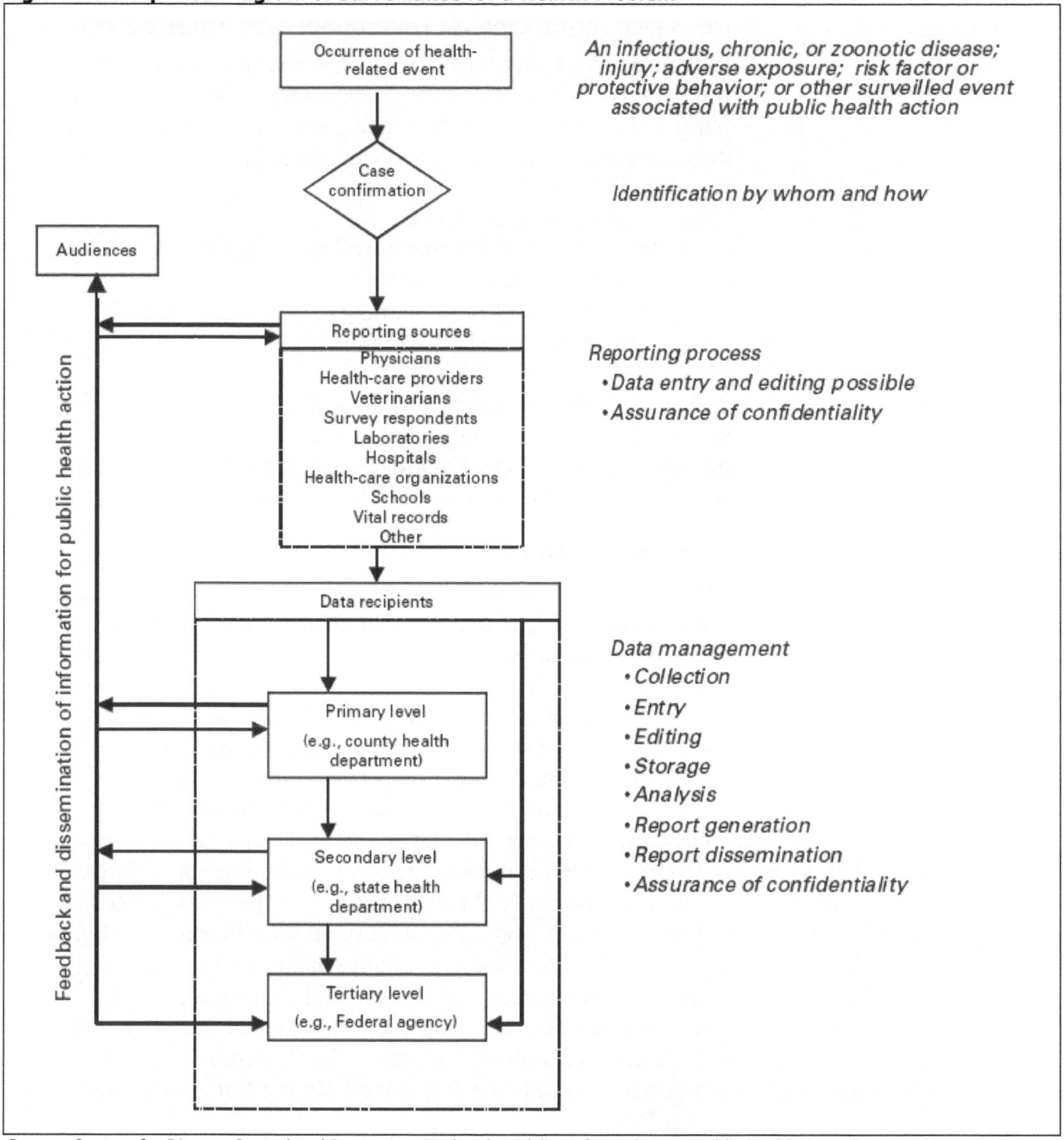

Source: Centers for Disease Control and Prevention. Updated guidelines for evaluating public health surveillance systems: recommendations from the guidelines working group. MMWR 2001;50(No. RR-13): p. 8.

Resource requirements (personnel and other costs)

In the context of surveillance evaluation, **resources** refers to finances, personnel, and other direct costs needed to operate all phases of surveillance, including any collection, analysis, and dissemination of data. The following should be identified and quantified:

- Funding sources and budget;
- Personnel requirements to collect, compile, edit, analyze, interpret, or disseminate data; and
- Other resources (e.g., training, travel, supplies, and computers and related equipment).

These costs are usually assessed in light of the objectives of surveillance and its usefulness and against the expected costs of possible modifications or alternatives to the way in which surveillance is conducted.

Recommendations

The purpose of evaluating surveillance for a specific disease is to draw conclusions and make recommendations about its present state and future potential. The conclusions should state whether surveillance as it is being conducted is meeting its objectives and whether it is operating efficiently. If it is not, recommendations should address what modifications should be made to do so. Recommendations must recognize that the characteristics and costs of conducting surveillance are interrelated and potentially conflicting. For example, improving sensitivity can reduce predictive value positive and increase costs. For surveillance, recommendations should be prioritized on the basis of needs and objectives. For example, for syndromic surveillance, timeliness and sensitivity are critical, but high sensitivity increases false alarms, which can drain limited public health resources. Each characteristic must be considered and balanced to ensure that the objectives of surveillance are met. (See Appendix E for an assessment of and recommendations for notifiable disease surveillance.)

Recommendations should be realistic, feasible, and clearly explained. Feedback to health facilities and stakeholders is an important, but sometimes neglected, part of the evaluation. Certain recommendations might be unpopular and will need convincing justification. When possible, include an estimate of the time and resources needed to implement the changes. Prioritizing plans and developing a timetable for surveillance improvements might be helpful. A method for ensuring that improvements are initiated in a timely fashion is critical to the evaluation's ultimate success.[9,29]

Summary

Surveillance has a long history of value to the health of populations and continues to evolve as new health-related problems arise. In this lesson, we have defined public health surveillance as continued watchfulness over health-related problems through systematic collection, consolidation, and evaluation of relevant data.[2] Data and interpretations derived from surveillance activities are useful in setting priorities, planning and conducting disease control programs, and assessing the effectiveness of control efforts. We have reviewed the identification and prioritization of health problems for surveillance; the need for a clear, functional definition of a health problem to facilitate surveillance for it; and various approaches for gathering data about health problems, including environmental monitoring, surveys, notifications, and registries. Sources of data are often available and used for surveillance at the national, state, and local levels.

We have described and illustrated basic methods for analyzing and interpreting data and have focused on time, place, and person as the foundation for characterizing a health-related problem through surveillance. Potential problems with surveillance data that can lead to errors in their analysis or interpretation have been presented. We have emphasized the importance of the timely, regular dissemination of basic data and their interpretation as a critical component of surveillance. These data and surveillance reports must be shared with those who supplied the data and those responsible for the control of health problems.

Critical to maintaining useful, cost-effective surveillance is periodic evaluation and implementation of recommended improvements. Stakeholders should be identified and included in evaluation processes; a clear description and diagram of surveillance activities should be developed; and the usefulness, resource requirements, and characteristics of optimal surveillance should be individually assessed. This lesson ends with examples of surveillance and recommendations for further reading.

Appendix A. Characteristics of Well-Conducted Surveillance

Acceptability reflects the willingness of individual persons and organizations to participate in surveillance. Acceptability is influenced substantially by the time and effort required to complete and submit reports or perform other surveillance tasks.

Flexibility refers to the ability of the method used for surveillance to accommodate changes in operating conditions or information needs with little additional cost in time, personnel, or funds. Flexibility might include the ability of an information system, whose data are used for surveillance of a particular health condition, to be used for surveillance of a new health problem.

Predictive Value Positive is the proportion of reported or identified cases that truly are cases, or the proportion of reported or identified epidemics that were actual epidemics. Conducting surveillance that has poor predictive value positive is wasteful, because the unsubstantiated or false-positive reports result in unnecessary investigations, wasteful allocation of resources, and especially for false reports of epidemics, unwarranted public anxiety (see Figure 5.10 for how to calculate predictive value positive.)

Quality reflects the completeness and validity of the data used for surveillance. One simple measure is the percentage of unknown or blank values for a particular variable (e.g., age) in the data used for surveillance.

Representativeness is the extent to which the findings of surveillance accurately portray the incidence of a health event among a population by person, place, or time. Representativeness is influenced by the acceptability and sensitivity (see the following) of the method used to obtain data for surveillance. Too often, epidemiologists who calculate incidence rates from surveillance data incorrectly assume that those data are representative of the population.

Sensitivity is the ability of surveillance to detect the health problem that it is intended to detect. (see Figure 5.10 for how to calculate sensitivity.) Surveillance for the majority of health problems might detect a relatively limited proportion of those that actually occur. The critical question is whether surveillance is sufficiently sensitive to be useful in preventing or controlling the health problem.

Simplicity refers to the ease of operation of surveillance as a whole and of each of its components (e.g., how easily case definitions can be applied or how easily data for surveillance can be obtained). The method for conducting surveillance typically should be as simple as possible while still meeting its objectives.

Stability refers to the reliability of the methods for obtaining and managing surveillance data and to the availability of those data. This characteristic is usually related to the reliability of computer systems that support surveillance but might also reflect the availability of resources and personnel for conducting surveillance.

Timeliness refers to the availability of data rapidly enough for public health authorities to take appropriate action. Any unnecessary delay in the collection, management, analysis, nterpretation, or dissemination of data for surveillance might affect a public health agency's ability to initiate prompt intervention or provide timely feedback.

Validity refers to whether surveillance data are measuring what they are intended to measure. As such, validity is related to sensitivity and predictive value positive: Is surveillance detecting the outbreaks it should? Is it detecting any nonoutbreaks?

Figure 5.10 Calculation of Predictive Value Positive, Sensitivity, and Specificity for Surveillance

		True case or outbreak		Total
		Yes	**No**	**Total**
Detected by surveillance?	**Yes**	True positive (A)	False positive (B)	Total detected by surveillance (A + B)
	No	False negative (C)	True negative (D)	Total missed by surveillance (C + D)
	Total	Total true cases or outbreaks (A + C)	Total noncases or non-outbreaks (B + D)	Total (A + B + C + D)

Predictive value positive = A / (A+B)
Sensitivity = A / (A+C)
Specificity = D / (B+D)

Adapted from: Centers for Disease Control and Prevention. Updated guidelines for evaluating public health surveillance systems: recommendations from the guidelines working group. MMWR 2001;50(No. RR-13): p. 18.
Protocol for the evaluation of epidemiological surveillance systems [monograph on the Internet]. Geneva: World Health Organization [updated 1997; cited 2006 Jan 20]. Available from: http://whqlibdoc.who.int/hq/1997/WHO_EMC_DIS_97.2.pdf.

Table 5.7 Relative Importance of Selected Surveillance Characteristics By Use of Surveillance Findings

Characteristic	Use of surveillance		
	Managing individual cases of disease	**Detecting outbreaks of disease**	**Planning and evaluating health programs**
Flexibility	***	****	*
Predictive value positive	****	***	****
Quality	*****	***	****
Representativeness	**	**	****
Sensitivity	****	****	***
Stability	****	*****	***
Timeliness	****	*****	*

The number of asterisks reflects the relative importance of each characteristic with more asterisks signifying greater importance.

Adapted from: Sosin DM, Hopkins RS. Monitoring disease and risk factors: surveillance. In: Pencheon D, Melzer D, Gray M, Guest C (editors). Oxford Handbook of Public Health, 2nd ed. Oxford: Oxford University Press; 2006 (in Press).

Appendix B. CDC Fact Sheet on Chlamydia

What is chlamydia? Chlamydia is a common sexually transmitted disease (STD) caused by the bacterium, *Chlamydia trachomatis*, which can damage a woman's reproductive organs. Even though symptoms of chlamydia are usually mild or absent, serious complications that can cause irreversible damage, including infertility, can occur without notice before a woman ever recognizes a problem. Chlamydia also can cause discharge from the penis of an infected man.

How common is chlamydia? Chlamydia is the most frequently reported bacterial STD in the United States. In 2002, a total of 834,555 chlamydial infections were reported to CDC from 50 states and the District of Columbia. Underreporting is substantial because the majority of persons with chlamydia are not aware of their infections and do not seek testing. Also, testing is not often performed if patients are treated for their symptoms. An estimated 2.8 million Americans are infected with chlamydia each year. Women are frequently re-infected if their sex partners are not treated.

How do people contract chlamydia? Chlamydia can be transmitted during vaginal, anal, or oral sex. Chlamydia can also be passed from an infected mother to her baby during vaginal childbirth. Any sexually active person can be infected with chlamydia. The greater the number of sex partners, the greater the risk for infection. Because the cervix (opening to the uterus) of teenage females and young women is not fully matured, they are at particularly high risk for infection if sexually active. Because chlamydia can be transmitted by oral or anal sex, men who have sex with men are also at risk for chlamydial infection.

What are the symptoms of chlamydia? Chlamydia is known as a "silent" disease because approximately three quarters of infected women and half of infected men have no symptoms. If symptoms do occur, they usually appear within 1–3 weeks after exposure.

Among women, the bacteria initially infect the cervix and the urethra (urine canal). Women who have symptoms might have an abnormal vaginal discharge or a burning sensation when urinating. When the infection spreads from the cervix to the fallopian tubes (the tubes that carry eggs from the ovaries to the uterus), certain women still have no signs or symptoms; others have lower abdominal pain, low back pain, nausea, fever, pain during intercourse, or bleeding between menstrual periods. Chlamydial infection of the cervix can spread to the rectum.

Men with signs or symptoms might have a discharge from their penis or a burning sensation when urinating. Men might also have burning and itching around the opening of the penis. Pain and swelling in the testicles are uncommon symptoms.

Men or women who have receptive anal intercourse might acquire chlamydial infection in the rectum, causing rectal pain, discharge, or bleeding. Chlamydia has also been identified in the throats of women and men having oral sex with an infected partner.

What complications can result from untreated chlamydia? If untreated, chlamydial infections can progress to serious reproductive and other health problems with both short- and long-term consequences. Similar to the disease itself, the damage that chlamydia causes is often asymptomatic.

Among women, untreated infection can spread into the uterus or fallopian tubes and cause pelvic inflammatory disease (PID). This happens among ≤40% of women with untreated chlamydia. PID can cause permanent damage to the fallopian tubes, uterus, and surrounding tissues. The damage can lead to chronic pelvic pain, infertility, and potentially fatal ectopic pregnancy (pregnancy outside the uterus). Women infected with chlamydia are ≤5 times more likely to become infected with HIV, if exposed.

To help prevent the serious consequences of chlamydia, screening at least annually for chlamydia is recommended for all sexually active women aged ≤25 years. An annual screening test also is recommended for women aged ≥25 years who have risk factors for chlamydia (a new sex partner or multiple sex partners). All pregnant women should have a screening test for chlamydia.

Complications among men are rare. Infection sometimes spreads to the epididymis (a tube that carries sperm from the testis), causing pain, fever, and, rarely, sterility. Rarely, genital chlamydial infection can cause arthritis that can be accompanied by skin lesions and inflammation of the eye and urethra (Reiter syndrome).

How does chlamydia affect a pregnant woman and her baby? Among pregnant women, evidence exists that untreated chlamydial infections can lead to premature delivery. Babies who are born to infected mothers can contract chlamydial infections in their eyes and respiratory tracts. Chlamydia is a leading cause of early infant pneumonia and conjunctivitis (pink eye) among newborns.

How is chlamydia diagnosed? Laboratory tests are used to diagnose chlamydia. Diagnostic tests can be performed on urine; other tests require that a specimen be collected from such sites as the penis or cervix.

What is the treatment for chlamydia? Chlamydia can be easily treated and cured with antibiotics. A single dose of azithromycin or a week of doxycycline (twice daily) are the most commonly used treatments. HIV-positive persons with chlamydia should receive the same treatment as those who are HIV-negative.

All sex partners should be evaluated, tested, and treated. Persons with chlamydia should abstain from sexual intercourse until they and their sex partners have completed treatment; otherwise re-infection is possible.

Women whose sex partners have not been appropriately treated are at high risk for re-infection. Having multiple infections increases a woman's risk for serious reproductive health complications, including infertility. Retesting should be considered for females, especially adolescents, 3–4 months after treatment. This is especially true if a woman does not know if her sex partner has received treatment.

How can chlamydia be prevented? The surest way to avoid transmission of STDs is to abstain from sexual contact or to be in a long-term mutually monogamous relationship with a partner who has been tested and is known to be uninfected. Latex male condoms, when used consistently and correctly, can reduce the risk of transmission of chlamydia.

Chlamydia screening is recommended annually for all sexually active women aged ≤25 years. An annual screening test also is recommended for older women with risk factors for chlamydia (a new sex partner or multiple sex partners). All pregnant women should have a screening test for chlamydia.

Any genital symptoms (e.g., discharge or burning during urination or unusual sores or rashes) should be a signal to stop having sex and to consult a health-care provider immediately. If a person has been treated for chlamydia (or any other STD), he or she should notify all recent sex partners so they can see a health-care provider and be treated. This will reduce the risk that the sex partners will experience serious complications from chlamydia and will also reduce the person's risk for becoming re-infected. The person and all of his or her sex partners should avoid sex until they have completed their treatment for chlamydia.

Adapted from: Chlamydia - CDC Fact Sheet [Internet]. Atlanta: CDC [updated 2006 April; cited 2006 May 17]. Available from: http://www.cdc.gov/std/chlamydia/STDFact-Chlamydia.htm.

Appendix C. Examples of Surveillance

Surveillance for Consumer Product-Related Injuries

The U.S. Consumer Product Safety Commission's (CPSC) National Electronic Injury Surveillance System (NEISS) is a national probability sample of hospitals in the United States and its territories (Figure 5.11). Patient information is collected from each NEISS hospital for every emergency department (ED) visit involving an injury associated with consumer products. From this sample, the total number of product-related injuries treated in hospital EDs nationwide can be estimated.

Figure 5.11 U.S. Consumer Product Safety Commission NEISS Hospitals, 2003

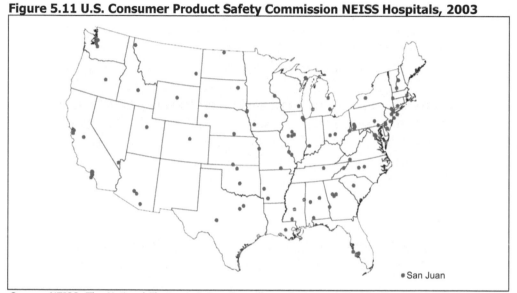

Source: NEISS: The National Electronic Injury Surveillance System - A Tool for Researchers [monograph on the Internet]. Washington (DC): U.S. Consumer Product Safety Commission, Division of Hazard and Injury Data Systems [updated 2000 Mar; cited 2005 Dec 2]. Available from: http://www.cpsc.gov/neiss/2000d015.pdf.

The data-collection process begins when a patient in the ED of an NEISS hospital relates to a clerk, nurse, or physician how the injury occurred. The ED staff enters this information in the patient's medical record. Each day, a person designated as an NEISS coordinator examines the records for within-scope cases. The NEISS coordinator is someone designated by the hospital who is given access to the ED records. NEISS coordinator duties are sometimes performed by an ED staff member and sometimes by a person under contract to CPSC. CPSC data-collection specialists train NEISS coordinators and conduct ED staff orientation during on-site hospital visits. For all within-scope cases, the NEISS coordinator abstracts information for the specified NEISS variables. The coordinator uses an NEISS coding manual to apply numerical codes to the NEISS variables. For CPSC, the key variable is the one that identifies any consumer product mentioned. The coordinator is trained to be as specific as possible in selecting among the approximately 900 product codes in the NEISS coding manual. Another essential variable is the free-text narrative description from the ED record of the incident scenario. Up to two lines of text are provided for this narrative that often describes what the patient was doing at the time of the accident. The specific NEISS variables are listed as follows:

Basic Surveillance Record Variables (before year 2000 expansion)
- Treatment date.
- Case record number.
- Patient's age.
- Patient's sex.
- Injury diagnosis.
- Body part affected.
- Disposition (e.g., treated and released or hospitalized).
- Product(s) mentioned.
- Locale.
- Fire or motor-vehicle involvement.
- Whether work-related.
- Race or ethnicity.
- Incident scenario.
- Whether intentionally inflicted (year 2000 expansion).

NEISS continuously monitors product-related injuries treated in the 100 hospital EDs that comprise the probability sample. Within-scope injuries examined in these EDs are reported to CPSC year-round on a daily basis. Thus, daily, weekly, monthly, seasonal, or episodic trends can be observed. Numerous published articles have used NEISS data to characterize consumer product-related injuries.[30-32]

Surveillance for Asthma

CDC conducts national surveillance for asthma, a chronic disease that affects the respiratory system among both children and adults. Because of its high prevalence and substantial morbidity, asthma has been the focus of clinical and public health interventions, and surveillance has been helpful in quantifying its prevalence and tracking its trend.

In conducting surveillance, CDC uses multiple sources of data because of asthma's broad spectrum of severity, which ranges from occasional, self-managed episodes to attacks requiring hospitalization, and rarely, resulting in death. Asthma-related health effects under surveillance and the data systems used to monitor them are as follows:
- Self-reported asthma prevalence, self-reported asthma episodes or attacks, school and work days lost because of asthma, and asthma-associated activity limitations are obtained from the National Health Interview Survey.
- Asthma-associated outpatient visits are obtained from the National Ambulatory Medical Care Survey.
- Asthma-associated ED and hospital outpatient visits are obtained from the National Hospital Ambulatory Medical Care Survey.
- Asthma-associated hospitalizations are obtained from the National Hospital Discharge Survey.
- Asthma-associated deaths are obtained from the Mortality Component of the National Vital Statistics System.

Data from these systems and from the U.S. Census Bureau are analyzed to produce national and regional estimates of asthma-related effects, including rates (see Figure 5.12 for examples of these estimates).

Two reports summarizing the findings of surveillance for asthma have been published; the first, in 1998[33] and the second in 2002[34]. The reports present findings in a series of tables and graphs. Efforts are under way to improve surveillance for asthma by obtaining state-level data on its prevalence, developing methods to estimate the incidence of asthma by using data from EDs, and improving the timeliness of reporting of asthma-related deaths so that they can be investigated to determine how such deaths might have been prevented.

Figure 5.12. Asthma Prevalence, Morbidity, and Mortality Rates — United States, 1960–1999

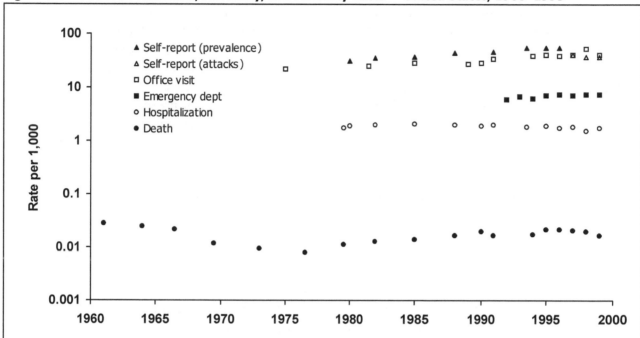

Data Sources: Mannino DM, Homa DM, Pertowski CA, et al. Surveillance for asthma—United States, 1960–1995. In: Surveillance Summaries, April 24, 1998. MMWR 1998;47(No. SS-1):1–28, and Mannino DM, Homa DM, Akinbami LJ, Moorman JE, Gwynn C, Redd SC. Surveillance for Asthma—United States, 1980–1999. In: Surveillance Summaries, March 29, 2002. MMWR 2002;51(No. SS-1):1–13.

Surveillance for Influenza

Reporting from states to the Centers for Disease Control and Prevention (CDC) is not limited to notifiable diseases. Surveillance for influenza is one such example. Because influenza can be widespread during the winter but its diagnosis is rarely confirmed by laboratory test, surveillance for influenza has presented challenges that have been met by using a combination of different sources of data.

At the state and local levels, health authorities receive reports of outbreaks of influenza-like illness, laboratory identification of influenza virus from nasopharyngeal swabs, and reports from schools of excess absenteeism (e.g., >10% of a school's student body). In addition, certain local systems monitor death certificates for pneumonia and influenza, arrange for selected physicians to report the number of patients they examine with influenza-like illness each week, and ask selected businesses and schools to report excessive employee absenteeism. At least one type of surveillance for influenza includes pharmacy reports of the number of prescriptions of antiviral drugs used to treat influenza. Another health department monitors the number of chest radiographs a mobile radiology group performs of nursing home patients; >50% of the total chest radiographs ordered is used as a marker of increased influenza activity.

At the national level, CDC collects and analyzes data weekly from seven different data systems to assess influenza activity.
- The laboratory-based system receives reports of the number of percentage of influenza isolates from approximately 125 laboratories located throughout the United States. Selected isolates are sent to CDC for additional testing.
- The U.S. Influenza Sentinel Providers Surveillance Network receives reports of the number and percentage of patients examined with influenza-like illness by age group from a network of approximately 1,000 health-care providers.
- The 122 City Mortality Reporting System receives counts of deaths and the proportion of those deaths attributable to pneumonia and influenza from 122 cities and counties across the country.
- Each state and territorial health department provides an assessment of influenza activity in the state as either "No Activity," "Sporadic," "Local," "Regional," or "Widespread."
- Influenza-associated pediatric mortality (defined as laboratory-confirmed influenza-associated death among children aged <18 years) is now a nationally notifiable condition and is reported through the National Notifiable Disease Surveillance System.
- Emerging Infections Program conducts surveillance for laboratory-confirmed influenza-related hospitalizations among persons aged <18 years in 11 metropolitan areas in 10 states.

By using multiple data sources at all levels — local, state, and national — public health officials are able to assess influenza activity reliably throughout the United States without asking every health-care provider to report each individual case.

Appendix D. Major Health Data Systems in the United States

Note: For additional information on data systems see the sources listed just below the table.

Title	Topic	Method	Approach	Geographic Level*
AirData	Air pollution	Environmental monitoring	Sampling and measurement	L
Behavioral Risk Factor Surveillance System	Behavior	Population survey	Telephone interview	N, S, Ci
Continuing Survey of Food Intake by Individuals	Nutrition	Population survey	Personal interview	N
Fatal Analysis Reporting System	Fatal traffic crashes	Agency and health-care provider survey	Police, driving, and health records review	N, S, L
HIV/AIDS Surveillance System	HIV/AIDS	Disease notification	Reports by physicians	N, S, L
Medical Expenditure Panel Survey	Health costs	Population and provider surveys	Personal interview Telephone interview	N
Monitoring the Future Study	Drug use	Population survey	School questionnaire	N, S, Ci
National Ambulatory Medical Care Survey	Ambulatory care	Health-care provider survey	Health record review	N, R
National Crime Victimization Survey	Victims of crime	Population survey	Telephone interview	N, S
National Electronic Injury Surveillance System	Consumer product-related injuries	Health-care provider survey	Reports by emergency department staff	N
National Health and Nutrition Examination Survey	General health	Population survey	Personal interview and exam	N
National Health Interview Survey	General health	Population survey	Personal Interview	N, R
National Hospital Ambulatory Medical Care Survey	Ambulatory care	Health-care provider survey	Health record review	N, R
National Hospital Discharge Survey	Hospitalizations	Health-care provider survey	Health record review	N, S
National Immunization Survey	Immunizations	Population survey	Telephone interview	N, S, L
National Notifiable Disease Surveillance System	Infectious diseases	Disease notification	Reports by physicians and laboratories	N, S, L
National Profile of Local Health Departments	Local public health agencies	Agency survey	Mailed questionnaire	N, L
National Program of Cancer Registries	Cancer incidence and mortality	Registry	Health record review	N, S
National Survey on Drug Use and Health	Drug use	Population survey	Personal interview	N
National Survey of Family Growth	Pregnancy and women's health	Population survey	Personal interview	
National Vital Statistics System	Birth and Death	Vital registration	Reports by physicians	N, S, Co
School Health Policies and Programs Study	School health policies and programs	Administrative data Population survey	Mailed questionnaire Personal interview	S, L
State and Local Area Integrated Telephone Survey	Health care	Population survey	Telephone interview	N, S, L
State Tobacco Activities Tracking and Evaluation System	Tobacco-related activities	Multiple		S
STD Case Surveillance Reporting System	Sexually transmitted diseases	Disease notification	Reports by physicians	N, S, L
STORET	Water quality	Environmental monitoring	Sampling and measurement	L
Surveillance, Epidemiology, and End Results	Cancer incidence and survival	Registry	Health record review	N, S, Ci
United States Renal Data System	End stage renal disease	Multiple		
Youth Risk Behavior Surveillance System	Behavior	Population survey	School questionnaire	N, S

*N = national; R = regional; S = state; L = local (county, city, or town); Co = county; Ci = city.

Sources: Healthy People 2010: Tracking Healthy People 2010 [Internet]. Washington, DC: Department of Health and Human Services; Part C. Major Data Sources for Healthy People 2010 [updated 2001 Jan 30; cited 2006 Jan 16]. Available from: http://www.healthypeople.gov/Document/html/tracking/THP_PartC.htm
Stroup DF, Brookmeyer R, Kalsbeek WD. Public health surveillance in action: a framework. In: Brookmeyer R, Stroup DF (editors). Monitoring the Health of Populations: Statistical Principles and Methods for Public Health Surveillance. Oxford: Oxford University Press; 2004, p. 1–35.

Appendix E. Limitations of Notifiable Disease Surveillance and Recommendations for Improvement

Surveillance need not be perfect to be useful. However, surveillance might have limitations, particularly as a result of underreporting, lack of representativeness, and lack of timeliness, that compromise its usefulness. Fortunately, health departments can implement measures to overcome these hurdles.

Although the intention of the laws and regulations of each state in the United States is that every case of a notifiable disease be reported, the reality is otherwise. For rare, serious diseases of public health importance (e.g., rabies, plague, or botulism), the percentage of cases actually reported might approach 100% of diagnosed cases. Reporting completeness for diseases that have local programs that specifically look for cases of the disease to aid in their prevention or control (e.g., AIDS, tuberculosis, and sexually transmitted diseases [STDs]) has been identified as being higher than for other, nonlife-threatening diseases.[35] For other diseases, reporting has been reported to be as low as 9%.[35] Table 5.8 illustrates this situation for the identification and reporting of shigellosis. The authors of the study from which these data are derived concluded that the number of *Shigella* cases reported nationally should be multiplied by 20 to obtain a more realistic estimate of the actual number of infections.[36] Others have proposed multiplication factors of 38 for infectious agents that cause nonbloody diarrhea, 20 for agents that cause bloody diarrhea, and two for pathogens that typically cause severe gastrointestinal illness.[37]

Table 5.8. Rosenberg's Shigellosis Cascade

Event	Percentage of Patients	Cumulative Days Elapsed from Onset of Symptoms
Infected	100	—
Symptomatic	76	—
Consulted physician	28	—
Culture obtained	9	7
Culture positive	7	10
Reported to local health department	***6***	***11***
Reported to CDC	6	29
Patient contacted	6	—
Negative follow-up culture obtained	2	39

Adapted from: Rosenberg MJ, Marr JS, Gangarosa EJ, Pollard RA, Wallace M, Brolnitsky O. Shigella surveillance in the United States, 1975. J Infect

Limitations

Underreporting. For the majority of notifiable diseases, data for surveillance are based on passive reporting by physicians and other health-care providers. Studies have demonstrated that in the majority of jurisdictions, only a fraction of cases of the notifiable diseases overall are ever reported.[37-39] The most obvious result of such underreporting is that effective action is delayed, and cases occur that might have been prevented by prompt reporting and prompt initiation of control measures. For example, if a case of hepatitis A in a food handler goes unreported, the opportunity to provide protective immune globulin to restaurant patrons will be missed, and cases or an outbreak of hepatitis A that should have been prevented will instead occur. However, underreported data might still be useful for assessing trends or other patterns reflecting the occurrence or burden of disease.

Health-care providers cite a number of reasons for not reporting.[40] Selected reasons are listed in the following text. Public health agencies must recognize these barriers to reporting, because the majority are within an agency's power to address or correct.

Lack of knowledge of reporting requirements:
- Lack of awareness of responsibility to report.
- Lack of awareness of which diseases must be reported.
- Lack of awareness of how or to whom to report.
- Assumption that someone else (e.g., the laboratory) will report.

Negative attitude toward reporting:
- Time consuming.
- Hassle (e.g., a lengthy or complex report form or procedure).
- Lack of incentive.
- Lack of feedback.
- Distrust of government.

Misconceptions that result from lack of knowledge or negative attitude:
- Compromises patient-physician relationship.
- Concern that report might result in a breach of confidentiality (e.g., HIPAA concerns).
- Disagreement with need to report.
- Judgment that the disease is not that serious.
- Belief that no effective public health measures exist.
- Perception that health department does not act on the reports.

Lack of representativeness of reported cases. Underreporting is not uniform or random. Two important biases distort the completeness of reporting. First, health-care providers are more likely to report a case that results in severe illness and hospitalization than a mild case, even though a person with mild illness might be more likely to transmit infection to others because the person might not be confined at home or in the hospital. This bias results in an inflated estimate of disease severity in such measures as the death-to-case ratio. Second, health-care providers are more likely to report cases when the disease is receiving media attention. This bias results in an underestimate of the baseline incidence of disease after media attention wanes.

Both biases were operating in 1981 during the national epidemic of tampon-associated toxic shock syndrome. Early reports indicated a death-to-case ratio much higher than the ratio determined by subsequent studies, and reported cases declined more than incident cases after the publicity waned.[41]

Lack of timeliness. Lack of timeliness can occur at almost any step in the collection, analysis, and dissemination of data on notifiable diseases. The reasons for the delays vary. Certain delays are disease-dependent. For example, physicians cannot diagnose certain diseases until confirmatory laboratory and other tests have been completed. Certain delays are caused by cumbersome or inefficient reporting procedures. Delays in analysis are common when surveillance is believed to be a rote function rather than as one that provides information for action. Finally, delays at any step might culminate in delays in dissemination, with the result that the medical and public health communities do not have the information they need to take prompt action.

Recommendations for Improving Notifiable Disease Surveillance

The preceding limitations of reporting systems demonstrate multiple steps that can be taken by a local or state health department to improve reporting.

Improving awareness of practitioners. Most important, all persons who have a responsibility to report must be aware of this responsibility. The health department should actively publicize the list of notifiable diseases and the reporting mechanisms. Certain states send the reporting requirements in a packet when a physician becomes licensed to practice in the state. Other state health officials visit hospitals and speak at medical presentations or seminars to increase the visibility of surveillance.

Incentives. Health-care providers might need services or therapeutic agents that are only available from the health department, which might be able to use this need to obtain reports of certain diseases. Services can include laboratory testing and consultation on diagnosis and treatment of certain diseases. Agents might include immune globulin for human rabies and hepatitis B and antitoxin for diphtheria and botulism. These services and agents might be particularly effective incentives if they are available promptly and delivered in a professional, authoritative manner.[10]

Simplify reporting. Reporting should be as simple as possible. Health departments often accept telephone reports or have toll-free telephone numbers. If paper forms are used, they should be widely available and easy to complete, and they should ask only for relevant information. Certain state health departments have arranged for electronic transfer of laboratory or other patient- or case-related data; therefore, reporting is accomplished automatically at scheduled times or at the push of a computer key.

Frequent feedback. The role of feedback cannot be overemphasized. Feedback can be written (e.g., a monthly newsletter) or oral (e.g., updates at regular meetings of medical staff or at rounds). The feedback should be timely, informative, interesting, and relevant to each reporter's practice. Feedback should include information about disease patterns and control activities to increase awareness and to reinforce the importance of participating in a meaningful public health activity.

Widening the net. Traditionally, surveillance for notifiable diseases has relied on reporting by physicians. Almost every state now requires reporting of positive cultures or diagnostic tests for notifiable diseases by commercial and hospital laboratories. For certain states, the number of laboratory reports exceeds the number of reports from physicians, hospitals, clinics, and other sources. Other health-care staff (e.g., infection control personnel and school nurses) can be used as sources of data for surveillance. Another way to widen the net is to develop alternative methods for conducting surveillance (e.g., using secondary sources of data). This method has been used effectively for surveillance of influenza and certain injuries.

Shifting the burden. Another effective approach is to shift the burden for gathering data from the health-care provider to the health department. In essence, this approach involves ongoing surveys of providers to more completely identify cases of disease, and it has been demonstrated to increase the number of cases and the proportion of identified-to-incident cases. Because health department staff contact health-care providers regularly, this approach also promotes closer personal ties among providers and health department staff. As with surveys in general, this approach is relatively expensive, and its cost-effectiveness is not entirely clear. In practice, it is usually limited to disease elimination programs, short-term intensive investigation and control activities, or seasonal problems (e.g., certain arboviral diseases).

Exercise Answers

Exercise 5.1

Public health importance of chlamydia

Incidence	Estimated to be 2.8 million new cases each year in the United States.
Severity	Approximately 40% of infected, untreated women experience pelvic inflammatory disease. Five-fold increase in risk among women of experiencing HIV infection, if exposed.
Mortality caused by chlamydia	Ectopic pregnancy, a potential complication of chlamydial infection, can cause death, but frequency is unknown.
Socioeconomic impact	Complications of chlamydial infections among women have impact on their reproductive ability and can cause chronic illness among certain women, resulting in an undue burden on them, their families, and the health-care system.
Communicability	Passed person to person through sexual contact or from mother to baby during birth.
Potential for an outbreak	Varies with population sexual activity and practices, as well as underlying prevalence.
Public perception and concern	Not described in fact sheet provided. Different readers might have differing perceptions of the level of public concern.
International requirements	None.

Ability to prevent, control, or treat chlamydia

Preventability	Preventable by sexual abstinence, sexual contact with uninfected partners, and use of latex male condoms.
Control measures and treatment	Secondary prevention through annual screening for chlamydia, which is recommended for all sexually active women aged ≤25 years. An annual screening test is also recommended for women aged ≥25 years who have risk factors for chlamydia (e.g., a new sex partner or multiple sex partners). All pregnant women should have a screening test for chlamydia. Chlamydia is highly responsive to antibiotic treatment. Sexual partners should be evaluated, tested, and treated, if infected.

Capacity of health-care system to implement control measures for Chlamydia

Speed of response	Disease is often asymptomatic, resulting in delayed diagnosis. Annual screening for chlamydia is recommended for all sexually active women aged ≤25 years and for women aged ≥25 years who have risk factors for chlamydia.
Economics	Treatment is typically through the health-care system, and the costs are paid by insurers, employers, or the government. Follow-up of patients to identify contacts is the responsibility of the health department. Given the frequency of the disease, this might require substantial resources that are not be available in certain places.
Availability of resources	Dependent on location.
What does surveillance for this event require?	Screening and diagnosis of men and women with chlamydial disease and then reporting of disease by health-care providers to the state health department by using a standard form. The percentage of women who actually receive recommended screening is unknown. Surveillance can also be conducted by using reporting of positive diagnostic tests by laboratory facilities.

Advantages
- Surveillance provides an estimate of the true prevalence of this important but often overlooked condition.
- Infection is treatable, and transmission is preventable.
- Untreated chlamydial infection is a major cause of pelvic inflammatory disease and infertility.
- Surveillance can be conducted through routine laboratory reporting of all positive tests for chlamydia, which might reduce the reporting burden on health-care providers.

Disadvantages
- Clinicians might ignore the requirement to report chlamydia, even if it is added to the list of notifiable diseases, if they believe the list is already too long. They might believe they should only be required to report communicable diseases with statistically significant morbidity or mortality that can lead to immediate intervention by the health department.
- Clinicians might not adhere to screening recommendations, and therefore, recognition of disease might be low.
- Adding chlamydia to the list will not lead to better diagnosis and treatment, because the majority of infections are asymptomatic.

Exercise 5.2

Asthma is a chronic illness that can vary in severity. Using just one source of data or just one dataset to monitor it provides limited knowledge of its extent and the potential effect of treatment and other interventions on it. Thus, using multiple sources of data with information on asthma's incidence, prevalence, morbidity, and mortality is the best way to conduct surveillance for this illness.

- Self-reported asthma prevalence or attacks provides information on its occurrence among the entire population, even those who might not seek or receive medical care for it.
- The majority of cases of asthma requiring medical attention are observed in physician offices, emergency departments, or outpatient clinics. Thus, obtaining information from these sources provides optimal knowledge of its occurrence and morbidity among the majority of persons.
- Severe episodes of illness can require hospitalization and be an indicator that routine treatment in outpatient settings is not being delivered effectively to the whole population. Thus, data on hospitalizations caused by asthma is helpful in monitoring effectiveness of interventions.
- Deaths from asthma are similar to hospitalizations and might represent a failure of the health-care system to deal effectively with the illness.

In addition to the usefulness of different sources, as described previously, certain advantages and disadvantages of different methods of gathering data from these sources are described in the following sections.

Surveys
Advantages
- More control over the quality of the data.
- More in-depth data possibly collected on each case than is usually possible with notifications.
- Can identify the spectrum of illness, including cases that do not warrant medical care.
- More accurate assessment of true incidence and prevalence.

Disadvantages
- More costly to perform because surveys usually require development of de-novo data-collection systems and hiring of interviewers who require training and supervision.
- Might represent only a single point in time ("snapshot"), if survey is not periodically repeated; might miss seasonal trends, rare diseases, or rapidly fatal diseases.
- Recall bias more likely to affect results because data collected retrospectively (notifications are usually prospective).

Notifications (Reporting of illness by health-care providers)
Advantages
- Cheaper (for the health department).
- Typically use existing systems and health-care personnel for collecting data.
- Allows monitoring of trends over time.
- Ongoing data collection might allow collection of an adequate number of cases to study those at risk. With surveys, an event might be too infrequent to gather enough cases for study; with notifications, the observation period can be extended until sufficient numbers of cases are collected.

Disadvantages

- Might not provide a representative picture of the incidence or prevalence unless care is taken in selecting reporting sites and ensuring complete reporting.
- Data that can be collected are limited by the skill, time, and willingness of the data collectors, who usually have other responsibilities.
- Quality control might be a major problem in data collection.
- The quality of data might vary among collection sites.
- As a result, notifications usually provide a substandard estimate of the true incidence and prevalence.

An alternative to notification might be to enroll interested and appropriate health-care providers and clinics in a sentinel system to gather case numbers of asthma.

Exercise 5.3

Factors that influence the choice of one source of data or one dataset over another include severity of illness (e.g., hospitalization and mortality); need for laboratory confirmation of diagnosis; rarity of the condition; specialization, if any, of the health-care providers who commonly examine patients with the condition under surveillance; quality, reliability, or availability of relevant data; and timeliness of the data in terms of need for response.

Listeriosis: A wide spectrum of nonspecific clinical illness and a low case fatality rate exists (except among newborns and immunocompromised persons). Therefore, surveillance should be based on morbidity rather than mortality data; diagnoses should be confirmed in the laboratory. Possible sources of surveillance data include laboratory reports, hospital discharge data (although patients with listeriosis are often not hospitalized), or adding listeriosis to the notifiable disease list.

Spinal cord injury: This is a severe health event with substantial mortality; almost all persons who sustain a spinal cord injury are brought to a hospital. Therefore, surveillance would most logically be based on hospital records and mortality data (e.g., death certificates or medical examiner data). Special efforts might be directed to obtaining data from regional trauma centers. Using data from emergency medical services and rehabilitation centers might also be explored.

Lung cancer among nonsmokers: Similar to spinal cord injury, lung cancer is a severe health event with high morbidity and mortality. Unfortunately, hospital discharge records and vital records do not routinely provide smoking information. For this condition, cancer registries might provide the best opportunity for surveillance, if smoking information is routinely collected. Alternatively, surveillance might be established by using interested internists, oncologists, and other health-care providers likely to interact with lung cancer patients.

Exercise 5.4

Possible explanations for the sudden increase include those listed in the following. Each possibility should be investigated before deciding that the increase is a true increase in incidence.

1. Change in surveillance system or policy of reporting.
2. Change in case definition.
3. Improved or incorrect diagnosis.
   - New laboratory test.
   - Increased physician awareness of the need to test for tuberculosis, new physician in town, and so forth.
   - Increase in publicity or public awareness that might have prompted persons or parents to seek medical attention for compatible illness.
   - New population subgroup (e.g., refugees) in state A who have previous recent vaccination against tuberculosis using the bacille de Calmette-Guérin (BCG) vaccine.
   - New or untrained staff conducting testing for tuberculosis and incorrect interpretation of skin reaction to tuberculin.
4. Increase in reporting (i.e., improved awareness of requirement to report).
5. Batch reporting (unlikely in this scenario).
6. True increase in incidence.

Exercise 5.5

No right answer exists, but one set of tables for health department staff might be as follows:

Table 1. Number of reported cases of each notifiable disease this week for each county in the state.

Table 2. Number of reported cases of each notifiable disease by week for the entire state for the current and the previous 6–8 weeks for comparison.

Table 3. Number of reported cases of each notifiable disease for the past 4 weeks (current week and previous 3 weeks) and for comparison, the number of cases during the same period during the previous 5 years.

Table 1 addresses disease occurrence by place. Tables 2 and 3 address disease occurrence by time. Together, these tables should provide an indication of whether an unusual cluster or pattern of disease is occurring. If such a pattern is detected, person characteristics might then be explored.

A report for health-care providers does not need to be distributed as frequently and does not need to include all of the notifiable diseases. One approach might be to distribute a report every 6 months and include notifiable diseases that have demonstrated substantial change since the last report, with a discussion of possible causes for the change. Maps of the geographic distribution and figures illustrating the trends over time of selected diseases might be more appealing and informative to health-care providers than tables of frequencies. Information on the diagnosis and treatment of highlighted diseases might also be of interest to health-care providers.

Reports for the media and public typically should be issued to inform them of outbreaks, of new diseases, or of diseases of particular concern. These reports should include basic information about the diseases, the location and frequency of their occurrence, and information on recognition, prevention, and treatment of the diseases.

Exercise 5.6

State health department newsletters do not always go to all those who have a need to know. Even among those who receive the newsletter, some do not read it, and many others skim the articles and ignore the tables. In addition, depending on the timing of the laboratory report and publication deadlines, the information might be delayed by weeks or months.

This information about finding rabid raccoons in a residential area is important for those who might be affected and for those who might be able to take preventive measures, including the following:

- Other public health agencies (e.g., neighboring local health departments or animal control staff) — Contact and inform by telephone or e-mail message.
- Health-care providers serving the population in the affected area — Contact and inform through a special mailing.
- Veterinarians — Inform through a mailing so that they can be on alert for pets that might have come into contact with rabid wildlife; veterinarians can provide specimens, as appropriate, of both wild animals and pets to the state laboratory for testing for rabies.
- The public — Inform by issuing press release to the media asking the public to avoid wild animals and to have their pets vaccinated.

SELF-ASSESSMENT QUIZ

Now that you have read Lesson 5 and have completed the exercises, you should be ready to take the self-assessment quiz. This quiz is designed to help you assess how well you have learned the content of this lesson. You may refer to the lesson text whenever you are unsure of the answer.

Unless instructed otherwise, choose ALL correct answers for each question.

1. As described in this lesson, public health surveillance includes which activities?
   A. Data collection.
   B. Data analysis.
   C. Data interpretation.
   D. Data dissemination.
   E. Disease control.

2. Current public health surveillance targets which of the following?
   A. Chronic diseases.
   B. Communicable diseases.
   C. Health-related behaviors.
   D. Occupational hazards.
   E. Presence of viruses in mosquitoes.

3. Public health surveillance can be described primarily as which of the following?
   A. A method to monitor occurrences of public health problems.
   B. A program to control disease outbreaks.
   C. A system for collecting health-related information.
   D. A system for monitoring persons who have been exposed to a communicable disease.

4. Public health surveillance is only conducted by public health agencies.
   A. True.
   B. False.

5. Common uses and applications of public health surveillance include which of the following?
   A. Detecting individual persons with malaria so that they can receive prompt and appropriate treatment.
   B. Helping public health officials decide how to allocate their disease control resources.
   C. Identifying changes over time in the proportion of children with elevated blood lead levels in a community.
   D. Documenting changes in the incidence of varicella (chickenpox), if any, after a law requiring varicella vaccination took effect.

6. Data collected through which of the following methods is commonly used for surveillance?
   A. Vital registration.
   B. Randomized clinical trials.
   C. Disease notifications.
   D. Population surveys.

7. Health-care providers might be important sources of surveillance data used by public health officials, and they should receive feedback to close the surveillance loop as a courtesy; however, the results almost never have any relevance to patient care provided by those health-care providers.
   A. True.
   B. False.

8. Vital statistics are important sources of data on which of the following?
   A. Morbidity.
   B. Mortality.
   C. Health-related behaviors.
   D. Injury and disability.
   E. Outpatient health-care usage.

9 Vital statistics provide an archive of certain health data. These data do not become surveillance data until they are analyzed, interpreted, and disseminated with the intent of influencing public health decision-making or action.
   A. True.
   B. False.

10. Key sources of morbidity data include which of the following?
   A. Environmental monitoring data.
   B. Hospital discharge data.
   C. Laboratory results.
   D. Notifiable disease reports.
   E. Vital records.

11 Notifiable disease surveillance usually focuses on morbidity from the diseases on the list and does not cover mortality from those diseases.
   A. True.
   B. False.

12. The list of diseases that a physician must report to the local health department is typically compiled by the . . .
   A. Local health department.
   B. State health department.
   C. Centers for Disease Control and Prevention (CDC).
   D. Council of State and Territorial Epidemiologists (CSTE).
   E. Medical licensing board.

13. A physician working in an emergency room in Town A, USA, has just examined a tourist from Southeast Asia with watery diarrhea. The physician suspects the man might have cholera. The physician should notify the . . .
   A. Local (town or county) health agency.
   B. State health department.
   C. Centers for Disease Control and Prevention (CDC).
   D. U.S. Department of State.
   E. Washington, D.C., embassy of country of origin (ask for health attaché).

14. Use the following choices for Questions 14a-e.
    A. Notifiable disease surveillance
    B. Surveillance for consumer product-related injuries
    C. Both.
    D. Neither.

    14a. _____ State-based, with subsequent reporting to CDC.

    14b. _____ Focused on identifying individual cases.

    14c. _____ Can monitor trends over time.

    14d. _____ Based on statistically valid sample.

    14e. _____ Complete, unbiased reporting.

15. Evaluating and improving surveillance should address which of the following?
    A. Purpose and objectives of surveillance.
    B. Resources needed to conduct surveillance.
    C. Effectiveness of measures for controlling the disease under surveillance.
    D. Presence of characteristics of well-conducted surveillance.

16. Criteria for prioritizing health problems for surveillance include which of the following?
    A. Incidence of the problem.
    B. Public concern about the problem.
    C. Number of previous studies of the problem.
    D. Social and economic impact of the problem.

17. Use the following choices for Questions 17a-d.
    A. Surveillance based on a specific case definition for a disease (e.g., listeriosis).
    B. Syndromic surveillance based on symptoms, signs, or other characteristics of a disease, rather than specific clinical or laboratory diagnostic criteria.
    C. Both.
    D. Neither.

    17a. _____ Watches for individual cases of disease of public health importance.

    17b. _____ Watches for diseases that might be caused by acts of biologic or chemical terrorism.

    17c. _____ Can watch for disease before a patient seeks care from a health-care provider.

    17d. _____ Requires little effort on the part of the health department.

18. Routine analysis of notifiable disease surveillance data at the state health department might include looking at the number of cases of a disease reported this week . . .
    A. and during the previous 2-4 weeks.
    B. and the number reported during the comparable weeks of the previous 2-5 years.
    C. simultaneously by age, race, and sex of the patient.
    D. by county.
    E. by county, divided by each county's population (i.e., county rates).

19. One week, a state health department received substantially more case reports of a disease in one county than had been reported during the previous 2 weeks. No increase was reported in neighboring counties. Possible explanations for this increase include which of the following?
    A. An outbreak in the county.
    B. Batch reports.
    C. Duplicate reports.
    D. Increase in the county's population.
    E. Laboratory error.

20. The primary reason for preparing and distributing periodic surveillance summaries is which of the following?
    A. Document recent epidemiologic investigations.
    B. Provide timely information on disease patterns and trends to those who need to know it.
    C. Provide reprints of *MMWR* articles, reports, and recommendations.
    D. Acknowledge the contributions of those who submitted case reports.

21. Use the following choices for Questions 21a-b.
    A. Predictive value positive.
    B. Sensitivity.
    C. Specificity.
    D. Validity.

    21a. _____ Surveillance detected 23 of 30 actual cases of a disease.

    21b. _____ Of 16 statistically significant aberrations (deviations from baseline) detected by syndromic surveillance, only one represented an actual outbreak of disease.

22. Underreporting is not a problem for detecting outbreaks of notifiable diseases because the proportion of cases reported tends to remain relatively stable over time.
    A. True.
    B. False.

23. Initiating surveillance for a public health problem or adding a disease to the notifiable disease list is justified for which of the following reasons?
    A. If it is a communicable disease with a high case-fatality rate.
    B. If the problem is new and systematically collected data are needed to characterize the disease and its impact on the public.
    C. If a program at CDC has recommended its addition to better understand national trends and patterns.
    D. To guide, monitor, and evaluate programs to prevent or control the problem.

24. The case definition used for surveillance of a health problem should be the same as the case definition used for clinical (treatment) purposes.
    A. True.
    B. False.

25. A state health department decides to strengthen its notifiable disease reporting. The one best action to take is to . . .
    A. allow reporting through use of the Internet.
    B. require more disease-specific forms from local health departments.
    C. ensure that all persons with a responsibility to report understand the requirements and reasons for reporting and how reports will be used.
    D. reduce the number of diseases on the list.

Answers to Self-Assessment Quiz

1. A, B, C, D. The term *public health surveillance* includes data collection, analysis, interpretation, and dissemination to help guide health officials and programs in directing and conducting disease control and prevention activities. However, surveillance does not include control or prevention activities themselves.

2. A, B, C, D, E. Current public health surveillance targets health-related conditions among humans, including chronic diseases (e.g., cancer), communicable diseases (e.g., those on the notifiable disease list), health-related behaviors, and occupationally related conditions (e.g., black lung disease and other pneumoconioses). Surveillance also focuses on indicators of disease potential (e.g., such diseases among animals as rabies) or presence of an infectious agent among animals or insects (e.g., West Nile virus among mosquitoes).

3. A. Public health surveillance can be thought of as one of the methods that a community has available to monitor the health among its population by detecting problems, communicating alerts as needed, guiding the appropriate response, and evaluating the effect of the response. Surveillance should not be confused with medical surveillance, which is monitoring of exposed persons to detect early evidence of disease. Public health surveillance is the continued watchfulness for public health problems; it is not a data-collection system.

4. B (False). The practice of surveillance is not limited to public health agencies. Hospitals, nursing homes, the military, and other institutions have long conducted surveillance of their populations.

5. A, B, C, D. Among the uses of surveillance are detecting individual cases of diseases of public health importance (e.g., malaria), supporting planning (e.g., priority setting), monitoring trends and patterns of health-related conditions (e.g., elevated blood lead levels), and supporting evaluation of prevention and control measures (e.g., a vaccination requirement).

6. A, C, D. Data collected through vital registration, disease notifications, and population surveys are commonly used for surveillance of health-related problems. Data from randomized clinical trials typically cover only a specially selected population and are used to answer specific questions about the effectiveness of a particular treatment. They are not useful for surveillance.

7. B (False). One of the important uses of surveillance data and one of the key reasons to close the surveillance loop by disseminating surveillance data back to health-care providers, is to provide clinically relevant information about disease occurrence, trends, and patterns. For example, health departments alert clinicians to the presence of new diseases (e.g., severe acute respiratory syndrome [SARS]) and provide information so that clinicians can make diagnoses. Health departments also advise clinicians about changing patterns of antibiotic resistance so that clinicians can choose the right treatment regimen.

8. B. Vital statistics refer to data on birth, death, marriage, and divorce. Therefore, vital statistics are the primary source of data on mortality, but not on morbidity (illness), behaviors, injury (other than fatal injuries), and health-care usage. Before development of population health surveys and disease registries and the use of health-care records to assess morbidity, vital statistics were the primary source of data on the health of populations. During recent years, administrative, financial, and other health-care–related records have supplemented the information from vital statistics, especially for assessing morbidity within populations. National, state, and local population-based health surveys, some of which are conducted on a regular or continuing basis, provide another important part of our view of the health of populations.

9. A (True). Vital statistics are usually thought of as an archive of births, deaths, marriages, and divorces. Vital statistics offices in health departments typically are not linked to disease prevention and control activities. However, surveillance for certain health problems might rely on vital statistics as its primary source of data. When these data undergo timely and systematic analysis, interpretation, and dissemination with the intent of influencing public health decision-making and action, they become surveillance data.

10. B, C, D. Sources of morbidity (illness) data include notifiable disease reports, laboratory data, hospital discharge data, outpatient health-care data, and surveillance for specific conditions (e.g., cancer). Vital records are an important source of mortality data, and even though a patient first gets sick from a disease before dying from it, vital records are not regarded as a source of data for the surveillance of morbidity from the disease. Environmental monitoring is used to evaluate disease potential or risk.

11. B (False). Notifiable disease surveillance targets occurrence or death from any of the diseases on the list.

12. B. The list of nationally notifiable diseases is compiled by the Council of State and Territorial Epidemiologists (CSTE) and the Centers for Disease Control and Prevention. The list of notifiable diseases that physicians must report to their state or local health department is set by the state, either by the state legislature, the state board of health, the state health department, the state health officer, or the state epidemiologist. CSTE votes on the diseases that should be nationally notifiable, but the states have the ultimate authority whether to add any newly voted diseases to their state list.

13. A or B, depending on the state. The agency that a physician should notify is determined by the state, just as the list of notifiable diseases is set by the state (see answer to question 12). The manner in which notification should occur and how rapidly reports should be made are also defined by the state and can vary by disease. For example, the state might require that a case of cholera be reported immediately by telephone or fax to the local or state health department, whereas reporting of varicella (chickenpox) might only be required monthly, by using a paper form. Regardless of the disease and reporting requirements, reporting should proceed through established channels. In certain states, physicians should notify the county health department, which will then notify the state health department, which will notify CDC, which will notify the World Health Organization. In states with no or limited local health departments, physicians are usually required to notify the state health department. The seriousness of the disease might influence how rapidly these communications take place but should not influence the sequence.

14a. A. Notifiable disease surveillance is state-based, with subsequent reporting to CDC. Surveillance for consumer product-related injuries is hospital emergency department-based with subsequent reporting to the Consumer Product Safety Commission.

14b. A. Notifiable disease surveillance attempts to identify every case of a notifiable disease. Surveillance for consumer product-related injuries relies on a sample of hospital emergency departments to characterize the incidence and types of these injuries.

14c. C. Because surveillance for notifiable diseases and surveillance for consumer product-related injuries are both ongoing, both can monitor trends over time.

14d. B. Surveillance for consumer product-related injuries is based on a statistically valid sample of hospital emergency departments in the United States. Notifiable disease surveillance covers the entire population.

14e. D. Neither approach to surveillance is perfect. Underreporting is a serious problem in the majority of states for notifiable disease surveillance. Surveillance for consumer product-related injuries is based on visits to a sample of emergency departments; therefore, persons who do not seek care at an emergency department are not represented.

15. A, B, D. Evaluation of surveillance for a health-related problem should include review of the purpose and objectives of surveillance, the resources needed to conduct surveillance for the problem, and whether the characteristics of well-conducted surveillance are present. Because surveillance does not have direct responsibility for the control of the health problem, this is not part of evaluating a surveillance system. Whether effective measures for preventing or controlling a health-related problem are available can be a useful criterion in prioritizing diseases for surveillance.

16. A, B, D. The incidence of, public concern about, and social and economic impact of a health problem are all important in assessing its suitability for surveillance. Although previous studies of the problem might have helped to characterize its natural history, cause, and impact, the number of such studies is not used as a criterion for prioritization.

17a. C (Both). Surveillance based on specific case definition for a disease attempts to identify individual cases of disease of public health importance, and syndromic surveillance, depending on its purpose, might also attempt to identify cases of disease of public health importance. In certain situations, the goal of syndromic surveillance might be to identify clusters or outbreaks (more cases than expected) of disease rather than individual cases.

17b. C (Both). Both syndromic surveillance and surveillance based on a specific case definition for a disease can be used to watch for diseases caused by acts of biologic or chemical terrorism. Which approach is used depends on the disease and the setting.

17c. B. Syndromic surveillance that targets sales of over-the-counter medications, calls to hotlines, and school or work absenteeism all watch for disease before a patient seeks care from a health-care provider. Surveillance based on a specific case definition for a disease is usually based on reporting by a health-care provider.

17d. D. Neither type of surveillance can function properly without attention and effort on the part of the health department. Health department staff should review the case report forms and conduct follow-up of cases reported through surveillance based on specific case definitions for diseases. Health department staff should review the cases identified by syndromic surveillance and determine whether they reflect true outbreaks or not. Additionally, health department staff should compile and communicate the results. These tasks are a minimum.

18. A, B, D, E. Analysis by time often includes comparison with previous weeks and previous years. Analysis by place can include analysis of both numbers and rates. Routine analysis by person includes age and sex, but a three-variable table of age by race and sex is probably too much stratification for routine analysis.

19. A, B, C, D, E. An increase in case reports during a single week might represent a true increase in disease (i.e., an outbreak). However, the increase can also represent an increase in the population (e.g., from an influx of tourists, migrant workers, refugees, or students); reporting of cases in a batch, particularly after a holiday season; duplicate reports of the same case; laboratory or computer error; a new clinic or health-care provider that is more likely to make a particular diagnosis or is more conscientious about reporting; or other sudden changes in the method of conducting surveillance.

20. B. The primary purpose of preparing and distributing surveillance summaries is to provide timely information about disease occurrence to those in the community who need to know. The report also serves to motivate those who report by demonstrating that their efforts are valued and to inform health-care providers and others in the community about health department activities and general public health concerns.

21a. B. Sensitivity is the ability of surveillance (or laboratory tests or case definitions) to detect a true case (or, for certain systems, a true outbreak). Specificity is the ability of surveillance (or laboratory tests or case definitions) to rule out disease among persons who do not have it.

21b. A. Predictive value positive is the proportion of patients (or outbreaks) detected by surveillance who truly have the disease (or are true outbreaks). Predictive value positive is a function of both the sensitivity of surveillance and the prevalence of the disease (or prevalence of real outbreaks).

22. B (False). Underreporting is a serious problem for surveillance that relies on notifications. Because the notifiable disease surveillance is supposed to identify individual cases of disease of public health importance, underreporting of even a single case of, for example, hepatitis A in a food handler, can result in an outbreak that should have been prevented. Similarly, if a limited number of cases are reported at all, even outbreaks can be missed.

23. B, D. Initiating surveillance for a health-related problem can be justified for multiple reasons. These reasons include if a disease is new and surveillance is the most effective means for collecting information on cases to learn more about its clinical and epidemiologic features (e.g., SARS); if a new prevention or control measure is about to be implemented and surveillance is the most effective means for assessing its impact (e.g., varicella vaccination regulations); or if surveillance is needed to guide, monitor,

and evaluate prevention or control measures. Surveillance is more difficult to justify if a disease does not occur locally, even if it is a communicable disease with a high case fatality rate (e.g., Ebola or Marburg virus infection), or simply because CDC requests it (without funding).

24. B (False). A case definition for surveillance should be clear, understandable, acceptable, and implementable by those who are required to apply it. However, it need not use the same criteria that are used for clinical purposes. For example, health-care providers might treat patients on the basis of clinical features without laboratory confirmation, whereas a surveillance case definition might require confirmation, or vice versa.

25. C. The most important way to improve notifiable disease surveillance is to ensure that everyone who is supposed to report knows
    - that they are supposed to report,
    - what to report (i.e., which diseases are on the list), and
    - how, to whom, and how quickly to report.
    In addition, they will be more likely to report if they know that the health department is actually doing something with the reports. No data are available that demonstrate that reporting through the Internet improves reporting; in fact, for certain health-care providers, reporting might involve extra work. Requiring more disease-specific forms tends to reduce reporting, because it requires more time and effort for those reporting. Reducing the number of diseases on the list might be part of a strategy to improve reporting, but it is not the most important way to do so.

References

1. Merriam-Webster. Merriam-Webster's Dictionary of English Usage. Springfield (MA): Merriam-Webster, Inc. 1976.

2. Langmuir AD. The surveillance of communicable diseases of national importance. N Engl J Med 1963;268:182–92.

3. Thacker SB, Berkelman RL. Public health surveillance in the United States. Epidemiol Rev 1988;10:164-190.

4. Communicable Disease Center. Communicable Disease Center Activities 1952-1953. Atlanta: Department of Health, Education, and Welfare; 1953. Public Health Service Publication Number 391, p. 17.

5. World Health Organization. Report of the technical discussions at the twenty-first World Health Assembly on 'national and global surveillance of communicable diseases.' Geneva: World Health Organization; 18 May 1968, p. A21.

6. Thacker SB, Stroup DF, Parrish RG, Anderson HA. Surveillance in environmental public health: issues, systems, and sources. Am J Public Health 1996;86:633–8.

7. Vaughan JP, Morrow RH. Manual of epidemiology for district health management. Geneva: World Health Organization; 1989.

8. Wegman DH. Hazard Surveillance. In: Halperin W, Baker E, Monson R (editors). Public Health Surveillance. New York: Van Nostrand Reinhold; 1992, pp. 62–75.

9. Protocol for the evaluation of epidemiological surveillance systems [monograph on the Internet]. Geneva: World Health Organization [updated 1997; cited 2006 Jan 20]. Available from: http://whqlibdoc.who.int/hq/1997/WHO_EMC_DIS_97.2.pdf.

10. Hopkins RS. Design and operation of state and local infectious disease surveillance systems. J Public Health Management Practice 2005;11(3):184–90.

11. Doherty JA. Establishing priorities for national communicable disease surveillance. Can J Infect Dis 2000;11(1):21–4.

12. Rushdy A, O'Mahony M. PHLS overview of communicable diseases 1997: results of a priority setting exercise. Commun Dis Rep CDR Suppl 1998;8 (suppl 5):S1–12.

13. Centers for Disease Control and Prevention. Case Definitions for Infectious Conditions Under Public Health Surveillance. MMWR 1997;46(No. RR-10):1–55. .

14. Parrish RG, McDonnell SM. Sources of health-related information. In: Teutsch SM, Churchill RE, editors. Principles and practice of Public Health Surveillance, 2nd ed. New York: Oxford University Press; 2000, pp. 30–75.

15. Groves RM, Fowler FJ, Couper MP, Lepkowski J, Singer E, Tourangeau R. Survey methodology. New York: John Wiley; 2004.

16. Hutwagner L, Thompson W, Seeman GM, Treadwell T. The bioterrorism preparedness and response Early Aberration Reporting System (EARS). J Urban Health 2003;80:89–96.

17. Croner CM. Public health GIS and the Internet. Annu Rev Public Health 2003;24:57–82.

18. Guerra M, Walker E, Jones C, Paskewitz S, Cortinas MR, Stancil A, Beck L, Bobo M, Kitron U. Predicting the risk of Lyme disease: habitat suitability for Ixodes scapularis in the north central United States. Emerg Infect Dis. 2002;8:289–97.

19. SaTScan [Internet]. Boston: SaTScan [updated 2006 Aug 14] Available from: http://www.satscan.org/.

20. Centers for Disease Control and Prevention [Internet]. Atlanta: CDC [updated 2005 Nov 8; cited 2006 Jan 31]. EpiInfo. Available from: http://www.cdc.gov/epiinfo/

21. The HealthMapper [Internet] Geneva: World Health Organization [updated 2006; cited 2006 Jan 31]. Available from: http://www.who.int/health_mapping/tools/healthmapper/en/.

22. Centers for Disease Control and Prevention. Current Trends Update: Impact of the expanded AIDS surveillance case definition for adolescents and adults on case reporting—United States, 1993a. MMWR 1994;43:160–1,167–70.

23. Ryan CA, Nickels MK, Hargrett-Bean NT, et al. Massive outbreak of antimicrobial-resistant salmonellosis traced to pasteurized milk. JAMA 1987;258:3269–74.

24. Friedman DJ, Parrish RG. Characteristics, desired functionalities, and datasets of state webbased data query systems. J Public Health Management Practice 2006;12(2):119–129. In press.

25. Henderson DA. Surveillance of smallpox. Int J Epidemiol 1976;5(1):19-28.

26. Centers for Disease Control and Prevention. Outbreak of West Nile-Like Viral Encephalitis-- New York, 1999. MMWR 1999;48(38):845–9.

27. Centers for Disease Control and Prevention. Updated guidelines for evaluating public health surveillance systems: recommendations from the guidelines working group. MMWR 2001;50(No. RR-13):1–35.

28. Centers for Disease Control and Prevention. Framework for evaluating public health surveillance systems for early detection of outbreaks; recommendations from the CDC Working Group. MMWR 2004;53(No. RR-5):1-13.

29. World Health Organization Regional Office for Africa and the Centers for Disease Control and Prevention. Technical Guidelines for Integrated Disease Surveillance and Response in the African Region. Harare, Zimbabwe and Atlanta, Georgia, USA. July 2001: 1–229.

30. Hopkins RS. Consumer product-related injuries in Athens, Ohio, 1980-85: assessment of emergency room-based surveillance. Am J Prev Med 1989 Mar-Apr;5(2):104–12.

31. Schrieber, R.A., Branche-Dorsey, C.M., Ryan, G.W. et al. Risk factors for injuries from in-line skating and the effectiveness of safety gear. N Engl J Med 1996;335:1630–1635.

32. NEISS: The National Electronic Injury Surveillance System - A Tool for Researchers [monograph on the Internet]. Washington (DC): U.S. Consumer Product Safety Commission, Division of Hazard and Injury Data Systems [updated 2000 Mar; cited 2005 Dec 2]. Available from: http://www.cpsc.gov/neiss/2000d015.pdf.

33. Mannino DM, Homa DM, Pertowski CA, et al. Surveillance for asthma—United States, 1960–1995. In: Surveillance Summaries, April 24, 1998. MMWR 1998;47(No. SS- 1):1–28.

34. Mannino DM, Homa DM, Akinbami LJ, Moorman JE, Gwynn C, Redd SC. Surveillance for Asthma—United States, 1980–1999. In: Surveillance Summaries, March 29, 2002. MMWR 2002;51(No. SS-1):1–13.

35. Doyle TJ, Glynn MK, Groseclose SL. Completeness of notifiable infectious disease reporting in the United States: an analytic literature review. Am J Epidemiol 2002;155:866–74.

36. Rosenberg MJ, Marr JS, Gangarosa EJ, Pollard RA, Wallace M, Brolnitsky O. *Shigella* surveillance in the United States, 1975. J Infect Dis 1977;136:458–60.

37. Mead PS, Slutsker L, Dietz V, et al. Food-related illness and death in the United States. Emerg Infect Dis 1999;5:607–25.

38. Campos-Outcalt D, England R, Porter B. Reporting of communicable diseases by university physicians. Public Health Rep 1991;106:579–83.

39. Marier R. The reporting of communicable diseases. Am J Epidemiol 1977;105:587–90.

40. Konowitz PM, Petrossian GA, Rose DN. The underreporting of disease and physicians' knowledge of reporting requirements. Public Health Rep 1984;99:31–5.

41. Hajjeh R, Reingold A, Weil A, Shutt K, Schuchat A, Perkins BA. Toxic shock syndrome in the United States: surveillance update, 1979–1996. Emerg Infect Dis 1999;5:807–10.

Further Reading

Buehler JW. Surveillance. In: Rothman KJ, Greenland S, editors. Modern Epidemiology, 2nd ed. Philadelphia: Williams and Wilkins; 1988, pp. 435–57.

Eylenbosch WJ, Noah ND, editors. Surveillance in health and disease. Oxford: Oxford University Press; 1988.

Langmuir AD. Evolution of the concept of surveillance in the United States. Proc R Soc Med. 1971;64:681–4.

Langmuir AD. William Farr: founder of modern concepts of surveillance. Int J Epidemiol 1976;5(1):13–8.

Orenstein WA, Bernier RH. Surveillance: information for action. Pediatr Clin N Amer 1990;37:709–734.

Rothman KJ. Lessons from John Graunt. Lancet. 1996;347(8993):37–9.

Sandiford P, Annett H, Cibulskis R. What can information systems do for primary health care? An international perspective. Soc Sci Med 1992:34(10):1077–87.

Teutsch SM, Churchill RE, editors. Principles and practice of public health surveillance, 2nd ed. New York: Oxford University Press; 2000.

Websites

For more information on:	Visit the following websites:
CDC Case Definitions	http://www.cdc.gov/epo/dphsi/casedef/case_definitions.htm
CPSC National Electronic Injury Surveillance System (NEISS) On-line	http://www.cpsc.gov/library/neiss.html
Emergency Preparedness & Response: Agents, Diseases, and Other Threats	http://www.bt.cdc.gov/agent/
FDA Adverse Event Reporting System (AERS)	http://www.fda.gov/cder/aers/default.htm
Healthy People 2010: Tracking Healthy People 2010: Part C. Major Data Sources for Healthy People 2010	http://www.healthypeople.gov/Document/html/tracking/THP_PartC.htm
MedWatch, The FDA Safety Information and Adverse Event Reporting Program	http://www.fda.gov/medwatch/index.html
National Health and Nutrition Examination Survey	http://www.cdc.gov/nchs/nhanes.htm
Nationally Notifiable Infectious Diseases	http://www.cdc.gov/epo/dphsi/phs/infdis.htm http://www.cdc.gov/epo/dphsi/nndsshis.htm
NCI cancer mortality maps & graphs	http://www3.cancer.gov/atlasplus/index.html
NCI SEER	http://seer.cancer.gov/faststats/
NIDA DAWN	http://www.drugabuse.gov/DESPR/Assessing/Guide7.html
NIDA Monitoring the Future Survey	http://www.drugabuse.gov/DrugPages/MTF.html
SAMHSA Office of Applied Studies Data Systems and Publications	http://www.drugabusestatistics.samhsa.gov/
Summary of notifiable diseases – United States, 2004	http://www.cdc.gov/mmwr/preview/mmwrhtml/mm5353a1.htm
World Health Organization International Classification of Diseases, 10th revision	http://www.who.int/classifications/icd/en/

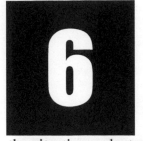

INVESTIGATING AN OUTBREAK

Public health department staff responsible for reviewing disease report forms notice that the number of forms for shigellosis seems higher than usual this week. Someone from a nursing home calls to report several cases of pneumonia among its residents. Is the number of cases in either of these situations actually higher than usual? What should be used to estimate "usual?" If it is higher than usual, should the health department staff call the situation a cluster, an outbreak, an epidemic? Is a field investigation needed? What criteria should they use to decide? And if they decide that a field investigation is indeed warranted, how do they go about conducting such an investigation? These and related questions will be addressed in this lesson.

Objectives

After studying this lesson and answering the questions in the exercises, you will be able to:
- *List the reasons that health agencies investigate reported outbreaks*
- *List the steps in the investigation of an outbreak*
- *Define cluster, outbreak, and epidemic*
- *Given the initial information of a possible disease outbreak, describe how to determine whether an epidemic exists*
- *State the purpose of a line listing*
- *Given information about a community outbreak of disease, list the initial steps of an investigation*
- *Given the appropriate information from the initial steps of an outbreak investigation, develop biologically plausible hypotheses*
- *Draw and interpret an epidemic curve*
- *Given data in a two-by-two table, calculate the appropriate measure of association*

Major Sections

Introduction to Investigating an Outbreak

Uncovering outbreaks

Outbreaks of disease — the occurrence of more cases than expected — occur frequently. Each day, health departments learn about cases or outbreaks that require investigation. While CDC recorded over 500 outbreaks of foodborne illness alone each year during the 1990s,[1] recognized outbreaks of respiratory and other diseases are also common, and many more outbreaks may go undetected.

So how are outbreaks uncovered? One way is to analyze surveillance data — reports of cases of communicable diseases that are routinely sent by laboratories and healthcare providers to health departments (see Lesson 5). Some health departments regularly review exposure information from individual case reports to look for common factors. For example, health department staff in Oregon uncovered an outbreak of *E. coli* O157:H7 in 1997 by noticing that three patients with the infection all had reported drinking raw milk.[2] Alternatively, outbreaks may be detected when health department staff conduct regular, timely analysis of surveillance data that reveals an increase in reported cases or an unusual clustering of cases by time and place. For example, by analyzing data from four different syndromic surveillance systems, health department staff in New York City noted a consistent increase in gastroenteritis in the days following a prolonged blackout in August 2003.[3] Investigation indicated that the increase in gastroenteritis was probably attributable to the consumption of meat that had spoiled during the power failure.

Review of surveillance data to detect outbreaks is not limited to health departments. Many hospital infection control practitioners review microbiologic isolates from patients by organism and ward each week to detect an increase in the number of, say, surgical wound infections or nosocomial (hospital-acquired) cases of legionellosis. In the same way, staff at CDC regularly review laboratory patterns of organisms and are able to detect clusters of illness caused by the same organism, even if the victims are geographically scattered.[4]

Nonetheless, most outbreaks come to the attention of health authorities because an alert clinician is concerned enough to call the health department. The emergence of West Nile virus infection in North America in 1999 was uncovered only after the New York City health department responded to a call from a physician who

---

To uncover outbreaks:

- Review routinely collected surveillance data
- Astutely observe single events or clusters by clinicians, infection control practitioners, or laboratorians
- Review reports by one or more patients or members of the public

had recently seen two patients with encephalitis.[5] Similarly, a single case of inhalational anthrax of suspicious origin in Florida in 2001 resulted in a massive investigation involving multiple government agencies, but it all started with an astute diagnosis and prompt report to the health department by a physician.[6]

Another reporting source for apparent clusters of both infectious and noninfectious disease is patients or other members of the community. For example, an individual may call the health department and report that she and some friends came down with severe gastroenteritis after attending a banquet a night or two earlier. Similarly, a local citizen may call about several cases of cancer diagnosed among his neighbors and express concern that these are more than coincidental. Most health departments have routine procedures for handling calls from the public regarding potential communicable disease outbreaks, and some states have guidelines for how to respond to noninfectious disease cluster reports.[7-9]

Deciding whether to investigate a possible outbreak

Different health departments respond to these reports in different ways. The decisions regarding whether and how extensively to investigate a potential outbreak depend on a variety of factors. These usually include some factors related to the health problem, some related to the health department, and some related to external concerns. Factors related to the problem itself include the severity of the illness, the number of cases, the source, mode or ease of transmission, and the availability of prevention and control measures. Most local health departments are more likely to investigate an apparent outbreak when the number of affected (or exposed) persons is large, when the disease is severe (serious illness with high risk of hospitalization, complications, or death), when effective control measures exist, and when the outbreak has the potential to affect others unless prompt control measures are taken. For example, a single case of gastroenteritis is unlikely to prompt a field investigation, but a cluster of cases may. On the other hand, even a single case of botulism is likely to be investigated immediately to identify and eliminate the source, because it is both potentially fatal and preventable, and the source can usually be identified. At the state or national level, the unusual presentation of disease may spur an investigation. Occurrence of a new or rare disease or a change in the pattern of disease in an area is more likely to prompt an investigation than occurrence of a common disease with well-established transmission patterns and control measures.

Epidemic: the occurrence of more cases of disease than expected in a given area or among a specific group of people over a particular period of time. Usually, the cases are presumed to have a common cause or to be related to one another in some way

Outbreak: epidemic limited to localized increase in the incidence of disease

Cluster: aggregation of cases in a given area over a particular period without regard to whether the number of cases is more than expected

However, field investigations place a burden on a health department, so the decision also hinges on the availability of staff and resources, and competing priorities. In addition, some health departments have a practice of aggressively investigating outbreaks and hence have experience in doing so, while other health departments may lack such experience.

Regardless, field investigations are usually justified for one or more of the following reasons:
- Control or prevention of the health problem
- Opportunity to learn (research opportunity)
- Public, political, or legal concerns
- Public health program considerations
- Training

Each of these reasons is discussed in more detail below.

Control and prevention

The most important public health reasons for investigating an outbreak are to help guide disease prevention and control strategies. These disease control efforts depend on several factors, including knowledge of the agent, the natural course of the outbreak, the usual transmission mechanism of the disease, and available control measures. For example, if a health department learns of an outbreak of hepatitis A (known agent) in which one of the victims is a restaurant cook, the department can offer immune globulin to the restaurant patrons to prevent a second wave of cases (control measure), but only if they are within 14 days of exposure (timing). On the other hand, if an outbreak appears to be almost over, the health agency may not need to implement control measures, but may be interested in identifying factors that contributed to the outbreak in order to develop strategies to prevent similar outbreaks in the future. For that outbreak of hepatitis A, investigators may find that the poor personal hygiene that led to the outbreak was the result of lack of soap or water in the workplace washroom, which could be addressed in public health messages to other worksites.

The balance between control measures and further investigation depends on how much is known about the cause, the source, and the mode of transmission of the agent.[10] Table 6.1 illustrates how public health emphasis on investigation versus control is influenced by these factors. In particular, if the source and/or mode of transmission are known, then control measures that target the source or interrupt transmission can be implemented. If the source and/or mode of transmission are not known, then you can't know what control measures to implement, so investigation takes priority.

Table 6.1 Relative Priority of Investigative and Control Efforts During an Outbreak, Based on Knowledge of the Source, Mode of Transmission, and Causative Agent

| | | Source/Mode of Transmission (How people are getting exposed to the agent) | |
		Known	Unknown
Causative Agent	Known	Investigation + Control +++	Investigation +++ Control +
	Unknown	Investigation +++ Control +++	Investigation +++ Control +

+++ = highest priority
+ = lowest priority

Source: Goodman RA, Buehler JW, Koplan JP. *The epidemiologic field investigation: science and judgment in public health practice. Am J Epidemiol 1990;132:9–16.*

Opportunity to learn (research opportunity)

Another important objective of many outbreak investigations is to advance research. For most public health problems, health officials cannot conduct randomized trials. We cannot randomize who eats the undercooked hamburger or sits near the ice resurfacing machine that emits carbon monoxide, nor should we randomize who receives preventive health benefits (e.g., mammogram screening). However, we can take advantage of what has already happened and learn from it. Some view an outbreak as an experiment of nature waiting to be analyzed and exploited. For a newly recognized disease, field investigation provides an opportunity to characterize the natural history — including agent, mode of transmission, and incubation period — and the clinical spectrum of disease. Investigators also attempt to characterize the populations at greatest risk and to identify specific risk factors. Acquiring such information was an important motivation for investigators studying such newly recognized diseases as Legionnaires' disease in Philadelphia in 1976, AIDS in the early 1980s, hantavirus in 1993, severe acute respiratory syndrome (SARS) in 2003, and avian flu in 2005.

Even for diseases that are well characterized, an outbreak may provide opportunities to gain additional knowledge by assessing the impact of control measures and the usefulness of new epidemiology and laboratory techniques. For example, outbreaks of varicella (chickenpox) in highly immunized communities allowed investigators to determine effectiveness of the new vaccine and immunization recommendations.[11,12] An outbreak of giardiasis provided the opportunity to study the appropriateness of a clinical case definition,[13] while an outbreak of rotavirus was used to study the performance of a novel diagnostic method.[14] With increased access to the Internet and e-mail in the 1990s, outbreak investigations were used to evaluate whether potential controls would respond to e-mail solicitations to participate.[15-17]

Public, political, or legal concerns

Public, political, or legal concerns can be the driving force behind the decision to conduct an investigation. A cluster of cancer cases in a neighborhood may prompt concerned residents to advocate for an investigation. Sometimes the public is concerned that the disease cluster is the result of an environmental exposure such as toxic waste. Investigations of such clusters almost never identify a causal link between exposure and disease.[18,19] Nevertheless, many health departments have learned that they must be "responsibly responsive" to public concerns, even if they think that an epidemiologic link is unlikely.[7,8,20] Similarly, the public may fear that an outbreak is the result of an intentional criminal or bioterrorist act. The health department may be able to allay those fears by documenting that the outbreak was the result of an inadvertent or naturally occurring exposure.

Some investigations are conducted because they are required by law. For example, CDC's National Institute for Occupational Safety and Health (NIOSH) is required to evaluate the risks to health and safety in a workplace if requested to do so by a union, three or more workers, or an employer.[21]

Program considerations

Many health departments run programs to control and prevent communicable diseases such as influenza, tuberculosis, vaccine-preventable diseases, and sexually transmitted diseases. An outbreak of a disease targeted by a public health program may reveal a weakness in that program and an opportunity to change or strengthen program efforts. Investigating the outbreak's causes may identify populations that have been overlooked, failures in intervention strategies, or changes in the agent. Using the outbreak to evaluate program effectiveness can help program directors improve future directions and strategies.

Training

Investigating an outbreak requires a combination of diplomacy, logical thinking, problem-solving ability, quantitative skills, epidemiologic know-how, and judgment. These skills improve with practice and experience. Thus, many investigative teams pair a seasoned epidemiologist with an epidemiologist-in-training. The latter gains valuable on-the-job training and experience while providing assistance in the investigation and control of the outbreak.

Exercise 6.1

During the previous year, nine residents of a community died from cervical cancer. List at least 4 reasons that might justify an investigation.

 Check your answers on page 6-59

Steps of an Outbreak Investigation

Once the decision to conduct a field investigation of an acute outbreak has been made, working quickly is essential — as is getting the right answer. In other words, epidemiologists cannot afford to conduct an investigation that is "quick and dirty." They must conduct investigations that are "quick and clean."[22] Under such circumstances, epidemiologists find it useful to have a systematic approach to follow, such as the sequence listed in Table 6.2. This approach ensures that the investigation proceeds without missing important steps along the way.

Table 6.2 Epidemiologic Steps of an Outbreak Investigation

1. Prepare for field work
2. Establish the existence of an outbreak
3. Verify the diagnosis
4. Construct a working case definition
5. Find cases systematically and record information
6. Perform descriptive epidemiology
7. Develop hypotheses
8. Evaluate hypotheses epidemiologically
9. As necessary, reconsider, refine, and re-evaluate hypotheses
10. Compare and reconcile with laboratory and/or environmental studies
11. Implement control and prevention measures
12. Initiate or maintain surveillance
13. Communicate findings

The steps listed in Table 6.2 are presented in conceptual order; in practice, however, several steps may be done at the same time, or the circumstances of the outbreak may dictate that a different order be followed. For example, the order of the first three listed steps is highly variable — a health department often verifies the diagnosis and establishes the existence of an outbreak before deciding that a field investigation is warranted. Conceptually, control measures come after hypotheses have been confirmed, but in practice control measures are usually implemented as soon as the source and mode of transmission are known, which may be early or late in any particular outbreak investigation.

Each of the steps is described below in more detail, based on the assumption that you are the health department staff member scheduled to conduct the next field investigation.

Step 1: Prepare for field work

The numbering scheme for this step is problematic, because preparing for field work often is not the first step. Only occasionally do public health officials decide to conduct a field investigation before confirming an increase in cases and verifying the diagnosis. More commonly, officials discover an increase in the number of cases of a particular disease and then decide that a field investigation is warranted. Sometimes investigators collect enough information to perform descriptive epidemiology without leaving their desks, and decide that a field investigation is necessary only if they cannot reach a convincing conclusion without one.

Regardless of when the decision to conduct a field investigation is made, you should be well prepared before leaving for the field. The preparations can be grouped into two broad categories: (a) scientific and investigative issues, and (b) management and operational issues. Good preparation in both categories is needed to facilitate a smooth field experience.

Scientific and investigative issues

As a field investigator, you must have the appropriate scientific knowledge, supplies, and equipment to carry out the investigation before departing for the field. Discuss the situation with someone knowledgeable about the disease and about field investigations, and review the applicable literature. In previous similar outbreaks, what have been the sources, modes of transmission, and risk factors for the disease? Assemble useful references such as journal articles and sample questionnaires.

Before leaving for a field investigation, consult laboratory staff to ensure that you take the proper laboratory material and know the proper collection, storage, and transportation techniques. By talking with the laboratory staff you are also informing them about the outbreak, and they can anticipate what type of laboratory resources will be needed.

You also need to know what supplies or equipment to bring to protect yourself. Some outbreak investigations require no special equipment while an investigation of SARS or Ebola hemorrhagic fever may require personal protective equipment such as masks, gowns, and gloves.

Finally, before departing, you should have a plan of action. What are the objectives of this investigation, i.e., what are you trying to accomplish? What will you do first, second, and third? Having a plan of action upon which everyone agrees will allow you to "hit the ground running" and avoid delays resulting from misunderstandings.

Management and operational issues

A good field investigator must be a good manager and collaborator as well as a good epidemiologist, because most investigations are conducted by a team rather than just one individual. The team members must be selected before departure and know their expected roles and responsibilities in the field. Does the team need a laboratorian, veterinarian, translator/interpreter, computer specialist, entomologist, or other specialist? What is the role of each? Who is in charge? If you have been invited to participate but do not work for the local health agency, are you expected to lead the investigation, provide consultation to the local staff who will conduct the investigation, or simply lend a hand to the local staff? And who are your local contacts?

Depending on the type of outbreak, the number of involved agencies may be quite large. The investigation of an outbreak from an animal source may include state and federal departments of agriculture and/or the Food and Drug Administration (FDA). If criminal or bioterrorist intent is suspected, law enforcement agencies and the Federal Bureau of Investigation (FBI) may be in charge, or at least involved. In a natural disaster (hurricane or flood), the Federal Emergency Management Agency (FEMA) may be the lead. Staff from different agencies have different perspectives, approaches, and priorities that must be reconciled. For example, whereas the public health investigation may focus on identifying a pathogen, source, and mode of transmission, a criminal investigation is likely to focus on finding the perpetrator. Sorting out roles and responsibilities in such multi-agency investigations is critical to accomplishing the disparate objectives of the different agencies.

A communications plan must be established. The need for communicating with the public health and clinical community has long been acknowledged, but the need for communicating quickly and effectively with elected officials and the public became obvious during the epidemics of West Nile Virus encephalitis, SARS, and anthrax. The plan should include how often and when to have conference calls with involved agencies, who will be the designated spokesperson, who will prepare health alerts and press releases, and the like. When a federal agency is involved in the survey of 10 or more individuals, the data collection instrument must first be cleared by the White House Office of Management and Budget (OMB).

In addition, operational and logistical details are important.

Arrange to bring a laptop computer, cell phone or phone card, camera, and other supplies. If you are arriving from outside the area, you should arrange in advance when and where you are to meet with local officials and contacts when you arrive in the field. You must arrange travel, lodging, and local transportation. Many agencies and organizations have strict approval processes and budgetary limits that you must follow. If you are traveling to another country, you will need a passport and often a visa. You should also take care of personal matters before you leave, especially if the investigation is likely to be lengthy.

Step 2: Establish the existence of an outbreak

An **outbreak** or an **epidemic** is the occurrence of more cases of disease than expected in a given area or among a specific group of people over a particular period of time. Usually, the cases are presumed to have a common cause or to be related to one another in some way. Many epidemiologists use the terms outbreak and epidemic interchangeably, but the public is more likely to think that epidemic implies a crisis situation. Some epidemiologists apply the term epidemic to situations involving larger numbers of people over a wide geographic area. Indeed, the Dictionary of Epidemiology defines outbreak as an epidemic limited to localized increase in the incidence of disease, e.g., village, town, or closed institution.[23]

In contrast to outbreak and epidemic, a **cluster** is an aggregation of cases in a given area over a particular period without regard to whether the number of cases is more than expected. This aggregation of cases seems to be unusual, but frequently the public (and sometimes the health agency) does not know the denominator. For example, the diagnosis in one neighborhood of four adults with cancer may be disturbing to residents but may well be within the expected level of cancer occurrence, depending on the size of the population, the types of cancer, and the prevalence of risk factors among the residents.

One of the first tasks of the field investigator is to verify that a cluster of cases is indeed an outbreak. Some clusters turn out to be true outbreaks with a common cause, some are sporadic and unrelated cases of the same disease, and others are unrelated cases of similar but unrelated diseases.

Even if the cases turn out to be the same disease, the number of cases may not exceed what the health department normally sees in a comparable time period. Here, as in other areas of epidemiology, the observed is compared with the expected. The expected number is usually the number from the previous few weeks or months, or from a comparable period during the previous few years. For a notifiable disease, the expected number is based on health department surveillance records. For other diseases and conditions, the expected number may be based on locally available data such as hospital discharge records, mortality statistics, or cancer or birth defect registries. When local data are not available, a health department may use rates from state or national data, or, alternatively, conduct a telephone survey of physicians to determine whether they are seeing more cases of the disease than usual. Finally, a survey of the community may be conducted to establish the background or historical level of disease.

Even if the current number of reported cases exceeds the expected number, the excess may not necessarily indicate an outbreak. Reporting may rise because of changes in local reporting procedures, changes in the case definition, increased interest because of local or national awareness, or improvements in diagnostic procedures. A new physician, infection control nurse, or healthcare facility may more consistently report cases, when in fact there has been no change in the actual occurrence of the disease. Some apparent increases are actually the result of misdiagnosis or laboratory error. Finally, particularly in areas with sudden changes in population size such as resort areas, college towns, and migrant farming areas, changes in the numerator (number of reported cases) may simply reflect changes in the denominator (size of the population).

Whether an apparent problem should be investigated further is not strictly tied to verifying the existence of an epidemic (more cases than expected). Sometimes, health agencies respond to small numbers of cases, or even a single case of disease, that may not exceed the expected or usual number of cases. As noted earlier, the severity of the illness, the potential for spread, availability of control measures, political considerations, public relations, available resources, and other factors all influence the decision to launch a field investigation.

Exercise 6.2

For the month of August, 12 new cases of tuberculosis and 12 new cases of West Nile virus infection were reported to a county health department. You are not sure if either group of cases is a cluster or an outbreak. What additional information might be helpful in making this determination?

 Check your answers on page 6-60

Step 3: Verify the diagnosis

The next step, verifying the diagnosis, is closely linked to verifying the existence of an outbreak. In fact, often these two steps are addressed at the same time. Verifying the diagnosis is important: (a) to ensure that the disease has been properly identified, since control measures are often disease-specific; and (b) to rule out laboratory error as the basis for the increase in reported cases.

First, review the clinical findings and laboratory results. If you have questions about the laboratory findings (for example, if the laboratory tests are inconsistent with the clinical and epidemiologic findings), ask a qualified laboratorian to review the laboratory techniques being used. If you need specialized laboratory work such as confirmation in a reference laboratory, DNA or other chemical or biological fingerprinting, or polymerase chain reaction, you must secure a sufficient number of appropriate specimens, isolates, and other laboratory material as soon as possible.

Second, many investigators — clinicians and non-clinicians — find it useful to visit one or more patients with the disease. If you do not have the clinical background to verify the diagnosis, bring a qualified clinician with you. Talking directly with some patients gives you a better understanding of the clinical features, and helps you to develop a mental image of the disease and the patients affected by it. In addition, conversations with patients are very useful in generating hypotheses about disease etiology and spread. They may be able to answer some critical questions: What were their exposures before becoming ill? What do **they** think caused their illness? Do they know anyone else with the disease? Do they have anything in common with others who have the disease?

Third, summarize the clinical features using frequency distributions. Are the clinical features consistent with the diagnosis? Frequency distributions of the clinical features are useful in characterizing the spectrum of illness, verifying the diagnosis, and developing case definitions. These clinical frequency distributions are considered so important in establishing the credibility of the diagnosis that they are frequently presented in the first table of an investigation's report or manuscript.

Step 4: Construct a working case definition

A case definition is a standard set of criteria for deciding whether an individual should be classified as having the health condition of interest. A case definition includes clinical criteria and — particularly in the setting of an outbreak investigation — restrictions by time, place, and person. The clinical criteria should be based on simple and objective measures such as "fever ≥ 40°C (101°F)," "three or more loose bowel movements per day," or "myalgias (muscle pain) severe enough to limit the patient's usual activities." The case definition may be restricted by time (for example, to persons with onset of illness within the past 2 months), by place (for example, to residents of the nine-county area or to employees of a particular plant) and by person (for example, to persons with no previous history of a positive tuberculin skin test, or to premenopausal women). Whatever the criteria, they must be applied consistently to all persons under investigation.

The case definition must not include the exposure or risk factor you are interested in evaluating. This is a common mistake. For example, if one of the hypotheses under consideration is that persons who worked in the west wing were at greater risk of disease, do not define a case as "illness among persons who worked in the west wing with onset between...." Instead, define a case as "illness among persons who worked in the facility with onset between...." Then conduct the appropriate analysis to determine whether those who worked in the west wing were at greater risk than those who worked elsewhere.

Diagnoses may be uncertain, particularly early in an investigation. As a result, investigators often create different categories of a case definition, such as confirmed, probable, and possible or suspect, that allow for uncertainty. To be classified as confirmed, a case usually must have laboratory verification. A case classified as probable usually has typical clinical features of the disease without laboratory confirmation. A case classified as possible usually has fewer of the typical clinical features. For example, in the box on page 6-16, you can see the Pan American Health Organization (PAHO) recommended case definition for meningococcal disease.[24] Here you can see the different categories that PAHO uses for this diagnosis.

> A case definition is a standard set of criteria for deciding whether an individual should be classified as having the health condition of interest.

> ## Meningococcal Disease — PAHO Case Definition
>
> **Clinical case definition**
> An illness with sudden onset of fever (>38.5°C rectal or >38.0°C axillary) and one or more of the following: neck stiffness, altered consciousness, other meningeal sign or petechial or puerperal rash.
>
> **Laboratory criteria for diagnosis**
> Positive cerebrospinal fluid (CSF) antigen detection or positive culture.
>
> **Case classification**
> *Suspected:* A case that meets the clinical case definition.
> *Probable:* A suspected case as defined above and turbid CSF (with or without positive Gram stain) or ongoing epidemic and epidemiological link to a confirmed case.
> *Confirmed:* A suspected or probable case with laboratory confirmation.
>
> *Source: Pan American Health Organization. Case Definitions Meningococcal Disease. Epidemiological Bulletin 2002; 22(4):14–5.*

In the outbreak setting, the investigators would need to specify time and place to complete the outbreak case definition. For example, if investigating an epidemic of meningococcal meningitis in Bamako, the case definition might be the clinical features as described in the box with onset between January and April of this year among residents and visitors of Bamako.

Classifications such as confirmed-probable-possible are helpful because they provide flexibility to the investigators. A case might be temporarily classified as probable or possible while laboratory results are pending. Alternatively, a case may be permanently classified as probable or possible if the patient's physician decided not to order the confirmatory laboratory test because the test is expensive, difficult to obtain, or unnecessary. For example, while investigating an outbreak of diarrhea on a cruise ship, investigators usually try to identify the causative organism from stool samples from a few afflicted persons. If the tests confirm that all of those case-patients were infected with the same organism, for example norovirus, the other persons with compatible clinical illness are all presumed to be part of the same outbreak and to be infected with the same organism. Note that while this approach is typical in the United States, some countries prefer to acquire laboratory samples from every affected person, and only those with a positive laboratory test are counted as true cases.

A case definition is a tool for classifying someone as having or not having the disease of interest, but few case definitions are 100% accurate in their classifications. Some persons with mild illness may be missed, and some persons with a similar but not identical illness may be included. Generally, epidemiologists strive to ensure that a case definition includes most if not all of the actual cases, but very few or no **false-positive** cases. However, this ideal is not always met. For example, case definitions often miss infected people who have mild or no symptoms, because they have little reason to be tested.

More About Case Definitions

Early in an investigation, investigators may use a "loose" or sensitive case definition that includes confirmed, probable, and possible cases to characterize the extent of the problem, identify the populations affected, and develop hypotheses about possible causes. The strategy of being more inclusive early on is especially useful in investigations that require travel to different hospitals, homes, or other sites to gather information, because collecting extra data while you are there is more efficient than having to return a second time. This illustrates an important axiom of field epidemiology: *Get it while you can*. Later on, when hypotheses have come into sharper focus, the investigator may tighten the case definition by dropping the "possible" and sometimes the "probable" category. In analytic epidemiology, inclusion of false-positive cases can produce misleading results. Therefore, to test these hypotheses by using analytic epidemiology (see Step 8), specific or tight case definitions are recommended.

Other investigations, particularly those of a newly recognized disease or syndrome, begin with a relatively specific or narrow case definition. For example, acquired immunodeficiency syndrome (AIDS) and severe acute respiratory syndrome (SARS) both began with relatively specific case definitions. This ensures that persons whose illness meets the case definition truly have the disease in question. As a result, investigators could accurately characterize the typical clinical features of the illness, risk factors for illness, and cause of the illness. After the cause was known and diagnostic tests were developed, investigators could use the laboratory test to learn about the true spectrum of illness, and could broaden the case definition to include those with early infection or mild symptoms.

Exercise 6.3

In 1989, a worldwide epidemic of a previously unrecognized syndrome occurred. This condition was characterized by severe myalgias (muscle pains) and an elevated number of a particular type of white blood cell called an eosinophil. The illness was given the name eosinophilia-myalgia syndrome. Public health officials initially used the following case definition:[25]

Eosinophil count ≥2,000 cells/mm³ in the absence of any other known cause of eosinophilia (in particular, parasitic or fungal infection, end-stage renal disease, leukemia, allergic disorder, or drug reaction)

Using the information in the line listing below, determine whether or not each should be classified as a case, according to the initial case definition above.

Table 6.3 Line Listing of 7 Persons with Suspected Eosinophilia-myalgia

Patient #	Eosinophils (per mm³)	Other Known Cause	Severe Myalgias	Myalgias*	Case? (Initial Def)	Case? (Revised Def)
1	535	No	Yes	No	_____	_____
2	12,100	No	Yes	Yes	_____	_____
3	2,310	No	Yes	Yes	_____	_____
4	2,064	No	Yes	No	_____	_____
5	2,250	No	Yes	Yes	_____	_____
6	1,670	No	Yes	Yes	_____	_____
7	2,115	Leukemia	Yes	Yes	_____	_____

* Severe enough to affect the patient's ability to pursue usual daily activities

Eventually, public health officials agreed on the following revised case definition:[26]

1. A peripheral eosinophil count of ≥1,000 cells/mm³;
2. Generalized myalgia at some point during the illness severe enough to affect the patient's ability to pursue usual daily activities;
3. No infection or neoplasm that could account for #1 or #2.

Reclassify each patient using the revised case definition.

 Check your answers on page 6-60

Exercise 6.4

In December 2003, an outbreak of gastroenteritis occurred among tenth-grade students who had participated in a city-wide field trip. Half of the students traveled from December 2 to December 7 (Tour A); the other half traveled from December 3 to December 8 (Tour B). The itineraries were similar. Although teachers and other adult chaperones accompanied the students on both tours, no adult reported illness. In addition, no illness was reported among students who did not go on the field trip, and no cases of E. coli O157 were reported in the community that week.

A line listing of 26 persons with symptoms of abdominal pain and/or diarrhea is presented below. Using the information in the line listing, develop a case definition that you might use for the outbreak investigation. [Note that persons infected with E. coli O157 typically experience severe abdominal cramps, bloody diarrhea, and low grade fever after a 1- to 8-day incubation period (usually 2-4 days).]

Table 6.4 Line Listing of 26 Persons with Symptoms — School District A, December 2003

Patient #	Grade & School	Age	Sex	Tour	Onset Date	Severe Abdominal Pain?	No. Times Diarrhea	Stool Testing
1	10 — 1	17	M	A	Dec. 8	Y	3	Not done
2	10 — 1	16	F	A	Dec. 6	N	1	Negative
3	10 — 2	16	M	A	Dec. 10	Y	2	*E. coli* O157
4	10 — 2	17	F	A	Dec. 8	Y	3	Not done
5	10 — 2	16	F	A	Dec. 5	Y	8	*E. coli* O157
6	10 — 2	16	M	A	Dec. 6	Y	3	Not done
7	10 — 3	17	M	A	Dec. 7	Y	4	Not done
8	10 — 3	17	F	A	Dec. 8	Y	2	*E. coli* O157
9	10 — 3	16	F	A	Dec. 7	Y	3	Negative
10	10 — 4	17	F	A	Dec. 7	Y	2	*E. coli* O157
11	10 — 4	16	M	A	Dec. 8	Y	3	Not done
12	10 — 4	16	M	A	Dec. 9	Y	3	Negative
13	10 — 5	16	F	A	Dec. 8	Y	3	Not done
14	10 — 6	17	F	B	Dec. 8	Y	3	*E. coli* O157
15	10 — 6	16	F	B	Dec. 9	Y	2	Negative
16	10 — 7	17	F	B	Dec. 6	Y	3	Not done
17	10 — 7	17	F	B	Dec. 7	Y	5	*E. coli* O157
18	10 — 7	16	F	B	Dec. 8	Y	2	Negative
19	10 — 8	17	F	B	Dec. 6	Y	5	*E. coli* O157
20	10 — 8	17	F	B	Dec. 7	Y	3	Negative
21	10 — 9	16	M	B	Dec. 8	Y	2	Not done
22	10 — 9	16	F	B	Dec. 7	Y	3	Negative
23	10 — 9	16	F	B	Dec. 7	Y	3	*E. coli* O157
24	10 — 10	17	F	B	Dec. 9	Y	3	*E. coli* O157
25	10 — 10	17	M	B	Dec. 7	N	1	Negative
26	10 — 10	16	M	B	Dec. 6	Y	3	Not done

 Check your answers on page 6-60

Step 5: Find cases systematically and record information

As noted earlier, many outbreaks are brought to the attention of health authorities by concerned healthcare providers or citizens. However, the cases that prompt the concern are often only a small and unrepresentative fraction of the total number of cases. Public health workers must therefore look for additional cases to determine the true geographic extent of the problem and the populations affected by it.

Usually, the first effort to identify cases is directed at healthcare practitioners and facilities — physicians' clinics, hospitals, and laboratories — where a diagnosis is likely to be made. Investigators may conduct what is sometimes called stimulated or enhanced **passive surveillance** by sending a letter describing the situation and asking for reports of similar cases. Alternatively, they may conduct **active surveillance** by telephoning or visiting the facilities to collect information on any additional cases.

In some outbreaks, public health officials may decide to alert the public directly, usually through the local media. In other situations, the media may have already spread the word. For example, in an outbreak of listeriosis in 2002 caused by contaminated sliceable turkey deli meat, announcements in the media alerted the public to avoid the implicated product and instructed them to see a physician if they developed symptoms compatible with the disease in question.[27]

If an outbreak affects a restricted population such as persons on a cruise ship, in a school, or at a work site, and if many cases are mild or asymptomatic and therefore undetected, a survey of the entire population is sometimes conducted to determine the extent of infection. A questionnaire could be distributed to determine the true occurrence of clinical symptoms, or laboratory specimens could be collected to determine the number of asymptomatic cases.

Finally, investigators should ask case-patients if they know anyone else with the same condition. Frequently, one person with an illness knows or hears of others with the same illness.

In some investigations, investigators develop a data collection form tailored to the specific details of that outbreak. In others, investigators use a generic case report form. Regardless of which form is used, the data collection form should include the following types of information about each case.

- **Identifying information**. A name, address, and telephone number is essential if investigators need to contact patients for additional questions and to notify them of laboratory results and the outcome of the investigation. Names also help in checking for duplicate records, while the addresses allow for mapping the geographic extent of the problem.
- **Demographic information**. Age, sex, race, occupation, etc. provide the **person** characteristics of descriptive epidemiology needed to characterize the populations at risk.
- **Clinical information**. Signs and symptoms allow investigators to verify that the case definition has been met. Date of onset is needed to chart the time course of the outbreak. Supplementary clinical information, such as duration of illness and whether hospitalization or death occurred, helps characterize the spectrum of illness.
- **Risk factor information**. This information must be tailored to the specific disease in question. For example, since food and water are common vehicles for hepatitis A but not hepatitis B, exposure to food and water sources must be ascertained in an outbreak of the former but not the latter.
- **Reporter information**. The case report must include the reporter or source of the report, usually a physician, clinic, hospital, or laboratory. Investigators will sometimes need to contact the reporter, either to seek additional clinical information or report back the results of the investigation.

Traditionally, the information described above is collected on a standard case report form, questionnaire, or data abstraction form. Examples of case report forms are shown in Figure 6.1 (in Exercise 6.5). Investigators then abstract selected critical items onto a form called a line listing (See Lesson 2 for more information on line listings.)

An example of the line listing from the 2001 anthrax investigation is shown in Table 6.5.[28] In a line listing, each column represents an important variable, such as name or identification number, age, sex, case classification, etc., while each row represents a different case. New cases are added to a line listing as they are identified. Thus, a line listing contains key information on every case and can be scanned and updated as necessary. Even in the era of computers, many epidemiologists still maintain a handwritten line listing of key data items, and turn to their computers for more complex manipulations and cross-tabulations.

Table 6.5 Line Listing of Demographic, Clinical, and Exposure Characteristics of 22 Cases of Bioterrorism-Related Anthrax—United States, 2001

Case No.	Onset Date, 2001	Date of Anthrax Diagnosis by Lab Testing	State[a]	Age (yrs)	Sex[a]	Race[a]	Occupation[a]	Case Status[b]	Anthrax Presentation[b]	Outcome	Diagnostic Tests[a]
1	9/22	10/19	NY	31	F	W	NY Post employee	Suspect	Cutaneous	Alive	Serum IgG reactive
2	9/25	10/12	NY	38	F	W	NBC anchor assistant	Confirmed	Cutaneous	Alive	Skin biopsy IHC+ / serum IgG reactive
3	9/26	10/18	NJ	39	M	W	USPS machine mechanic	Suspect	Cutaneous	Alive	Serum IgG reactive
4	9/28	10/15	FL	73	M	W, H	AMI mailroom worker	Confirmed	Inhalational	Alive	Pleural biopsy IHC+ / serum IgG reactive
5	9/28	10/18	NJ	45	F	W	USPS mail carrier	Confirmed	Cutaneous	Alive	Skin biopsy IHC+ and PCR+ / serum IgG reac.
6	9/28	10/12	NY	23	F	W	NBC TV news intern	Suspect	Cutaneous	Alive	Serum IgG reactive
7	9/29	10/15	NY	0.6	M	W	Child of ABC employee	Confirmed	Cutaneous	Alive	Skin biopsy IHC+ / blood PCR+
8	9/30	10/4	FL	63	M	W	AMI photo editor	Confirmed	Inhalational	Dead	Cerebrospinal fluid culture +
9	10/1	10/18	NY	27	F	W	CBS anchor assistant	Confirmed	Cutaneous	Alive	Skin biopsy IHC+ / serum IgG reactive
10	10/14	10/19	PA	35	M	W	USPS mail processor	Confirmed	Cutaneous	Alive	Blood culture + / serum IgG reactive
11	10/14	10/28	NJ	56	F	B	USPS mail processor	Confirmed	Inhalational	Alive	Blood PCR+ / pleural fluid cytology IHC+ / serum IgG reactive
12	10/15	10/29	NJ	43	F	A	USPS mail processor	Confirmed	Inhalational	Alive	Pleural fluid IHC+ / bronchial biopsy IHC+ / serum IgG reactive
13	10/16	10/21	VA	56	M	B	USPS mail worker	Confirmed	Inhalational	Alive	Blood culture +
14	10/16	10/23	MD	55	M	B	USPS mail worker	Confirmed	Inhalational	Dead	Blood culture +
15	10/16	10/26	MD	47	M	B	USPS mail worker	Confirmed	Inhalational	Dead	Blood culture +
16	10/16	10/22	MD	56	M	B	USPS mail worker	Confirmed	Inhalational	Alive	Blood culture +
17	10/17	10/29	NJ	51	F	W	Bookkeeper	Confirmed	Cutaneous	Alive	Skin biopsy IHC+ and PCR+ / serum IgG reactive
18	10/19	10/22	NY	34	M	W, H	NY Post mail handler	Suspect	Cutaneous	Alive	Skin biopsy IHC+
19	10/22	10/25	VA	59	M	W	Government mail processor	Confirmed	Inhalational	Alive	Blood culture +
20	10/23	10/28	NY	38	M	W	NY Post employee	Confirmed	Cutaneous	Alive	Skin biopsy culture +
21	10/25	10/30	NY	61	F	A	Hospital supply worker	Confirmed	Inhalational	Dead	Pleural fluid and blood culture +
22	11/14	11/21	CT	94	F	W	Retired at home	Confirmed	Inhalational	Dead	Blood culture +

[a]NY, New York; FL, Florida; NJ, New Jersey; PA, Pennsylvania; VA, Virginia; DC, District of Columbia; MD, Maryland; CT, Connecticut; F, female; M, male; W, white; B, black; A, Asian; W,H, white with Hispanic ethnicity; NY, New York; NBC, National Broadcasting Company; AMI, American Media Inc.; USPS, United States Postal Service; CBS, Columbia Broadcasting System; PCR, polymerase chain reaction; IHC, immunohistochemical staining; + positive; IgG, immunoglobulin G.
[b]Case status and anthrax presentation are described in the anthrax surveillance case definition in the Methods section.

Source: Jernigan DB, Raghunathan PL, Bell BP, Brechner R, Bresnitz EA, Butler JC, et al. Investigation of bioterrorism-related anthrax, United States, 2001: epidemiologic findings. Emerg Infect Dis 2002;8:1019–28.

Exercise 6.5

Review the six case report forms in Figure 6.1. Create a line listing based on this information.

Figure 6.1

STATE DISEASE REPORT FORM		
NAME Clifton, R.	AGE 46	PHONE 555-2110
ADDRESS 361 Chander St.	SEX Male	RACE White
CITY, STATE Springdale, VA	COUNTY Columbia	
DISEASE Lyme Disease	DATE OF ONSET 8/1/2006	LAB CONFIRMED? Yes
HOSPITAL ALERTED? HOSPITAL NAME Yes	ADMISSION DATE	DISCHARGE DATE
LAB TEST RESULTS WB IgM+ COMMENTS (CLINICAL DESCRIPTION, IMMUNIZATION THEORY, ETC.) Erythema migrans, fatigue, sweats, chills POSSIBLE EXPOSURE		
PHYSICIAN REPORTING Dr. Snow	PHONE 555-1200	DATE OF REPORT 11/24/06

STATE DISEASE REPORT FORM		
NAME Houston, M.	AGE 56	PHONE 555-4897
ADDRESS 4890 Pleasant St.	SEX Female	RACE White
CITY, STATE Arlington, VA	COUNTY Columbia	
DISEASE Lyme Disease	DATE OF ONSET 8/2/2006	LAB CONFIRMED? Yes
HOSPITAL ALERTED? HOSPITAL NAME Yes	ADMISSION DATE	DISCHARGE DATE
LAB TEST RESULTS WB IgM+; WB IgG+ COMMENTS (CLINICAL DESCRIPTION, IMMUNIZATION THEORY, ETC.) Erythema migrans, arthritis, fatigue, sweats, fever POSSIBLE EXPOSURE		
PHYSICIAN REPORTING Dr. Farr	PHONE 555-1313	DATE OF REPORT 11/24/06

STATE DISEASE REPORT FORM		
NAME Mason, M.	AGE 40	PHONE 555-3756
ADDRESS 34 Winifred Ave.	SEX Female	RACE White
CITY, STATE Brookville, VA	COUNTY Columbia	
DISEASE Lyme Disease	DATE OF ONSET 8/17/2006	LAB CONFIRMED? Yes
HOSPITAL ALERTED? HOSPITAL NAME Yes	ADMISSION DATE	DISCHARGE DATE
LAB TEST RESULTS WB IgM+; WB IgG+ COMMENTS (CLINICAL DESCRIPTION, IMMUNIZATION THEORY, ETC.) Erythema migrans POSSIBLE EXPOSURE		
PHYSICIAN REPORTING Dr. Howard	PHONE 555-1950	DATE OF REPORT 11/24/06

STATE DISEASE REPORT FORM

NAME		AGE	PHONE
Michael, S.		53	555-4899
ADDRESS		SEX	RACE
48 Valley Hill Dr.		Male	Black
CITY, STATE Brookville, VA		COUNTY Columbia	
DISEASE Lyme Disease	DATE OF ONSET 9/02/2006	LAB CONFIRMED? Yes	
HOSPITAL ALERTED? HOSPITAL NAME Yes – Columbia Medical Ctr	ADMISSION DATE 9/18/06	DISCHARGE DATE	
LAB TEST RESULTS WB IgM+; WB IgG-			
COMMENTS (CLINICAL DESCRIPTION, IMMUNIZATION THEORY, ETC.) Erythema migrans			
POSSIBLE EXPOSURE			
PHYSICIAN REPORTING Dr. Fine		PHONE 555-1951	DATE OF REPORT 11/24/06

STATE DISEASE REPORT FORM

NAME		AGE	PHONE
Rollins, W.		45	555-4771
ADDRESS		SEX	RACE
127 Midland St.		Male	White
CITY, STATE Portland, VA		COUNTY Columbia	
DISEASE Lyme Disease	DATE OF ONSET Mid May 2006	LAB CONFIRMED? Yes	
HOSPITAL ALERTED? HOSPITAL NAME	ADMISSION DATE	DISCHARGE DATE	
LAB TEST RESULTS WB IgG+			
COMMENTS (CLINICAL DESCRIPTION, IMMUNIZATION THEORY, ETC.) Arthritis, arthralgias, headache, fatigue, sweats, chills			
POSSIBLE EXPOSURE			
PHYSICIAN REPORTING Dr. Howard		PHONE 555-1950	DATE OF REPORT 11/24/06

STATE DISEASE REPORT FORM

NAME		AGE	PHONE
Turner, L.		13	555-1539
ADDRESS		SEX	RACE
12 Elmwood Rd.		Male	Black
CITY, STATE Salem, VA		COUNTY Columbia	
DISEASE Lyme Disease	DATE OF ONSET 2005	LAB CONFIRMED? No	
HOSPITAL ALERTED? HOSPITAL NAME	ADMISSION DATE	DISCHARGE DATE	
LAB TEST RESULTS			
COMMENTS (CLINICAL DESCRIPTION, IMMUNIZATION THEORY, ETC.) Arthritis, arthralgias, fatigue			
POSSIBLE EXPOSURE			
PHYSICIAN REPORTING Dr. Steere		PHONE 555-1234	DATE OF REPORT 11/24/06

 Check your answers on page 6-61

Step 6: Perform descriptive epidemiology

Conceptually, the next step after identifying and gathering basic information on the persons with the disease is to systematically describe some of the key characteristics of those persons. This process, in which the outbreak is characterized by time, place, and person, is called **descriptive epidemiology**. It may be repeated several times during the course of an investigation as additional cases are identified or as new information becomes available.

This step is critical for several reasons.

- Summarizing data by key demographic variables provides a comprehensive characterization of the outbreak — trends over time, geographic distribution (place), and the populations (persons) affected by the disease.
- From this characterization you can identify or infer the population at risk for the disease.
- The characterization often provides clues about etiology, source, and modes of transmission that can be turned into testable hypotheses (see Step 7).
- Descriptive epidemiology describes the where and whom of the disease, allowing you to begin intervention and prevention measures.
- Early (and continuing) analysis of descriptive data helps you to become familiar with those data, enabling you to identify and correct errors and missing values.

Time

Traditionally, a special type of histogram is used to depict the time course of an epidemic. This graph, called an **epidemic curve**, or **epi curve** for short, provides a simple visual display of the outbreak's magnitude and time trend. The classic epidemic curve, such as the one shown in Figure 6.2a from an outbreak of *Salmonella enterica* serotype Enteritidis, graphs the number of cases by date or time of onset of illness.

**Figure 6.2a Outbreak of _Salmonella_ Enteritidis Gastroenteritis —
Maryland, 2003 (Epidemic Curve by 12-Hour Intervals)**

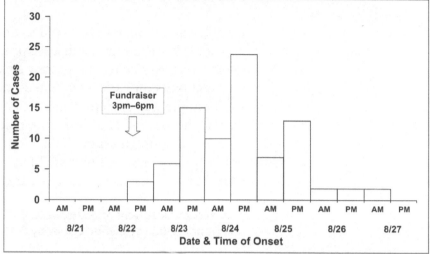

Source: Castel AD, Blythe D, Edwards L, Totaro J, Shah D, Moore M. A large outbreak of
Salmonella Enteritidis infections associated with crabcakes at a church fundraiser–
Maryland, 2003. Presented at 53rd Annual Epidemic Intelligence Service Conference, April
19-23, 2004, Atlanta.

Epidemic curves are a basic investigative tool because they are so informative (see Lesson 4).

- The epi curve shows the magnitude of the epidemic over time as a simple, easily understood visual. It permits the investigator to distinguish epidemic from endemic disease. Potentially correlated events can be noted on the graph.
- The shape of the epidemic curve may provide clues about the pattern of spread in the population, e.g., point versus intermittent source versus propagated.
- The curve shows where you are in the course of the epidemic — still on the upswing, on the down slope, or after the epidemic has ended. This information forms the basis for predicting whether more or fewer cases will occur in the near future.
- The curve can be used for evaluation, answering questions like: How long did it take for the health department to identify a problem? Are intervention measures working?
- Outliers — cases that don't fit into the body of the curve — may provide important clues.
- If the disease and its incubation period are known, the epi curve can be used to deduce a probable time of exposure and help develop a questionnaire focused on that time period.

Drawing an epidemic curve. To draw an epidemic curve, you first must know the time of onset of illness for each case. For some diseases, date of onset is sufficient. For other diseases, particularly those with a relatively short incubation period, hour of onset may be more suitable (see Lesson 4).

Occasionally, you may be asked to draw an epidemic curve when you don't know either the disease or its incubation time. In that situation, it may be useful to draw several epidemic curves with different units on the *x*-axis to find one that best portrays the data. For example, the epidemic curves shown in Figures 6.2b and 6.2c display the same data as in Figure 6.2a; the x-axis is measured in units of 12 hours in Figure 6.2a, 6 hours in Figure 6.2b, and 24 hours (1 day) in 6.2c. Figure 6.2d shows the same data one more time, but with stacks of squares that each represent one case.

Figure 6.2b Outbreak of *Salmonella* Enteritidis Gastroenteritis — Maryland, 2003 (Epidemic Curve by 6-Hour Intervals)

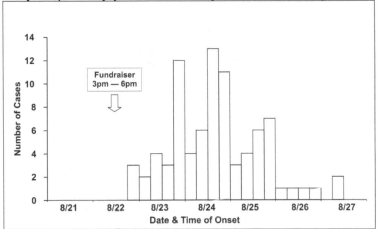

Source: Castel AD, Blythe D, Edwards L, Totaro J, Shah D, Moore M. A large outbreak of Salmonella Enteritidis infections associated with crabcakes at a church fundraiser– Maryland, 2003. Presented at 53rd Annual Epidemic Intelligence Service Conference, April 19-23, 2004, Atlanta.

Figure 6.2c Outbreak of *Salmonella* Enteritidis Gastroenteritis — Maryland, 2003 (Epidemic Curve by One Day Intervals)

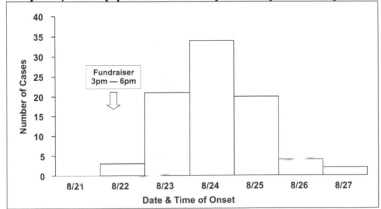

Source: Castel AD, Blythe D, Edwards L, Totaro J, Shah D, Moore M. A large outbreak of Salmonella Enteritidis infections associated with crabcakes at a church fundraiser– Maryland, 2003. Presented at 53rd Annual Epidemic Intelligence Service Conference, April 19-23, 2004, Atlanta.

**Figure 6.2d Outbreak of *Salmonella* Enteritidis Gastroenteritis —
Maryland, 2003 (Epidemic Curve by 6-Hour Intervals)**

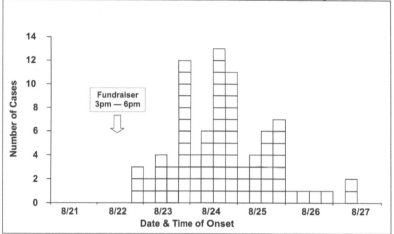

Source: Castel AD, Blythe D, Edwards L, Totaro J, Shah D, Moore M. A large outbreak of
Salmonella Enteritidis infections associated with crabcakes at a church fundraiser–
Maryland, 2003. Presented at 53rd Annual Epidemic Intelligence Service Conference, April
19-23, 2004, Atlanta.

Interpreting an epidemic curve. The first step in interpreting an
epidemic curve is to consider its overall shape. The shape of the
epidemic curve is determined by the epidemic pattern (for
example, common source versus propagated), the period of time
over which susceptible persons are exposed, and the minimum,
average, and maximum incubation periods for the disease.

An epidemic curve that has a steep upslope and a more gradual
down slope (a so-called **log-normal** curve) is characteristic of a
point-source epidemic in which persons are exposed to the same
source over a relative brief period. In fact, any sudden rise in the
number of cases suggests sudden exposure to a common source
one incubation period earlier (Figure 6.3).

In a point-source epidemic, all the cases occur within one
incubation period. If the duration of exposure is prolonged, the
epidemic is called a **continuous common-source epidemic**, and
the epidemic curve has a plateau instead of a peak. An intermittent
common-source epidemic (in which exposure to the causative
agent is sporadic over time) usually produces an irregularly jagged
epidemic curve reflecting the intermittence and duration of
exposure and the number of persons exposed. In theory, a
propagated epidemic — one spread from person-to-person with
increasing numbers of cases in each generation — should have a
series of progressively taller peaks one incubation period apart, but
in reality few produce this classic pattern.

Figure 6.3 Typical Epi Curves for Different Types of Spread

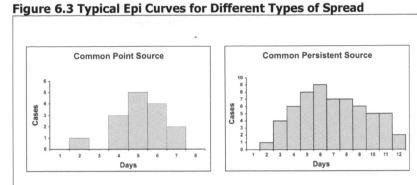

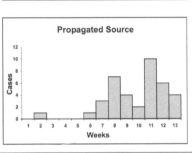

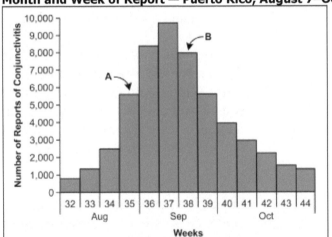

Adapted from: European Programme for Intervention Epidemiology Training [Internet]. Solna, Sweden: Smittskyddsinstitutet [updated 2004 Sep 27; cited 2006 Sep 22] Available from: http://www.epiet.org/course/Presentations/2004/04-Outbreak investigation/03-Outbreak investigation-filer/frame.htm

Figure 6.4 Number of Cases of Acute Hemorrhagic Conjunctivitis, By Month and Week of Report — Puerto Rico, August 7–October 30, 2003

Adapted from: Acute hemorrhagic conjunctivitis outbreak caused by Coxsackievirus A24– Puerto Rico, 2003. MMWR 2004;53:632–4.

As noted above, the epidemic curve shows where you are in the natural course of the epidemic. Consider the epidemic curve of acute hemorrhagic conjunctivitis in Puerto Rico, shown in Figure 6.4. If you only had data through Week 35, that is, through point A, you might conclude that the outbreak is still on the upswing, with more cases to come. On the other hand, if you had data through point B, you might judge that the outbreak has peaked and may soon be over.

The cases that stand apart may be just as informative as the overall pattern. An early case may represent a background or unrelated case, a source of the epidemic, or a person who was exposed earlier than most of the cases (for example, the cook who tasted a dish hours before bringing it to the big picnic). Similarly, late cases may represent unrelated cases, cases with long incubation periods, secondary cases, or persons exposed later than most others (for example, someone eating leftovers). On the other hand, these outlying cases sometimes represent miscoded or erroneous data. All outliers are worth examining carefully because if they are part of the outbreak, they may have an easily identifiable exposure that may point directly to the source.

In a point-source epidemic of a known disease with a known incubation period, the epidemic curve can be used to identify a likely period of exposure. Knowing the likely period of exposure allows you to ask questions about the appropriate period of time so you can identify the source of the epidemic.

To identify the likely period of exposure from an epidemic curve of an apparent point source epidemic:

1. Look up the average and minimum incubation periods of the disease. This information can be found on disease fact sheets available on the Internet or in the *Control of Communicable Diseases Manual.*[29]
2. Identify the peak of the outbreak or the median case and count back on the *x*-axis one average incubation period. Note the date.
3. Start at the earliest case of the epidemic and count back the minimum incubation period, and note this date as well.

Ideally, the two dates will be similar, and represent the probable period of exposure. Since this technique is not precise, widen the probable period of exposure by, say, 20% to 50% on either side of these dates, and then ask about exposures during this widened period in an attempt to identify the source.

In a similar fashion, if the time of exposure and the times of onset of illness are known but the cause has not yet been identified, the incubation period can be estimated from the epidemic curve. Subtract the time of onset of the earliest cases from the time of exposure to estimate the minimum incubation period. Subtract the time of onset of the median case from the time of exposure to estimate the median incubation period. These incubation periods can be compared with a list of incubation periods of known diseases to narrow the possibilities.

EXAMPLE: Interpreting an Epidemic Curve

Consider, for example, the outbreak of hepatitis A illustrated by the epidemic curve in Figure 6.5. The incubation period for hepatitis A ranges from 15 to 50 days (roughly 2 to 7 weeks), with an average incubation period of 28–30 days (roughly one month). Because cases can occur from 15 to 50 days after exposure, all cases from a point source exposure should occur within a span of 50 − 15 = 35 days.

Figure 6.5 Hepatitis A from Sub Shop — Massachusetts, 2001

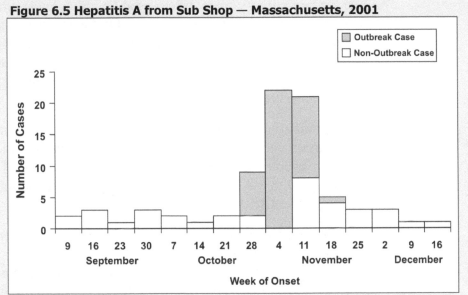

Adapted from: Foodborne transmission of hepatitis A–Massachusetts, 2001. MMWR 2003;52:565–7.

Is this epidemic curve consistent with a point-source epidemic? (That is, do all of the cases occur with one incubation period?)

> Yes. The date of onset of the first case was during the week of October 28. The date of onset of the last known case was during the week of November 18, less than one month later. All of the cases occur within the range of incubation periods expected for a point source exposure. Therefore, the epidemic curve can be used to identify the likely period of exposure.

What is the peak of the outbreak or the median date of onset?

> Both the peak of the outbreak and the median case occurred during the week of November 4.

When is the likely date(s) of exposure, based on one average incubation period prior to the peak (median date) of the outbreak?

> Since both the peak and the median of the outbreak occurred during the week of November 4, the most likely period of exposure was a month earlier, in early October.

When is the beginning of the outbreak?

> The earliest case occurred during the week of October 28.

When is the likely dates of exposure, based on the minimum incubation period before the first case?

> Subtracting 2 weeks from the week of October 28 points to the week of October 14.

Thus you would look for exposures during the weeks of October 7 and 14, plus or minus a few days. This turned out to be the exact period during which a restaurant employee, diagnosed with hepatitis A in mid-October, would have been shedding virus while still working. In summary, the graph reflects an outbreak (number of cases clearly in excess of usual) beginning during the week of October 28, peaking during the week of November 4, and ending during the week of November 18. Based on these data and knowledge of the incubation period of hepatitis A, the period of exposure was probably in early to mid-October.

Exercise 6.6

An outbreak of an acute respiratory disease, coccidioidomycosis, occurred among volunteers, group leaders, and archaeologists who began working at a Native American archaeological site in Utah on June 18.[30]

1. *Using the dates of onset listed below, draw an epidemic curve. Graph paper is provided at the end of this lesson.*

Case #	Date of Onset	Case #	Date of Onset
1	6/28	6	6/29
2	6/28	7	6/29
3	6/29	8	6/30
4	6/29	9	7/1
5	6/29	10	7/1

2. *The average incubation period for coccidioidomycosis is 12 days, with a minimum incubation period of 7 days. Using your epidemic curve and the average and minimum incubation periods for coccidioidomycosis, identify the likely exposure period.*

 Check your answers on page 6-62

Place

Assessment of an outbreak by place not only provides information on the geographic extent of a problem, but may also demonstrate clusters or patterns that provide important etiologic clues. A spot map is a simple and useful technique for illustrating where cases live, work, or may have been exposed.

Some spot maps indicate each patient's residence. If the map shows a cluster or other pattern (such as cases along a road), the investigator must consider possible explanations — perhaps water supplies, wind currents, or proximity to a restaurant or grocery. A spot map, like that used by John Snow in London in 1854 (see Lesson 1, Figure 1.1), can give clues about mode of spread.[31] For example, clustering of cases in a wing of a nursing home is consistent with either a focal source or person-to-person spread, whereas scattering of cases throughout the facility is more consistent with a widely disseminated vehicle or a source common to the residents that is not associated with room assignment, such as a common dining hall or water supply. In an outbreak of pneumococcal pneumonia in a nursing home in New Jersey, cases were more common in the north wing than in the south wing (Figure 6.6). Nursing home staff did report that the 2 residents of the south wing who developed pneumonia did spend much of their time in the north wing.[32]

Figure 6.6 Cases of Pneumonia by Room, Nursing Home A — New Jersey, 2001

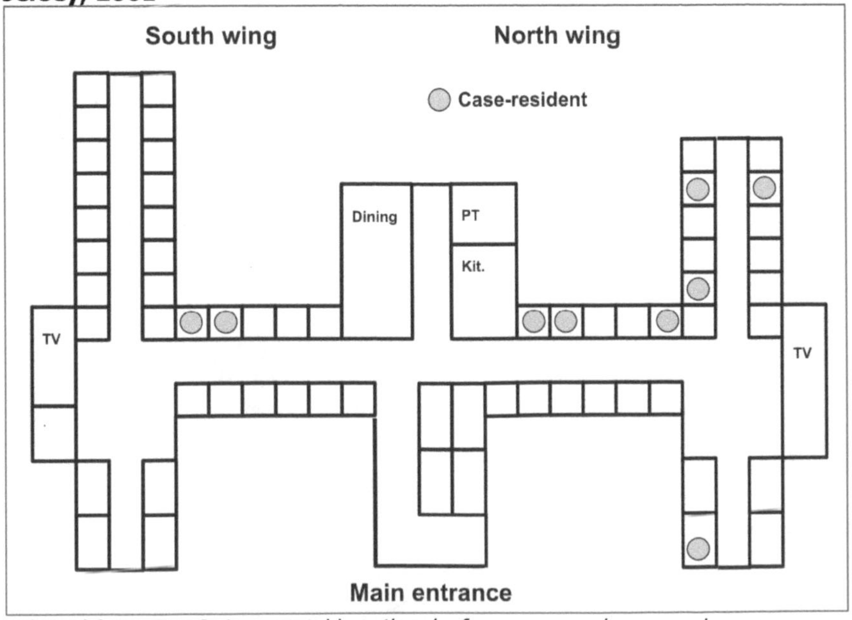

Adapted from: Tan C. A preventable outbreak of pneumococcal pneumonia among unvaccinated nursing home residents in New Jersey during 2001. Infect Control Hosp Epidemiol 2003;24:848–52.

Often, a spot map by site of presumed exposure is more informative than one by residence. Figure 6.7 shows the location of staff in two offices in the U.S. Senate's Hart Building who had nasal swabs positive for *B. anthracis* after an envelope containing anthrax spores was opened in their presence.[33]

To look for clustering in an outbreak of surgical wound infections in a hospital, cases may be plotted by operating room, recovery room, and ward room. In studying "sick-building syndrome" and other disorders related to air-flow patterns in buildings, cases should be plotted by work location. A spot map may even plot sites of recreational or other outdoor exposures.

Figure 6.7 Desk Locations of Persons with Nasal Swabs Positive for
***Bacillus anthracis*, Hart Building — Washington, DC, 2001**

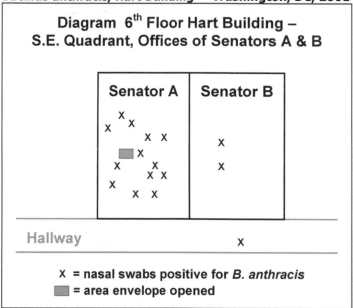

Adapted from: Lukacs SL, Hsu V, Harper S, Handzel T, Hayslett J, Khabbaz R,,et al. Anthrax outbreak averted: public health response to a contaminated envelope on Capital Hill–Washington, DC, 2001. Presented at 51st Annual Epidemic Intelligence Service Conference, April 22-26, 2004, Atlanta.

Spot maps are useful for demonstrating cases within a geographic area, but they do not take the size of the underlying population into account. To compare incidence between different areas with different population densities, an area map showing area-specific rates is preferable. Figure 6.8 shows the number of cases of human granulocytic ehrlichiosis by county in Wisconsin during 1996–1998.[34] The most cases occurred in Washburn (n=21) and Chippewa (n=17) Counties. By dividing the number of cases by the size of the population, county-specific rates of ehrlichiosis can be calculated (Figure 6.9). While Jackson (n=11) and Rusk (n=9) Counties had fewer cases than Chippewa, their populations are much smaller, and they turned out to have higher rates of disease.

**Figure 6.8 Cases of Human Granulocytic Ehrlichiosis by County —
Wisconsin, May 1996–December 1998**

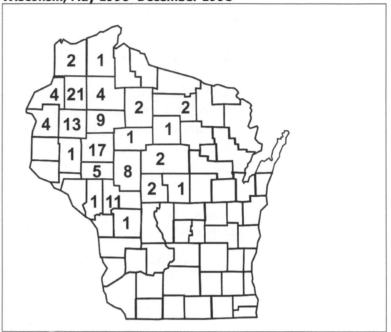

*Source: Ramsey AH, Belongia EA, Gale CM, Davis JP. Outcomes of treated human
granulocytic ehrlichiosis cases. Emerg Infect Dis 2002;8:398-401.*

**Figure 6.9 Rates of Human Granulocytic Ehrlichiosis by County —
Wisconsin, May 1996–December 1998**

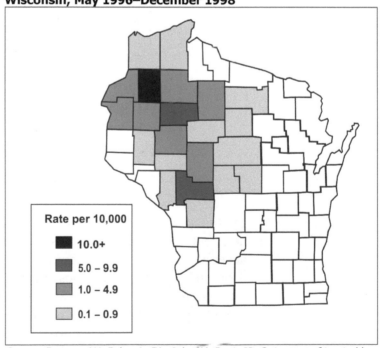

*Source: Ramsey AH, Belongia EA, Gale CM, Davis JP. Outcomes of treated human
granulocytic ehrlichiosis cases. Emerg Infect Dis 2002;8:398-401.*

Person

Characterization of the outbreak by person provides a description of whom the case-patients are and who is at risk. Person characteristics that are usually described include both host characteristics (age, race, sex, and medical status) and possible exposures (occupation, leisure activities, and use of medications, tobacco, and drugs). Both of these influence susceptibility to disease and opportunities for exposure.

The two most commonly described host characteristics are age and sex because they are easily collected and because they are often related to exposure and to the risk of disease. Depending on the outbreak, occupation, race, or other personal characteristics specific to the disease under investigation and the setting of the outbreak may also be important. For example, investigators of an outbreak of hepatitis B might characterize the cases by intravenous drug use and sexual contacts, two of the high risk exposures for that disease. Investigators of a school-based gastroenteritis outbreak might describe occurrence by grade or classroom, and by student versus teacher or other staff.

Early in an investigation, investigators may restrict the descriptive epidemiology to numbers of cases. However, in many circumstances the investigators also calculate rates (number of cases divided by the population or number of people at risk). Numbers indicate the burden of disease and are useful for planning and service delivery. Rates are essential for identifying groups with elevated risk of disease.

Summarizing by time, place, and person

After characterizing an outbreak by time, place, and person, it is useful to summarize what you know. For example, during an investigation of an outbreak of Legionnaires' disease in Louisiana, members of the investigative team discussed what they knew based on the descriptive epidemiology.[35] Specifically, the epidemic curve indicated that the outbreak was basically over, because no new case had been reported in the previous two weeks. The affected population had a greater proportion of persons who were black, female, young, and less likely to smoke than persons in a typical Legionnaires' outbreak. There appeared to be no clustering by either residence or worksite, and no connection with exposure to the town's cooling towers. Thus, the investigators were forced to develop new hypotheses about a source of Legionnaires' disease to explain this outbreak.

Step 7: Develop hypotheses

Although the next conceptual step in an investigation is formulating hypotheses, in reality, investigators usually begin to generate hypotheses at the time of the initial telephone call. Depending on the outbreak, the hypotheses may address the source of the agent, the mode (and vehicle or vector) of transmission, and the exposures that caused the disease. The hypotheses should be testable, since evaluating hypotheses is the next step in the investigation.

In an outbreak context, hypotheses are generated in a variety of ways. First, consider what you know about the disease itself: What is the agent's usual reservoir? How is it usually transmitted? What vehicles are commonly implicated? What are the known risk factors? In other words, by being familiar with the disease, you can, at the very least, "round up the usual suspects."

Another useful way to generate hypotheses is to talk to a few of the case-patients, as discussed in Step 3. The conversations about possible exposures should be open-ended and wide-ranging, not necessarily confined to the known sources and vehicles. In some challenging investigations that yielded few clues, investigators have convened a meeting of several case-patients to search for common exposures. In addition, investigators have sometimes found it useful to visit the homes of case-patients and look through their refrigerators and shelves for clues to an apparent foodborne outbreak.

Just as case-patients may have important insights into causes, so too may the local health department staff. The local staff know the people in the community and their practices, and often have hypotheses based on their knowledge.

The descriptive epidemiology may provide useful clues that can be turned into hypotheses. If the epidemic curve points to a narrow period of exposure, what events occurred around that time? Why do the people living in one particular area have the highest attack rate? Why are some groups with particular age, sex, or other person characteristics at greater risk than other groups with different person characteristics? Such questions about the data may lead to hypotheses that can be tested by appropriate analytic techniques.

Given recent concerns about bioterrorism, investigators should consider intentional dissemination of an infectious or chemical agent when trying to determine the cause of an outbreak. An intentional act, one with either terrorist or criminal intent, should be considered under a variety of circumstances listed in Table 6.6. Investigators of an outbreak of salmonellosis in The Dalles, Oregon, were stumped when they were able to implicate salad bars in several local restaurants, but could not identify any common ingredients or distribution system.[36] A year later, a member of a local cult admitted that the cult had intentionally contaminated the salads bars with *Salmonella* organisms. The lesson learned is that when the epidemiology does not fit the usual or natural patterns of transmission, investigators should think about intentional modes of transmission.

> When the epidemiology does not fit the natural pattern, think unnatural, i.e., intentional.

Table 6.6 Epidemiologic Clues to Bioterrorism

1. Single case of disease caused by an uncommon agent (e.g., glanders, smallpox, viral hemorrhagic fever, inhalational or cutaneous anthrax) without adequate epidemiologic explanation
2. Unusual, atypical, genetically engineered, or antiquated strain of an agent (or antibiotic-resistance pattern)
3. Higher morbidity and mortality in association with a common disease or syndrome or failure of such patients to respond to usual therapy
4. Unusual disease presentation (e.g., inhalational anthrax or pneumonic plague)
5. Disease with an unusual geographic or seasonal distribution (e.g., tularemia in a non-endemic area, influenza in the summer)
6. Stable endemic disease with an unexplained increase in incidence (e.g., tularemia, plague)
7. Atypical disease transmission through aerosols, food, or water, in a mode suggesting deliberate sabotage (i.e., no other physical explanation)
8. No illness in persons who are not exposed to common ventilation systems (have separate closed ventilation systems) when illness is seen in persons in close proximity who have a common ventilation system
9. Several unusual or unexplained diseases coexisting in the same patient without any other explanation
10. Unusual illness that affects a large, disparate population (e.g., respiratory disease in a large population may suggest exposure to an inhalational pathogen or chemical agent)
11. Illness that is unusual (or atypical) for a given population or age group (e.g., outbreak of measles-like rash in adults)
12. Unusual pattern of death or illness among animals (which may be unexplained or attributed to an agent of bioterrorism) that precedes or accompanies illness or death in humans
13. Unusual pattern of death or illness among humans (which may be unexplained or attributed to an agent of bioterrorism) that precedes or accompanies illness or death in animals
14. Ill persons who seek treatment at about the same time (point source with compressed epidemic curve)
15. Similar genetic type among agents isolated from temporally or spatially distinct sources
16. Simultaneous clusters of similar illness in noncontiguous areas, domestic or foreign
17. Large number of cases of unexplained diseases or deaths

Source: Treadwell TA, Koo D, Kuker K, Khan AS. Epidemiologic clues to bioterrorism. Public Health Reports 2003; 118:92–8.

Outliers also can provide important clues. In an outbreak of thyrotoxicosis in 1985, most cases came from Luverne, Minnesota, and the surrounding areas. Only one case was identified in Sioux Falls, South Dakota, 60 miles away. Did this person ever go to Luverne? *Yes.* Was she a friend or acquaintance of any of the Luverne cases? *Not really.* What does she do when she goes to Luverne? *Visit my father and buy the locally produced ground beef that he sells in his store.* Aha! The hypothesis that the locally produced ground beef was the vehicle could easily be tested by asking case-patients and controls (persons without thyrotoxicosis or other thyroid disease) whether they ate ground beef from the same source. Case-patients did, controls did not.[37]

Step 8: Evaluate hypotheses epidemiologically

After a hypothesis that might explain an outbreak has been developed, the next step is to evaluate the plausibility of that hypothesis. Typically, hypotheses in a field investigation are evaluated using a combination of environmental evidence, laboratory science, and epidemiology. From an epidemiologic point of view, hypotheses are evaluated in one of two ways: either by comparing the hypotheses with the established facts or by using analytic epidemiology to quantify relationships and assess the role of chance.

The first method is likely to be used when the clinical, laboratory, environmental, and/or epidemiologic evidence so obviously supports the hypotheses that formal hypothesis testing is unnecessary. For example, in an outbreak of hypervitaminosis D that occurred in Massachusetts in 1991, investigators found that all of the case-patients drank milk delivered to their homes by a local dairy. Therefore, investigators hypothesized that the dairy was the source and the milk was the vehicle. When they visited the dairy, they quickly recognized that the dairy was inadvertently adding far more than the recommended dose of vitamin D to the milk. No analytic epidemiology was really necessary to evaluate the basic hypothesis in this setting or to implement appropriate control measures, although investigators did conduct additional studies to identify additional risk factors.[38,39]

In many other investigations, however, the circumstances are not as straightforward, and information from the series of cases is not sufficiently compelling or convincing. In such investigations, epidemiologists use analytic epidemiology to test their hypotheses. The key feature of analytic epidemiology is a comparison group. The comparison group allows epidemiologists to compare the **observed** pattern among case-patients or a group of exposed persons with the **expected** pattern among noncases or unexposed persons. By comparing the observed with expected patterns, epidemiologists can determine whether the observed pattern differs substantially from what should be expected and, if so, by what degree. In other words, epidemiologists can use analytic epidemiology with its hallmark comparison group to quantify relationships between exposures and disease, and to test hypotheses about causal relationships. The two most common types of analytic epidemiology studies used in field investigations are retrospective cohort studies and case-control studies, as described in the following sections.

Retrospective cohort studies

A retrospective cohort study is the study of choice for an outbreak in a small, well-defined population, such as an outbreak of gastroenteritis among wedding guests for which a complete list of guests is available. In a cohort study, the investigator contacts each member of the defined population (e.g., wedding guests), determines each person's exposure to possible sources and vehicles (e.g., what food and drinks each guest consumed), and notes whether the person later became ill with the disease in question (e.g., gastroenteritis).

After collecting similar information from each attendee, the investigator calculates an attack rate for those exposed to (e.g., who ate) a particular item and an attack rate for those who were not exposed. Generally, an exposure that has the following three characteristics or criteria is considered a strong suspect:

1. The attack rate is high among those exposed to the item.
2. The attack rate is low among those not exposed, so the difference or ratio between attack rates is high.
3. Most of the case-patients were exposed to the item, so that the exposure could "explain" or account for most, if not all, of the cases.

Method for calculating risk ratio:

$$\frac{\text{Attack rate (risk)}}{\text{in exposed group}} \div \frac{\text{Attack rate (risk)}}{\text{in unexposed group}}$$

Relative and attributable risk. Commonly, the investigator compares the attack rate in the exposed group to the attack rate in the unexposed group to measure the association between the exposure (e.g., the food item) and disease. This is called the **risk ratio** or the **relative risk**. When the attack rate for the exposed group is the same as the attack rate for the unexposed group, the relative risk is equal to 1.0, and the exposure is said not to be associated with disease. The greater the difference in attack rates between the exposed and unexposed groups, the larger the relative risk, and the stronger the association between exposure and disease.

Table 6.7 includes data from an investigation of an outbreak of *Salmonella* Typhimurium gastroenteritis following a company's holiday banquet in December 2003.[40] Approximately 135 persons attended the party, and of 116 who were interviewed, 57 (49%) met the case definition. Food-specific attack rates for those who did and did not eat each of 9 items served only at this banquet are presented.

Scan the column of attack rates among those who ate the specified items and consider the three criteria listed on the previous page. Which item shows the highest attack rate? Is the attack rate low among persons not exposed to that item? Were most of the 57 case-patients exposed to that food item?

Table 6.7 Attack Rates By Items Served at Company A's Holiday Banquet — Virginia, December 2003

Food Items Served	Number of Persons who ATE Specified Food				Number of Persons who DID NOT EAT Specified Food				Risk Ratio
	Ill	Not Ill	Total	Attack Rate	Ill	Not Ill	Total	Attack Rate	
Beef	53	28	81	65%	4	31	35	11%	5.7
Ravioli	43	35	78	55%	14	24	38	37%	1.5
Cajun sauce*	19	11	30	63%	37	48	85	44%	1.5
Pesto cream*	37	29	66	56%	19	30	49	39%	1.4
California rolls*	21	14	35	60%	34	44	78	44%	1.4
Mushrooms*	32	26	58	55%	24	31	55	44%	1.3
Broccoli*	34	30	64	53%	22	29	51	43%	1.2
Carrots*	34	30	64	53%	23	28	51	43%	1.2
Potatoes*	39	41	80	49%	17	17	34	50%	1.0

*Excludes 1 or more persons with indefinite history of consumption of that food.

Source; Jani AA, Barrett E, Murphy J, Norton D, Novak C, Painter J, Toney D. A steamship full of trouble: an outbreak of Salmonella Typhimurium DT 104 gastroenteritis at a holiday banquet–Virginia, 2003. Presented at 53rd Annual Epidemic Intelligence Service Conference, April 19-23, 2004, Atlanta.

Beef, which had the highest attack rate among those who ate it, the lowest attack rate among those who did not eat it, and could account for almost all (53 of 57) of the cases, was indeed the culprit. The data showing the relationship between an exposure and disease are often displayed in a two-by-two table. The following two-by-two table shows the data for beef and gastroenteritis.

Table 6.8 Risk of Gastroenteritis By Consumption of Beef — Virginia, December 2003

		Ill	Not Ill	Total	Attack Rate (Risk)
Ate beef?	Yes	53	28	81	65.4%
	No	4	31	35	11.4%
	Total	57	59	116	49.1%

Risk ratio = 65.4 / 11.4 = 5.7

Proportion of cases exposed = 53 / 57 = 93.0%
Population attributable risk percent = (49.1 - 11.4) / 49.1 = 76.7%

Source; Jani AA, Barrett E, Murphy J, Norton D, Novak C, Painter J, Toney D. A steamship full of trouble: an outbreak of Salmonella Typhimurium DT 104 gastroenteritis at a holiday banquet–Virginia, 2003. Presented at 53rd Annual Epidemic Intelligence Service Conference, April 19-23, 2004, Atlanta.

The risk ratio is calculated as the ratio of the attack rates or risks, i.e., 65.4% divided by 11.4%, which equals 5.7. This risk ratio indicates that persons who ate the beef were 5.7 times more likely to become ill than those who did not eat the beef.

Considering the third criterion listed earlier, notice that almost all (53 out of 57) of the cases could be accounted for by the beef. Some investigators use a more quantitative approach and calculate a population attributable risk percent for each food. The population attributable risk percent describes the proportion of illness in the entire study population that could be attributable to a given exposure, assuming that those who became ill in the unexposed group and a similar proportion in the exposed group must be attributable to something else. The population attributable risk percent may actually be an underestimate in many outbreaks, since it does not take into account such common occurrences as cross-contamination of foods or sampling of a spouse's dish. The population attributable risk percent for beef was 76.7% (see Table 6.8), much higher than that for any other food.

Statistical significance testing. When an exposure is found to have a relative risk different from 1.0, many investigators calculate a chi-square or other test of statistical significance to determine the likelihood of finding an association as large or larger on the basis of chance alone. A detailed description of statistical testing is beyond the scope of this lesson, but the following text presents some key features and formulas.

To test an association for statistical significance, assume first that the exposure is not related to disease, i.e., the relative risk (RR) equals 1.0. This assumption is known as the **null hypothesis**. The **alternative hypothesis**, which will be adopted if the null hypothesis proves to be implausible, is that exposure is associated with disease. Next, compute a measure of association, such as a risk ratio or odds ratio. Then calculate a chi-square or other statistical test. This test indicates the probability of finding an association as strong as or stronger than the one you have observed if the null hypothesis were really true, that is, if in reality the exposure being tested was not related to the disease. This probability is called the **p-value**. A very small p-value means that the observed association occurs only rarely if the null hypothesis is true. If the p-value is smaller than some cutoff that has been specified in advance, commonly 0.05 or 5%, you discard or reject the null hypothesis in favor of the alternative hypothesis.

Table 6.9 shows the standard notation for a two-by-two table.

Table 6.9 Standard Notation of a Two-By-Two Table

	Ill	Well	Total	Attack Rate (Risk)
Exposed	a	b	$a+b = H_1$	$a / a+b$
Unexposed	c	d	$c+d = H_0$	$c / c+d$
Total	$a+c=V_1$	$b+d=V_2$	T	V_1 / T

The most common statistical test for data in a two-by-two table from an outbreak is the chi-square test. To apply this test, calculate the chi-square statistic, then look up its corresponding p-value in a table of chi-squares, such as Table 6.10. Since a two-by-two table has 1 degree of freedom, a chi-square larger than 3.84 corresponds to a p-value smaller than 0.05. This means that if you planned to reject the null hypothesis if the p-value is less than 0.05, you can do so if your value for chi-square is greater than 3.84. Recognize, however, that the chi-square and similar tests are guides to help you make a decision about a hypothesis. Whichever decision you make, you may be right or you may be wrong. You could calculate a p-value that is not less than 0.05 and consequently fail to reject the null hypothesis, which may turn out to be true. This often occurs when a study has relatively few people. The opposite can also occur — a p-value less than 0.05 can actually be a chance finding rather than the true explanation of the outbreak.

One formula for the chi-square test:

$$\frac{T(ad-bc)^2}{H_1 \times H_0 \times V_1 \times V_2}$$

Table 6.10 Table of Chi-Squares

Degrees of Freedom	Probability						
	.50	.20	.10	.05	.02	.01	.001
1	.455	1.642	2.706	3.841	5.412	6.635	10.827
2	1.386	3.219	4.605	5.991	7.824	9.210	13.815
3	2.366	4.642	6.251	7.815	9.837	11.345	16.268
4	3.357	5.989	7.779	9.488	11.668	13.277	18.465
5	4.351	7.289	9.236	11.070	13.388	15.086	20.517
10	9.342	13.442	15.987	18.307	21.161	23.209	29.588
15	14.339	19.311	22.307	24.996	28.259	30.578	37.697
20	19.337	25.038	28.412	31.410	35.020	37.566	43.315
25	24.337	30.675	34.382	37.652	41.566	44.314	52.620
30	29.336	36.250	40.256	43.773	47.962	50.892	59.703

Consider the gastroenteritis and beef consumption data presented in Table 6.8. The relative risk is 5.7, which most epidemiologists would deem a "strong" association between exposure and disease. In addition, the p-value is exceedingly small, less than 0.001, and far less than the commonly used cutoff of 0.05. So the investigators rejected the null hypothesis (that beef was not associated with illness) and adopted the alternative hypothesis (that beef was indeed associated with illness). In this outbreak, the association between eating beef at the banquet and gastroenteritis was both strong (RR=5.7) and statistically significant (p < 0.001).

The chi-square test works well if the number of people in the study is greater than about 30. For smaller studies, a test called the Fisher Exact Test may be more appropriate. Because the Fisher Exact Test is tedious to calculate, let Epi Info or another computer program perform the calculations for you.

Confidence intervals. An alternative to calculating a p-value is calculating a confidence interval. A 95% confidence interval, the interval used most commonly by epidemiologists, corresponds to a p=0.05 cut-off. In non-technical terms, a confidence interval for a risk ratio is the range of values of the risk ratio consistent with the data in a study. A wide confidence interval indicates that the study is consistent with a wide range of values, i.e., the study is not very precise in describing the strength of the association (risk ratio) between exposure and disease. A narrow confidence interval indicates that the risk ratio is fairly precise. Consider again the gastroenteritis data in Table 6.8. The 95% confidence interval for the risk ratio of 5.7 ranged from 2.2 to 14.6. This confidence interval indicates that the study is consistent with risk ratios for the beef/gastroenteritis association in that range.

Because a confidence interval provides more information than a p-value does, many medical and epidemiologic journals now prefer confidence intervals to p-values. However, in the outbreak setting, the difference may be irrelevant. If the objective of an outbreak investigation is to identify the culprit such as a contaminated food, a relative risk and p-value may do just as well as a relative risk and confidence interval.

Case-control studies

A cohort study is feasible only when the population is well defined and can be followed over a period of time. However, in many outbreak settings, the population is not well defined and speed of investigation is important. In such settings, the case-control study becomes the study design of choice.

In a case-control study, the investigator asks both case-patients and a comparison group of persons without disease ("controls") about their exposures. Using the information about disease and exposure status, the investigator then calculates an **odds ratio** to quantify the relationship between exposure and disease. Finally, a p-value or confidence interval is calculated to assess statistical significance.

Choosing controls. When designing a case-control study, one of the most important decisions is deciding who the controls should be. The controls must not have the disease being studied, but should represent the population in which the cases occurred. In other words, they should be similar to the cases except that they don't have the disease. The controls provide the level of exposure you would expect to find among the case-patients if the null hypothesis were true. If exposure is much more common among the case-patients than among the controls, i.e., the observed exposure among case-patients is greater than expected exposure provided by the controls, then exposure is said to be associated with illness.

In practice, choosing who the most appropriate control group is may be quite difficult. In addition, investigators must consider logistical issues, such as how to contact potential controls, gain their cooperation, ensure that they are free of disease, and obtain appropriate exposure data from them. In a community outbreak, a random sample of the healthy population may, in theory, be the best control group. In practice, however, persons in a random sample may be difficult to contact and enroll. Nonetheless, many investigators attempt to enroll such "population-based" controls through dialing of random telephone numbers in the community or through a household survey.

Other common control groups consist of:
- Neighbors of case-patients,
- Patients from the same physician practice or hospital who do not have the disease in question,
- Friends of case-patients.

While controls from these groups may be more likely to participate in the study than randomly identified population-based controls, they may not be as representative of the population. If the control group is systematically different from the case group in certain ways, a true association between exposure and disease may be missed or a spurious association may be observed between a non-causal exposure and disease. A systematic difference between cases and controls that results in a mistaken estimate of the association between exposure and disease is called a **bias**.

When designing a case-control study, you must consider a variety of other issues about controls, including how many to use. Sample size formulas are available to help you make this decision. In general, the more subjects (case-patients and controls) in a study, the easier it will be to find a statistically significant association.

Often, the number of case-patients that can be enrolled in a study is limited by the size of the outbreak. For example, in a hospital, four or five cases may constitute an outbreak. Fortunately, potential controls are usually plentiful. In an outbreak of 50 or more cases, one control per case will usually suffice. In smaller outbreaks, you might use two, three, or four controls per case. Including more than four controls per case is rarely worth the effort in terms of increasing the statistical power of your investigation.

As an example, consider again the outbreak of Legionnaires' disease that occurred in Louisiana described at the end of Step 6. Investigators enrolled 27 case-patients into a case-control study. They also enrolled two controls per case, a total of 54 controls. Using descriptive epidemiology, the investigators did not see any connection with the town's various cooling towers. Using analytic epidemiology, the investigators determined quantitatively that case-patients and controls were about equally exposed to cooling towers. However, case-patients were far more likely to shop at a particular grocery store, as shown in the following two-by-two table.[35]

Table 6.11 Exposure to Grocery Store A Among Cases and Controls, Legionellosis Outbreak — Louisiana, 1990

	Cases	Controls	Total
Exposed	25	28	53
Unexposed	2	26	28

Data Source: Mahoney FJ, Hoge CW, Farley TA, Barbaree JM, Breiman RF, Benson RF, McFarland LM. Communitywide outbreak of Legionnaires' disease associated with a grocery store mist machine. J Infect Dis 1992;165:736–9.

Method for calculating the odds ratio:

$$\frac{\left(\begin{array}{c} \text{Number of exposed cases} \\ X \\ \text{Number of unexposed controls} \end{array}\right)}{\left(\begin{array}{c} \text{Number of exposed controls} \\ X \\ \text{Number of unexposed cases} \end{array}\right)}$$

OR

$$ad / bc$$

Odds ratios. In most case-control studies, the population is not well defined, and the total number of people exposed (or unexposed) to a suspected vehicle or source is not known. Without a proper denominator, attack rates cannot be calculated. In the example above, since the investigators did not know how many community residents did or did not shop at Grocery Store A, they could not calculate attack rates or a risk ratio. For a case-control study, the measure of association of choice is the **odds ratio**. Fortunately, for a rare disease such as legionellosis and most other outbreak-associated diseases, the odds ratio from a case-control study approximates the relative risk that would have been found if a cohort study had been feasible.

The odds ratio for Grocery Store A is calculated as:

$$25 \times 26 / 28 \times 2 = 11.6$$

An odds ratio of 11 is quite large, indicating that shopping at Grocery Store A was strongly associated with developing legionellosis. These data would seem to indicate that persons exposed to Grocery Store A had 11.6 times the odds of developing legionellosis than persons not exposed to that store.

To test the statistical significance of this finding, a chi-square test can be computed using the formula shown earlier.

For Grocery Store A, the chi-square is:

$$= \frac{81 \times (25 \times 26 - 28 \times 2)^2}{53 \times 28 \times 27 \times 54}$$

$$= 28{,}579{,}716 \, / \, 2{,}163{,}672$$

$$= 13.02$$

Referring to Table 6.10, a chi-square of 13.02 corresponds to a p-value less than 0.001. A p-value this small indicates that the null hypothesis is highly improbable, and the investigators rejected the null hypothesis. The 95% confidence interval ranged from 2.3 to 78.7. Although this confidence interval is quite wide and includes a wide range of values compatible with the data in the study, it does not include the null hypothesis value of 1.0.

Exercise 6.7

You are called to help investigate a cluster of 17 persons who developed brain cancer in an area over the past couple of years. Most, perhaps all, used cell phones. Which study design would you choose to investigate a possible association between cell phone use and brain cancer?

 Check your answers on page 6-62

Exercise 6.8

Investigators conducted a case-control study of histoplasmosis among industrial plant workers in Nebraska.[41] The following table shows the number of case-patients and controls who worked in Building X, near a recently excavated site.

	Cases	Controls	Total
Building X	15	8	23
Other Building	7	23	30
Total	22	31	53

1. *What is the appropriate measure of association?*

2. *Calculate this measure.*

3. *The chi-square is 9.41, and the 95% confidence interval is 1.6-25.1. How would you interpret your results?*

✔ **Check your answers on page 6-63**

Exercise 6.9

Consider the following data from an outbreak of gastroenteritis among college football players.[42] At which meal do you think the critical exposure occurred?

Meal	Ate Meal			Did Not Eat Meal		
	#Ill	(% Ill)	Total	#Ill	(% Ill)	Total
9/18 Breakfast	9	(90)	10	45	(46)	98
9/18 Lunch	50	(62)	81	4	(15)	27
9/18 Dinner	45	(52)	87	9	(43)	21
9/18 Late dinner	34	(54)	63	20	(44)	45
9/19 Breakfast	42	(49)	85	12	(52)	23
9/19 Lunch	39	(51)	76	15	(47)	32

 Check your answers on page 6-63

Step 9: Reconsider, refine, and re-evaluate hypotheses

Unfortunately, analytic studies sometimes are unrevealing. This is particularly true if the hypotheses were not well founded at the outset. It is an axiom of field epidemiology that if you cannot generate good hypotheses (for example, by talking to some case-patients or local staff and examining the descriptive epidemiology and outliers), then proceeding to analytic epidemiology, such as a case-control study, is likely to be a waste of time.

When analytic epidemiology is unrevealing, rethink your hypotheses. Consider convening a meeting of the case-patients to look for common links or visiting their homes to look at the products on their shelves. Consider new vehicles or modes of transmission.

An investigation of an outbreak of *Salmonella* Muenchen in Ohio illustrates how a reexamination of hypotheses can be productive. In that investigation, a case-control study failed to implicate any plausible food source as a common vehicle. Interestingly, all case-households but only 41% of control households included persons aged 15–35 years. The investigators thus began to consider vehicles of transmission to which young adults were commonly exposed. By asking about drug use in a second case-control study, the investigators implicated marijuana as the likely vehicle. Laboratory analysts subsequently isolated the outbreak strain of *S.* Muenchen from several samples of marijuana provided by case-patients.[43]

Even when an analytic study identifies an association between an exposure and disease, the hypothesis may need to be honed. For example, in the investigation of Legionnaires' disease (Table 6.11), what about Grocery Store A linked it to disease? The investigators asked case-patients and controls how much time they spent in the store and where they went in the store. Using the epidemiologic data, the investigators were able to implicate the ultrasonic mist machine that sprayed the fruits and vegetables. This association was confirmed in the laboratory, where the outbreak subtype of the Legionnaires' disease bacillus was isolated from the water in the mist machine's reservoir.[35]

Sometimes a more specific control group is needed to test a more specific hypothesis. For example, in many hospital outbreaks, investigators use an initial study to narrow their focus. They then conduct a second study, with more closely matched controls, to identify a more specific exposure or vehicle. In a large community outbreak of botulism in Illinois, investigators used three sequential case-control studies to identify the vehicle. In the first study, investigators compared exposures of case-patients and controls from the general public to implicate a restaurant. In a second study they compared restaurant exposures of case-patients and healthy restaurant patrons to identify a specific menu item, a meat and cheese sandwich. In a third study, investigators used radio broadcast appeals to identify healthy restaurant patrons who had eaten the implicated sandwich. Compared to case-patients who had also eaten the sandwich, controls were more likely to have avoided the onions that came with the sandwich. Type A *Clostridium botulinum* was then identified from a pan of leftover sautéed onions used to make only that particular sandwich.[44]

Finally, recall that one reason to investigate outbreaks is research. An outbreak may provide an "experiment of nature" that would be unethical to set up deliberately but from which the scientific community can learn when it does happen to occur. For example, the outbreak of West Nile virus in Queens, New York, in 1999 was promptly investigated to determine the extent of the outbreak and risk factors for disease so appropriate control measures could be developed and implemented.[45] However, capitalizing on this unfortunate "experiment of nature," investigators continued to follow the patients to determine the persistence of IgM and the prognosis of patients up to two years after infection.[46,47] Thus, the investigations resulted not only in the development of appropriate control and prevention strategies, but also in increased knowledge about a health problem not previously seen or studied in the Western hemisphere.

When an outbreak occurs, whether it is routine or unusual, consider what questions remain unanswered about that particular disease and what kind of study you might do in this setting to answer some of those questions. The circumstances may allow you to learn more about the disease, its modes of transmission, the characteristics of the agent, host factors, and the like.

Step 10: Compare and reconcile with laboratory and environmental studies

While epidemiology can implicate vehicles and guide appropriate public health action, laboratory evidence can confirm the findings. The laboratory was essential in both the outbreak of salmonellosis linked to marijuana and in the Legionellosis outbreak traced to the grocery store mist machine. You may recall that the investigation of pneumonia among attendees of an American Legion conference in Philadelphia in 1976 that gave Legionnaires' disease its name was not considered complete until a new organism was isolated in the laboratory some six months later.[48]

Environmental studies are equally important in some settings. They are often helpful in explaining why an outbreak occurred. For example, in the investigation of the outbreak of *E. coli* O157:H7 among visitors to a county fair, the epidemiologists were able to identify one very strong risk factor — consumption of beverages with ice purchased from a vendor in zone 6. Environmental inspection of the fairgrounds identified lack of chlorination of the well supplying water to that zone. Furthermore, the well was found to be close to the manure pits and a septic tank for the worker's dormitory. Flourescein dye poured into the bathroom of the dorm found its way into the well water, revealing cross-contamination. Finally, laboratorians were able to culture *E. coli* from the well, the supply line, and the tap at zone 6.[49] Thus the epidemiologic, environmental, and laboratory arms of the investigation complemented one another, and led to an inescapable conclusion that the well had been contaminated and was the source of the outbreak.

While you may not be an expert in these other areas, you can help. Use a camera to photograph working or environmental conditions. Coordinate with the laboratory, and bring back physical evidence to be analyzed.

Step 11: Implement control and prevention measures

In most outbreak investigations, the primary goal is control of the outbreak and prevention of additional cases. Indeed, although implementing control and prevention measures is listed as Step 11 in the conceptual sequence, in practice control and prevention activities should be implemented as early as possible. The health department's first responsibility is to protect the public's health, so if appropriate control measures are known and available, they should be initiated even before an epidemiologic investigation is launched. For example, a child with measles in a community with other susceptible children may prompt a vaccination campaign before an investigation of how that child became infected.

Confidentiality is an important issue in implementing control measures. Healthcare workers need to be aware of the confidentiality issues relevant to collection, management and sharing of data. For example, in the treatment of tuberculosis (TB), the relationship between the patient and the healthcare worker is extremely important because of the serious consequences of treatment failure. If patient information is disclosed to unauthorized persons without the patient's permission, the patient may be stigmatized or experience rejection from family and friends, lose a job, or be evicted from housing. Moreover, the healthcare worker may lose the trust of the patient, which can affect adherence to TB treatment. Therefore, confidentiality — the responsibility to protect a patient's private information — is critical in TB control and many other situations.[50]

In general, control measures are usually directed against one or more segments in the chain of transmission (agent, source, mode of transmission, portal of entry, or host) that are susceptible to intervention. For some diseases, the most appropriate intervention may be directed at controlling or eliminating the agent at its source. A patient with a communicable disease such as tuberculosis, whether symptomatic or asymptomatic, may be treated with antibiotics both to clear the infection and to reduce the risk of transmission to others. For an environmental toxin or infectious agent that resides in soil, the soil may be decontaminated or covered to prevent escape of the agent.

Some interventions are aimed at blocking the mode of transmission. Interruption of direct transmission may be accomplished by isolation of someone with infection, or counseling persons to avoid the specific type of contact associated with transmission. Similarly, to control an outbreak of influenza-like illness in a nursing home, affected residents could be **cohorted**, that is, put together in a separate area to prevent transmission to others. Vehicle borne transmission may be interrupted by elimination or decontamination of the vehicle. For example, contaminated foods should be discarded, and surgical equipment is routinely sterilized to prevent transmission. Efforts to prevent fecal-oral transmission often focus on rearranging the environment to reduce the risk of contamination in the future and on changing behaviors, such as promoting hand washing. For airborne diseases, strategies may be directed at modifying ventilation or air pressure, and filtering or treating the air. To interrupt vector borne transmission, measures may be directed toward controlling the vector population, such as spraying to reduce the mosquito population that may carry West Nile virus.

Some simple and effective strategies protect portals of entry. For example, bed nets are used to protect sleeping persons from being bitten by mosquitoes that may transmit malaria. A dentist's mask and gloves are intended to protect the dentist from a patient's blood, secretions, and droplets, as well to protect the patient from the dentist. Wearing of long pants and sleeves and use of insect repellent are recommended to reduce the risk of Lyme disease and West Nile virus infection.

Some interventions aim to increase a host's defenses. Vaccinations promote development of specific antibodies that protect against infection. Similarly, prophylactic use of antimalarial drugs, recommended for visitors to malaria-endemic areas, does not prevent exposure through mosquito bites but does prevent infection from taking root.

Step 12: Initiate or maintain surveillance

Once control and prevention measures have been implemented, they must continue to be monitored. If surveillance has not been ongoing, now is the time to initiate active surveillance. If active surveillance was initiated as part of case finding efforts, it should be continued. The reasons for conducting active surveillance at this time are twofold. First, you must continue to monitor the situation and determine whether the prevention and control measures are working. Is the number of new cases slowing down or, better yet, stopping? Or are new cases continuing to occur? If so, where are the new cases? Are they occurring throughout the area, indicating that the interventions are generally ineffective, or are they occurring only in pockets, indicating that the interventions may be effective but that some areas were missed?

Second, you need to know whether the outbreak has spread outside its original area or the area where the interventions were targeted. If so, effective disease control and prevention measures must be implemented in these new areas.

Step 13: Communicate findings

As noted in Step 1, development of a communications plan and communicating with those who need to know during the investigation is critical. The final task is to summarize the investigation, its findings, and its outcome in a report, and to communicate this report in an effective manner. This communication usually takes two forms:

- **An oral briefing for local authorities**. If the field investigator is responsible for the epidemiology but not disease control, then the oral briefing should be attended by the local health authorities and persons responsible for implementing control and prevention measures. Often these persons are not epidemiologists, so findings must be presented in clear and convincing fashion with appropriate and justifiable recommendations for action. This presentation is an opportunity for the investigators to

Epi-X is the CDC's Web-based communications solution for public health professionals. Through Epi-X, CDC officials, state and local health departments, poison control centers, and other public health professionals can access and share preliminary health surveillance information quickly and securely. Users can also be actively notified of breaking health events as they occur. Key features of Epi-X include:

- Scientific and editorial support
- Controlled user access
- Digital credentials and authentication
- Rapid outbreak reporting
- Peer-to-peer consultation.

describe what they did, what they found, and what they think should be done about it. They should present their findings in a scientifically objective fashion, and they should be able to defend their conclusions and recommendations.

- **A written report**. Investigators should also prepare a written report that follows the usual scientific format of introduction, background, methods, results, discussion, and recommendations. By formally presenting recommendations, the report provides a blueprint for action. It also serves as a record of performance and a document for potential legal issues. It serves as a reference if the health department encounters a similar situation in the future. Finally, a report that finds its way into the public health literature serves the broader purpose of contributing to the knowledge base of epidemiology and public health.

In recent years, the public has become more aware of and interested in public health. In response, health departments have made great strides in attempting to keep the public informed. Many health departments strive to communicate directly with the public, usually through the media, both during an investigation and when the investigation is concluded.

Summary

Outbreaks occur frequently. Not every outbreak comes to light, but of those that do, public health agencies must decide whether to handle them without leaving the office, or spend the time, energy, and resources to conduct field investigations. The most important reason to investigate is to learn enough about the situation to implement appropriate control and prevention measures. Other reasons include taking the opportunity to advance knowledge about the disease, agent, risk factors, interventions and other scientific issues; responding to public, political, or legal concerns; evaluating a health program's effectiveness and weaknesses; and to provide training.

Outbreaks are almost always unexpected events. Sometimes they are the subject of media attention and public concern, so investigators feel pressured to work quickly to find answers. When multiple agencies are involved, coordination and communication become even more essential but are more complicated than usual. Often the investigation takes place in the field, far from the conveniences and routines one counts on in the office. Under these circumstances, it is essential to have a systematic plan for conducting the investigation.

The steps listed in Table 6.2 comprise one such plan. Note that the order of the steps is conceptual, and investigators may decide that a different order is best suited for any given outbreak. To summarize, these are the steps of an outbreak investigation:

- Planning for field work, establishing the existence of an outbreak, and verifying the diagnosis are usually the first steps, sometimes done in that order, sometimes done in reverse order, sometimes done simultaneously. (Steps 1-3)
- After the diagnosis has been confirmed investigators create a workable case definition, then go out and look for additional cases. Information about these cases is organized either in a line listing or in a computer database that allows staffers to check for duplicate records, update records as additional information comes in, and perform descriptive epidemiology. (Steps 4-6)
- Descriptive epidemiology — organizing the data by time, place, and person — is essential for characterizing the outbreak, identifying populations at risk, developing hypotheses about risk factors, and targeting control/prevention strategies. An epidemic curve — a histogram of number of cases by time of onset of illness — provides a handy visual display of the outbreak's magnitude and time trend. (Step 6)
- Hypotheses, based on what is known about the disease, descriptive epidemiology, and what others have postulated, must be developed before conducting any kind of epidemiologic study (what are you going to study if you don't know what you are looking for?). (Step 7)
- While not every outbreak requires an analytic study, those that do are usually addressed by either a cohort study or a case-control study. Both types of study attempt to identify associations between exposures (risk factors or causes) and the disease of interest. In a cohort study, best suited for an outbreak in a well-defined population such as guests at a wedding, investigators usually attempt to enroll everyone, determine exposures and outcomes, calculate attack rates, and compare attack rates with a risk ratio or relative risk to identify associations. In a case-control study, which is well suited for outbreaks without a well-defined population, investigators usually enroll all of the case-patients plus a

sample of persons who did not get ill, then ask about exposures and compute an odds ratio to look for associations. (Step 8)

- If needed, hypotheses can be refined and re-evaluated. In many investigations, while the epidemiologists are conducting their epidemiologic investigations, environmental health specialists and laboratorians are conducting studies and tests of their own. Ideally, this multidisciplinary approach points to a single conclusion. (Steps 9 and 10)

- While implementing control and prevention measures is listed as Step 11, it is the primary goal of most outbreak investigations and usually occurs early in the investigation. Such measures can be implemented as soon as any link in the chain of disease transmission that is susceptible to intervention can be identified. If the source and mode of transmission is known, disease control measures need not wait. However, there is no guarantee that these measures will work, so continued surveillance is essential. (Steps 11 and 12)

- Finally, communicating what was found and what should be or was done in a written report provides key public health, scientific, and legal documentation. (Step 13)

Exercise Answers

Exercise 6.1

Nine cases of cancer in a community represents a cluster — a group of cases in a given area over a particular period of time that seems to be unusual, although we do not actually know the size of the community, the background rate of cancer, and the number of cases that might be expected. Nonetheless, either the health department or the community or both is concerned enough to raise the issue. Under these circumstances, an investigation may be justified for several reasons.

1. Because the number of expected cases is not known (or at least not stated), one reason to investigate is to determine how many cases to expect in the community. In a large community, nine cases of a common cancer (for example, lung, breast, or colon cancer) would not be unusual. If the particular cancer is a rare type, nine cases even in a large community may be unusual. And in a very small community, nine cases of even a common cancer may be unusual.

2. If the number of cancer cases turns out to be high for that community, public health officials might choose to investigate further. They may have a research agenda — perhaps they can identify a new risk factor (workers exposed to a particular chemical) or predisposition (persons with a particular genetic trait) for the cancer.

3. Control and prevention may be the justification for additional investigation. If modifiable risk factors are known or identified, control and prevention measures can be developed. Alternatively, if the cancer is one that can treated successfully if found early, and a screening test is available, then investigation might focus on why these persons died from a treatable disease. If, for example, the nine cases were cancers of the cervix (detectable by Pap smear and generally nonfatal if identified and treated early), a study might identify: a) lack of access to healthcare; b) physicians not following the recommendations to screen women at appropriate intervals; and/or c) laboratory error in reading or reporting the test results. Measures to correct these problems, such as public screening clinics, physician education, and laboratory quality assurance, could then be developed.

4. If new staff need to gain experience in conducting cluster investigations, training might be a justification for investigating these cases. More commonly, cancer clusters generate public concern, which, in turn, often results in political pressure. Perhaps one of the affected persons is a member of the mayor's family. A health department needs to be responsive to such concerns, and should investigate enough to address the concerns with facts. Finally, legal concerns may prompt an investigation, especially if a particular site (manufacturing plant, houses built on an old dump site, etc.) is accused of causing the cancers.

Exercise 6.2

First, you should check the dates of onset rather than dates of report. The 12 reports could represent 12 recent cases, but could represent 12 cases scattered in time that were sent in as a batch.

However, assuming that all 12 reports of tuberculosis and the 12 of West Nile virus infection represent recent cases in a single county, both situations could be called clusters (several new cases seen in a particular area during a relatively brief period of time). Classifying the cases as an outbreak depends on whether the 12 cases exceed the usual number of cases reported in August in that county.

Tuberculosis does not have a striking seasonal distribution. The number of cases during August could be compared with: a) the numbers reported during the preceding several months; and b) the numbers reported during August of the preceding few years.

West Nile virus infection is a highly seasonal disease that peaks during August-September-October. As a result, the number of cases in August is expected to be higher than the numbers reported during the preceding several months. To determine whether the number of cases reported in August is greater than expected, the number must be compared with the numbers reported during August of the preceding few years.

Exercise 6.3

Initial Case Definition	**Revised Case Definition**
Patient 1: No, eosinophil count < 2,000 cells/mm3	Patient 1: No, eosinophil count < 1,000 cells/mm3 and myalgias not severe
Patient 2: Yes	Patient 2: Yes
Patient 3: Yes	Patient 3: Yes
Patient 4: Yes	Patient 4: No, myalgias not severe
Patient 5: Yes	Patient 5: Yes
Patient 6: No, eosinophil count < 2,000 cells/mm3	Patient 6: Yes
Patient 7: No, other known cancer of eosinophilia	Patient 7: No, other known cancer of eosinophilia

This illustrates that a case definition is a method for deciding whether to classify someone as having the disease of interest or not, not whether they actually do or do not have the disease. Patients 1 and 4 may have mild cases, and Patient 7 may have leukemia and eosinophilia-myalgia syndrome, but are classified as non-cases under the revised definition.

Exercise 6.4

A case definition is a set of standard criteria for determining whether an individual should be categorized as having a particular disease or health-related condition. For an outbreak, a case definition consists of clinical criteria and specification of time, place, and person. A case definition can have degrees of certainty, e.g., suspect case (usually based on clinical and sometimes epidemiologic criteria) versus confirmed case (based on laboratory confirmation).

The outbreak appeared to be limited to students (no adults reported illness), but included both tour groups. Some students had severe abdominal pain and diarrhea and stool cultures positive for *E. coli* O157. Clearly these should be counted as case-patients. Some students had the same symptoms but negative cultures. Should they be counted as case-patients? Still others had the same symptoms but no stool testing. Should they be counted as case-patients? Finally, two students had single bouts of diarrhea, but no abdominal pain and negative cultures.

No one case definition is the absolutely correct case definition. One investigator could decide to include those with symptoms but without testing as suspect or probable cases, while another investigator could exclude them. Similarly, one investigator might put a great deal of faith in the stool culture and exclude those who tested negative, regardless of the presence of compatible symptoms, while another investigator might allow that some stool cultures could be "false negatives" (test negative even though the person actually has the infection) and include them in a suspect or probable or possible category. The two students with single bouts of diarrhea but no abdominal pain and negative cultures seem least likely to have true cases of *E. coli* infection.

Similarly, the beginning time limit could be set on December 2, the date that Tour A departed, or could be set later, to account for the minimum incubation period.

So, one case definition might be:

PERSON:	Any tenth-grade student who went on either tour
PLACE:	Limited to students at city high schools
TIME:	Onset since December 2? 3? 4?
CLINICAL:	Confirmed stool sample positive for *E. coli* O157:H7, regardless of symptoms
SUSPECT:	Self-reported severe abdominal pain and diarrhea >2 episodes/day, with stool culture not done; or self-reported abdominal pain and diarrhea >2 episodes/day and stool culture negative

Exercise 6.5

ID #	Age	Sex	Race	Disease	Date of Onset	Lab Results	Signs, Symptoms	Physician
1	46	M	W	Lyme disease	8/1/2004	WB IgM+	EM,Fat,S,C	Snow
2	56	F	W	Lyme disease	8/2/2006	WB IgM+, WB IgG+	EM,A,Fat,S,Fev	Farr
3	40	F	W	Lyme disease	8/17/2006	WB IgM+, WB IgG+	EM	Howard
4	53	M	B	Lyme disease	9/18/2006	WB IgM+, WB IgG-	EM	Fine
5	45	M	W	Lyme disease	mid-May 2006	WB IgG+	A,Arthral, HA,Fat,S,C	Howard
6	13	M	B	Lyme disease	2005		A,Arthral,Fat	Steere

A = arthritis	C = chills	Fat = fatigue	HA = headache
Arthral = arthralgias	*EM = erythema migrans*	Fev = fever	S = sweats

Exercise 6.6

1.

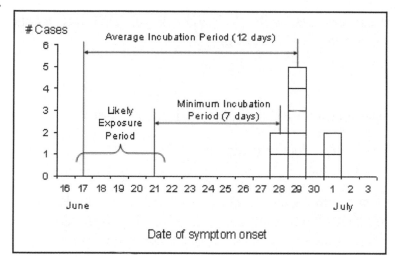

2. The date of onset of the earliest case was June 28. Subtracting the minimum incubation period (7 days) from June 28 points to June 21. The median and modal date of onset was June 29. Subtracting the average (say, 12 days) from June 29 points to June 17. So the most likely exposure period was sometime around June 17 through June 21, give or take a day or two on either side. Indeed, the investigators determined that exposure most likely occurred on June 19, when all ill persons either actively participated in or were nearby the sifting of dirt that probably harbored the organism.

Exercise 6.7

Cell phones are quite popular. Noting that most if not all of the 17 patients had used cell phones does not indicate that cell phones are the cause of brain cancer. An epidemiologic study that compares the exposure experience of the case-patients with the exposure experience of persons without brain cancer is necessary. A case-control study is the design of choice, since 17 persons with the disease of interest have already been identified.

As many as possible of the 17 persons with brain cancer should be enrolled in the case-control study as the case group. A group of persons without brain cancer need to be identified and enrolled as the control group. Whom would you enroll as controls? Remember that controls are supposed to represent the general exposure experience in the population from which the case-patients came. Controls could come from the same community (randomly selected telephone numbers, neighbors, friends) or the same healthcare providers (e.g., patients treated by the same neurologist but who do not have brain cancer). Once case-patients and controls are identified and enrolled, each would be questioned about exposure to cell phones. Finally, the exposure experience of case-patients and controls would be compared to determine whether case-patients were more likely to use cell phones, or use particular types of phones, or used them more frequently, or for longer cumulative time, etc.

The alternative to a case-control study is a cohort study. For a cohort study you would have to enroll a group of cell phone users ("exposed group") and a group of persons who do not use cell phones ("unexposed group"). You would then have to determine how many in each group develop brain cancer. Since brain cancer is a relatively rare event, you would need rather large groups in order to have enough brain cancer cases for the study to be useful. Therefore, a cohort study is less practical than a case-control study in this setting.

Exercise 6.8

1. The appropriate measure of association for a case-control study is the odds ratio.

2. The odds ratio is calculated as the cross-product ratio: ad / bc.
    Odds ratio = 15 x 23 / 8 x 7 = 6.16 = 6.2

3. With a chi-square of 9.41 and a 95% confidence interval of 1.6–25.1, this study shows a very strong (odds ratio = 6.2) association between histoplasmosis and working in Building X. This finding is quite statistically significant (chi-square = 9.41 corresponds to a p-value between 0.01 and 0.001). And although the 95% confidence interval indicates that the study is compatible with a seemingly relatively wide range of values (1.6–25.1), most of these values indicate a strong if not stronger association than the one observed.

Exercise 6.9

The first step in answering this question is to compare the attack rates (% ill) among those who ate the meal and those who did not eat the meal. Since the % ill is a measure of risk of illness, you could calculate a risk ratio for each meal.

	Risk Ratio		
9/18	Breakfast	90% vs. 46%	= 2.0
9/18	Lunch	62% vs. 15%	= 4.1
9/18	Dinner	52% vs. 43%	= 1.2
9/18	Late dinner	54% vs. 44%	= 1.2
9/19	Breakfast	49% vs. 52%	= 0.9
9/19	Lunch	51% vs. 47%	= 1.1

Clearly, the September 18 lunch has the highest risk ratio. It has a relatively high attack rate (though not the highest) among those who ate the meal, and the lowest attack rate among those who did not eat the meal. Furthermore, almost all of the cases (50 out of 54) could be "accounted for" by that lunch.

In contrast, although the September 18 breakfast has a high attack rate among those who ate that meal, it has a relatively high attack rate among those who did not eat that breakfast, and most importantly, it can only account for one-sixth (9 out of 54) of the cases. Perhaps the September 18 breakfast was a minor contributor, but most of the illness probably resulted from exposure that occurred at the September 18 lunch.

SELF-ASSESSMENT QUIZ

Now that you have read Lesson 1 and have completed the exercises, you should be ready to take the self-assessment quiz. This quiz is designed to help you assess how well you have learned the content of this lesson. You may refer to the lesson text whenever you are unsure of the answer.

Unless instructed otherwise, choose ALL correct answers for each question.

1. Which are the most common ways that a local health department uncovers outbreaks?
    A. Performing descriptive analysis of surveillance data each week
    B. Performing time series analysis to detect deviations from expected values based on the previous few weeks and comparable periods during the previous few years
    C. Receiving calls from affected residents
    D. Receiving calls from healthcare providers
    E. Reviewing all case reports received each week to detect common features

2. Factors that influence a health department's decision whether or not to conduct a field investigation in response to one or more cases of disease include:
    A. The nature of the disease
    B. The number of cases
    C. Resources available
    D. Health department's traditional attitude toward conducting field investigations

3. If a particular outbreak presents an unusual opportunity to learn more about the disease and its epidemiology by conducting a study, but early disease control measures would interfere with the study, one should conduct the study quickly, then implement control measures immediately afterwards.
    A. True
    B. False

4. Use the following choices for Questions 14a–c.
    A. Disease control and prevention efforts take priority over investigation efforts
    B. Investigation efforts take priority over disease control and prevention efforts

    4a. _____ Outbreak with known causative agent, source, and mode of transmission

    4b. _____ Outbreak with known causative agent, but unknown source and mode of transmission

    4c. _____ Outbreak with unknown causative agent, source, and mode of transmission

Use the following steps of an outbreak investigation for Question 5:
1. Analyze data by time, place, and person
2. Conduct a case-control study
3. Generate hypotheses
4. Conduct active surveillance for additional cases
5. Verify the diagnosis
6. Confirm that the number of cases exceeds the expected number
7. Talk with laboratorians about specimen collection

5. For an investigation of an outbreak, what is the logical conceptual order of the steps listed above?
   A. 1-2-3-4-5-6-7
   B. 5-6-4-1-2-3-7
   C. 6-5-3-1-2-7-4
   D. 6-5-7-4-1-3-2

6. To avoid skipping a critical step, investigators should conduct the steps of an outbreak investigation in the precise order you answered in Question 5.
   A. True
   B. False

7. Use the following choices for Questions 7a–c.
   A. Cluster
   B. Epidemic
   C. Outbreak

   7a. _____ 200 cases of Marburg virus infection in several districts in Angola over several months (usually none)

   7b. _____ 40 cases of *Salmonella* Enteritidis in 1 week traced to a single meal served at a cafeteria (usually none)

   7c. _____ 10 cases of cancer diagnosed over 2 years among residents of a single neighborhood (previous data not available)

8. Why should an investigator who has no clinical background nonetheless talk to a patient or two as an early step in the outbreak investigation?
   A. To advise the patient about common risk factors and the usual course of the illness, after reviewing such information in appropriate reference material
   B. To develop hypotheses about the cause of the outbreak
   C. To learn more about the clinical manifestations of the disease
   D. To verify the clinical findings as part of verifying the diagnosis
   E. To verify the laboratory findings as part of verifying the diagnosis

9. A case definition during an outbreak investigation should specify:
   A. Clinical features
   B. Time
   C. Place
   D. Person
   E. Hypothesized exposure

10. Ideally, a case definition is 100% accurate in identifying who does and does not have the disease in question, but in reality few case definitions achieve this ideal.
    A. True
    B. False

11. Once a case definition for an outbreak investigation has been established, it should not be changed.
    A. True
    B. False

12. Common methods of identifying additional cases (expanding surveillance) as part of an outbreak investigation include:
    A. Advising the public through newspapers, TV, radio, and the health department's website to contact the local health department
    B. Asking case-patients who they were with at the time of exposure (if known)
    C. Sending a fax to healthcare providers
    D. Telephoning the infection control practitioners at local hospitals

13. A case report form devised for an outbreak investigation usually includes which of the following types of information?
    A. Identifying information
    B. Demographic information
    C. Clinical information
    D. Risk factor information
    E. Reporter, interviewer, or data abstractor information

14. Descriptive epidemiology is essential for "characterizing the outbreak" by time, place, and person, but has little bearing on the analytic epidemiology.
    A. True
    B. False

Use the following epi curves as choices for Questions 15a–c.

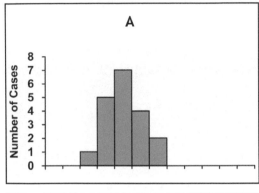

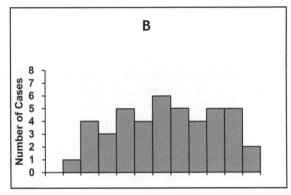

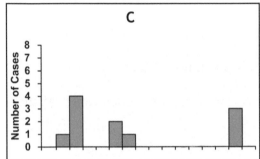

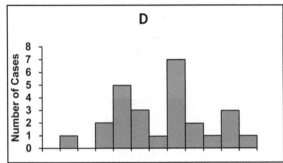

15. Match the epi curve with the outbreak description.

15a._____ A malfunctioning space heater was used each time the outside temperature dropped below freezing

15b._____ At the Eclipse Restaurant, sodium nitrite was mistaken for table salt in the preparation of breakfast one morning only

15c._____ Common cold passed from classmate to classmate

Use the following epidemic curve for Question 16.

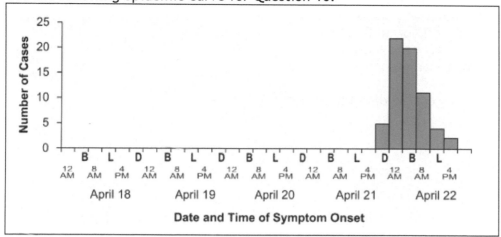

16. A group of tourists on a weeklong bus tour of a European country experienced an outbreak of norovirus. The group had followed a consistent meal time pattern: each morning they had breakfast together in whichever hotel they had stayed from 6:00 a.m. to 7:00 a.m., stopped for lunch from 1:00 p.m. to 2:00 p.m., then had dinner together either at the next hotel or at a restaurant at about 7:00 p.m. The incubation period for norovirus is about 24-48 hours, with a median of about 33 hours. On which day and at which meal was exposure most likely?

A. April 19 Dinner
B. April 20 Breakfast
C. April 20 Lunch
D. April 20 Dinner
E. April 21 Breakfast

17. Possible explanations for a case that occurs substantially later than the other cases in an outbreak include:
A. Similar but unrelated disease
B. Secondary case
C. Case with unusually long incubation period
D. Time of exposure later than others
E. Error in recording date

18. A spot map is particularly useful for displaying:
A. Geographic location of exposure of each case-patient
B. Residence of each case-patient
C. Incidence rate of disease by area
D. Prevalence rate of disease by area

19. Which of the following may be useful in generating hypotheses in an outbreak setting?
A. Review the literature
B. Look at the descriptive epidemiology
C. Look at the outliers
D. Talk with the local health authorities
E. Talk with a few of the case-patients
F. Talk with subject matter experts

20. The key feature of an analytic (epidemiologic) study is: (Select only one answer)
    A. Analysis by time, place, and person
    B. Calculation of a risk ratio or odds ratio
    C. Use of Epi Info to analyze the data
    D. Presence of a comparison group

21. Disease control measures can be directed at the:
    A. Agent
    B. Source
    C. Mode of transmission
    D. Portal of entry
    E. Host susceptibility

Use the information in the following paragraph and data in the table for Questions 22-25.

An outbreak of gastrointestinal disease occurred 24-36 hours after people had attended a wedding. Of the 203 attendees (including the bride and groom), 200 completed questionnaires, and 50 reported illness compatible with the case definition. Tabulated food consumption histories are presented in the table below.

Food Item	Ate Specified Food			Did Not Eat Specified Food		
	Ill	Well	Total	Ill	Well	Total
Punch	46 (25%)	138	184	4 (25%)	12	16
Wedding Cake	45 (45%)	55	100	5 (5%)	95	100
Sushi	10 (91%)	1	11	40 (21%)	149	189

22. This study is an example of a retrospective cohort study.
    A. True
    B. False

23. The most appropriate measure of association for these data is the:
    A. Attributable risk percent
    B. Chi-square
    C. Odds ratio
    D. Risk ratio

24. Which food is the most likely culprit?
    A. Punch
    B. Wedding cake
    C. Sushi
    D. Can't determine from the data presented.
    E. Must be more than one food.

25. Results of this outbreak investigation should be communicated to:
    A. The caterer
    B. Local officials
    C. Wedding party family and attendees
    D. World Health Organization

Answers to Self-Assessment Quiz

1. C, D. Most outbreaks come to the attention of health authorities because an alert clinician or a concerned case-patient (or parent of a case-patient) calls. The other methods listed occasionally detect outbreaks, but less frequently.

2. A, B, C, D. Factors influencing a health department's decision to conduct a field investigation include some related to the health problem itself (e.g., severity of illness, number of cases, availability of prevention / control measures), some relate to the health department (e.g., "corporate culture" for conducting field investigations versus handling it by telephone, available staff and resources), and some relate to external concerns (e.g., public or political pressure).

3. B (False). The most important public health reason for investigating an outbreak is disease control and prevention. Protecting and promoting the public's health is our primary mission, even if it interferes with our ability to conduct research.

4a. A. As in Answer 3, our primary mission is to protect the public's health, so disease control and prevention measures should take priority whenever possible. Because disease prevention and control measures are often aimed at interrupting transmission, such measures can be implemented if the source and mode of transmission are known.

4b. B. If the agent is known but the source and mode of transmission are not known (example: *Salmonella* eventually traced to marijuana), then the health department does not know how to target its intervention. Investigation to learn the source and/or mode is necessary.

4c. B. As in Answer 4b, If the agent, source, and mode of transmission are not known (examples: Legionnaires' Disease in Philadelphia in 1976; Kawasaki Syndrome — if it turns out to be an infectious disease), then the health department does not know how to target its intervention. Investigation to learn the source and/or mode is necessary.

5. D. Early steps include confirming that the number of cases exceeds the expected number, verifying the diagnosis, and preparing for field work (which includes talking with laboratorians about specimen collection). Next steps include conducting surveillance to identify additional cases; analyzing the data by time, place, and person; generating hypotheses; and evaluating those hypotheses (for example, by conducting a case-control study).

6. B (False). The order presented in this text is conceptual. In practice, the order can be different. For example, preparing for field work often follows establishing the existence of an outbreak and verifying the diagnosis. When possible, control measures are initiated at the same time the field investigation begins, or even earlier.

7a. B. **Epidemic**, the occurrence of more cases of disease than expected in a given area or among a specific group of people over a particular period of time, tends to refer to more widespread occurrence than **outbreak**.

7b. C. **Outbreak** tends to be used for an increase that is localized.

7c. A Cluster is an aggregation of cases in a given area over a particular period of time that **seems** unusual or suspicious, but often the usual or expected number of cases is not known.

8. B, C. Even an investigator without a clinical background should, if possible, see and talk to a patient or two to gain a better understanding of the clinical features of the disease (needed for developing a case definition) and to generate hypotheses by asking about possible exposures.

9. A, B, C, D. A case definition for an outbreak should specify clinical criteria as well as appropriate time, place, and person characteristics. The case definition should NOT include the hypothesized exposure of interest. First, the hypothesized exposure may not turn out to be the true exposure, so inclusion of the hypothesized exposure as part of the case definition during the case-finding step may result in missed cases. Second, during the analytic step, disease status and exposure must be determined independently to avoid bias. Including exposure as part of the case definition means that all cases will, by definition, be exposed, while only some of the controls will likely be exposed. As a result, the exposure will appear to be associated with disease, not necessarily because it is the true exposure, but because of the case definition.

10. A (True). A case definition is a decision making tool. It provides criteria for classifying illness as a "case" or "not a case." However, few case definitions are 100% accurate, because people with mild or atypical or asymptomatic disease are likely to be missed, and people with similar but not the same disease may be included. Even a case definition that requires a laboratory test is not 100% perfect, because laboratory tests themselves are not perfect.

11. B (False). On the one hand, case definitions need to be applied consistently, so that everyone involved in an investigation defines a case in the same way. On the other hand, case definitions can change during the course of an outbreak. For example, for case finding purposes, a case definition might include categories such as confirmed, probable, and possible, to try to include as many cases as possible. Later on, in the analytic phase, the case definition may be restricted to the confirmed cases. As another example, a case definition may initially be restricted to a particular community. If the outbreak spreads beyond that geographic area, the "place" component of the case definition also would need to be expanded.

12. A, B, C, D. To identify additional cases as part of an outbreak investigation, health department staff contact (by telephone, broadcast fax, or e-mail) physicians' offices, clinics, hospitals, and laboratories. Depending on the affected age group, staff might also contact day care centers, schools, employers, or nursing homes. Sometimes a press release is issued to local media outlets that inform the public and suggest that persons with particular symptoms or exposures contact their healthcare providers or health department. In addition, health department staff routinely interview case-patients and ask whether they know any persons with the same exposure, if known, or with the same illness.

13. A, B, C, D, E. A data collection form for an outbreak investigation should include patient identifying information (e.g., name, telephone number), demographic information (e.g., age, sex), clinical information (e.g., date of onset, laboratory confirmation, whether

hospitalized), risk factor information (disease-specific, e.g., attended sports banquet (yes/no), previously vaccinated?), and information about who collected the data (e.g., interviewer or abstracter initials, date of collection).

14. B (False). Descriptive epidemiology is essential not only for characterizing the pattern and distribution of the outbreak, but also for generating testable hypotheses about the source, mode of transmission, and risk factors for illness. Two of the suggested ways for generating hypotheses are to review the descriptive epidemiology, particularly (1) the overall pattern of cases and develop hypotheses about what they have in common, and (2) the outliers to determine how they might be linked to the other cases. These hypotheses, in turn, are the ones that are tested using analytic epidemiology.

15a. C. This scenario represents an intermittent exposure. The resulting epidemic curve has cases that appear to be occurring sporadically, but in fact occur when the malfunctioning heater is turned on at irregular intervals.

15b. A. This scenario represents a point source exposure. The epidemic curve has a single peak, and all cases occur during a single incubation period.

15c. D. This scenario represents person-to-person transmission. The epidemic curve has a succession of "waves" of cases.

16 D. Subtracting 24 hours (the minimum incubation period) from the time of onset of the first case puts you in the April 20 Dinner interval. Subtracting 33 hours from the median case (which occurred in the 4-8 AM interval) on April 22), puts you in the April 20 4-7 pm interval, near both lunch and dinner that day. While the minimum method points to dinner on April 20, thorough investigators would probably investigate possible exposures at lunch that day, too.

17. A, B, C, D, E. A late case on an epidemic curve has several possible explanations, including a case of a similar but unrelated disease, a secondary case (assuming it occurs one incubation period after another case), a case with an unusually long incubation period, a case that resulted from exposure at a different time (for example, someone who ate leftovers the next day), or an error in recall or in recording the date.

18. A, B. A spot map is useful for pinpointing the geographic location of exposures, residences, employment sites, and the like. The spots represent occurrences, either of exposure or disease. Spot maps are not used to display rates. Rather, area maps (also called shaded or chloropleth maps) are used to display incidence and prevalence rates.

19. A, B, C, D, E, F. Hypotheses can be generated in a variety of ways. One way is based on subject matter knowledge derived by reviewing the literature or talking with experts – what are the usual causes, sources, vehicles, or modes of transmission? Other ways include reviewing the overall pattern and the outliers from the descriptive epidemiology, by asking case-patients if they have any suspicions about the cause of their illness, and by asking the same question of local authorities (if you are from out of town).

20. D. The key feature that characterizes an analytic (epidemiologic) study is presence of a comparison group. Single case reports and case series do not have comparison groups and are not analytic studies. Cohort studies (compares disease experience among exposed and

unexposed groups) and case-control studies (compares exposure experience among persons with and without disease) have comparison groups and are analytic studies.

21. A, B, C, D, E. Disease control measures can be directed at the eliminating the agent (e.g., by sterilizing surgical equipment), interrupting transmission (e.g., reducing mosquito population, covering one's mouth when coughing), preventing entry into a host (e.g., wearing a mask, using insect repellant), or improving host defenses (e.g., by immunization).

22. A. A retrospective cohort study is one in which disease has already occurred (hence, retrospective) and the investigator enrolls all (or almost all) of a population (hence, cohort). The investigator then determines exposures and calculates risks (attack rates) for different exposures and risk ratios (relative risks) for those exposed and unexposed. The study described for Questions 22-25 meets this characterization.

23. D. The measure of association recommended for a retrospective cohort study is a risk ratio, calculated as the ratio of the risk of disease among those exposed divided by the risk of disease among those not exposed. The attributable risk percent is a supplemental measure that quantifies how much of the disease could be "explained" or accounted for by a particular exposure. The chi-square is not a measure of association, but a test of statistical significance (which is affected both by the strength of association and number of subjects in the study). The odds ratio is used primarily as a measure of association in case-control studies.

24. B. The wedding cake (risk ratio = 45% / 5% – 9.0) is the most likely culprit. It has a high attack rate among the exposed group, a low attack rate among the unexposed group, and can account for 45 out of the 50 cases. The five "unaccounted for" cases are within the range that can be "explained away," for example by misreporting (for example, a man takes a bite of his partner's cake but reports "no" for cake because he didn't take a whole piece himself), poor recall, etc. Punch is not associated with illness at all (risk ratio = 25% / 25% = 1.0). Sushi has an extremely high attack rate among those exposed (91%), but a relatively high attack rate among those unexposed (21%), and most importantly, could only account for 10 of the 50 cases.

25. A, B, C. The results should be communicated to all those who need or want to know, including the concerned family and wedding attendees, local governmental officials, the caterer, the church or facility where the wedding was held, et al. The outbreak is also reportable to the state health department, who in turn is likely to report it to CDC. However, local outbreaks do not need to be reported to the World Health Organization.

References

1. Olsen SJ, MacKinon LC, Goulding JS, Bean NH, Slutsker L. Surveillance for foodborne disease outbreaks–United States, 1993-1997. In: Surveillance Summaries, March 27, 2000. MMWR 2000; 49(No. SS-1):1–59.

2. Keene WE, Hedberg K, Herriott DE, Hancock DD, McKay R, Barrett T, Fleming D. A prolonged outbreak of *Escherichia coli* O157:H7 infections caused by commercially distributed raw milk. J Infect Dis 1997;176:815–8.

3. Marx M. Diarrheal illness detected through syndromic surveillance after a massive blackout, New York City. Presented at 2003 National Syndromic Surveillance Conference.

4. Swaminathan B, Barrett TJ, Hunter SB, Tauxe RV. PulseNet: the molecular subtyping network for foodborne bacterial disease surveillance, United States. Emerg Infect Dis 2001; 7:382–9.

5. Preston R. West Nile mystery. The New Yorker, October 18–25,1999;90–107.

6. Bush LM, Abrams BH, Beall A, Johnson CC. Index case of fatal inhalational anthrax due to bioterrorism in the United States, N Engl J Med 2001;345:1607–10.

7. Bender AP, Williams AN, Johnson RA, Jagger HG. Appropriate public health responses to clusters: the art of being responsibly responsive. Am J Epidemiol 1990;132:S48–S52.

8. Fiore BJ, Hanrahan LP, Anderson HA. State health department response to disease cluster reports: a protocol for investigation. Am J Epidemiol 1990;132:S14–22.

9. Washington State Department of Health. Guidelines for investigating clusters of chronic disease and adverse birth outcomes [monograph on the Internet]. Olympia, Washington; 2001 [cited 2006 Sep 19]. Available from: http://www.doh.wa.gov/EHSPHL/Epidemiology/NICE/publications/ClusterProt.pdf.

10. Goodman RA, Buehler JW, Koplan JP. The epidemiologic field investigation: science and judgment in public health practice. Am J Epidemiol 1990;132:9–16.

11. Galil K, Lee B, Strine T, Carraher C, Baughman AL, Eaton M, et al. Outbreak of varicella at a day-care center despite vaccination. New Engl J Med 2002;347:1909–15.

12. Tugwell BD, Lee LE, Gillette H, Lorber EM, Hedberg K, Cieslak PR. Chickenpox outbreak in a highly vaccinated school population. Pediatrics. 2004;113:455–9.

13. Hopkins RS, Juranek DD. Acute giardiasis: an improved clinical case definition for epidemiologic studies. Am J Epidemiol 1991;133:402–7.

14. Fischer TK, Gentsch J, Ashley D, et al. Evaluation and utility of a novel diagnostic method in the investigation of an unusual outbreak of rotavirus diarrhea among children–Jamaica, 2003. Presented at: 53rd Annual EIS Conference, CDC, Atlanta, Georgia, April 19-23, 2004.

15. Raupach JC, Hundy RL. An outbreak of *Campylobacter jejuni* infection among conference delegates. Commun Dis Intell 2003;27:380–3.

16. Kuusi M, Nuorti JP, Maunula L, Miettinen I, Pesonen H, von Bonsdorff C-H. Internet use and epidemiologic investigation of gastroenteritis outbreak. Emerg Infect Dis 2004;10:447–50.

17. Pryor JH, Martin MT, Whitney CG, Turco JH, Baumgartner YY, Zegans ME. Rapid response to a conjunctivitis outbreak: the use of technology to leverage information. J Am Coll Health 2002;50:267–71.

18. Caldwell GG. Twenty-two years of cancer cluster investigations at the Centers for Disease Control. Am J Epidemiol 1990;132:S43–S47.

19. Schulte PA, Ehrenberg RL, Singal M. Investigation of occupational cancer clusters: theory and practice. Am J Public Health 1987;77:52–6.

20. Cartwright RA. Cluster investigations: are they worth it? Med J Aust 1999;171:p. 172.

21. Centers for Disease Control and Prevention. NIOSH health hazard evaluation program. Cincinnati, Ohio: Department of Health and Human Services (NIOSH) Publication No. 2000-132: p. 3

22. Palmer SR. Epidemiology in search of infectious diseases: methods in outbreak investigation. J Epidemiol Comm Health 1989;43:311-4.

23. Last JM. A dictionary of epidemiology, 4th ed. New York: Oxford U Press, 2001:129.

24. PAHO. Case definitions: meningococcal disease and viral meningitis. Epidemiol Bull 2001;22(4):14–6.

25. Centers for Disease Control and Prevention. Eosinophilia — myalgia syndrome — New Mexico. MMWR 1989;38:765–7.

26. Centers for Disease Control and Prevention. Eosinophilia-myalgia syndrome and L-tryptophan-containing products — New Mexico, Minnesota, Oregon, and New York, 1989. MMWR 1989;38:785–8.

27. Centers for Disease Control and Prevention. Public health dispatch: outbreak of listeriosis — northeastern United States, 2002. MMWR 2002;51:950–1.

28. Jernigan DB, Raghunathan PL, Bell BP, Brechner R, Bresnitz EA, Butler JC, et al. Investigation of bioterrorism-related anthrax, United States, 2001: epidemiologic findings. Emerg Infect Dis 2002;8:1019–28.

29. Heyman DL, ed. Control of communicable diseases manual, 18th ed. Washington, DC: American Public Health Association, 2004.

30. Peterson LR, Marshall SL, Barton-Dickson C, Hajjeh RA, Lindsley MD, Warnock DW, et al. Coccidioidomycosis among workers at an archaeologic site, northeast Utah. Emerg Infect Dis 2004;10:637–42.

31. Snow J. Snow on cholera. London: Humphrey Milford: Oxford U Press, 1936.

32. Tan C. A preventable outbreak of pneumococcal pneumonia among unvaccinated nursing home residents–New Jersey, 2001. Presented at Northeast Regional Epidemic Intelligence Service Conference, March 14, 2002, New York City.

33. Lukacs SL, Hsu V, Harper S, Handzel T, Hayslett J, Khabbaz R, et al. Anthrax outbreak averted: public health response to a contaminated envelope on Capital Hill–Washington, DC, 2001. Presented at 51st Annual Epidemic Intelligence Service Conference, April 22-26, 2004, Atlanta.

34. Ramsey AH, Belongia EA, Gale CM, Davis JP. Outcomes of treated human granulocytic ehrlichiosis cases. Emerg Infect Dis 2002;8:383–401.

35. Mahoney FJ, Hoge CW, Farley TA, Barbaree JM, Breiman RF, Benson RF, McFarland LM. Communitywide outbreak of Legionnaires' disease associated with a grocery store mist machine. J Infect Dis 1992;165: 736–9.

36. Torok TJ, Tauxe RV, Wise RP, Livengood JR, Sokolow R, Mauvais S, et al. A large community outbreak of salmonellosis caused by intentional contamination of restaurant salad bars. JAMA 1997;278:389–95.

37. Hedberg CW, Fishbein DB, Janssen RS, Meyers B, McMillen JM, MacDonald KL, et al. An outbreak of thyrotoxicosis caused by the consumption of bovine thyroid gland in ground beef. N Engl J Med 1987;316:993–8.

38. Jacobus CH, Holick MF, Shao Q, Chen TC, Holm IA, Kolodny JM, et al. Hypervitaminosis D associated with drinking milk. New Engl J Med 1992;326:1173–7.

39. Blank S, Scanlon KS, Sinks TH, Lett S, Falk H. An outbreak of hypervitaminosis D associated with the overfortication of milk from a home-delivery dairy. Am J Public Health 1995;85:656–9.

40. Jani AA, Barrett E, Murphy J, Norton D, Novak C, Painter J, Toney D. A steamship full of trouble: an outbreak of Salmonella Typhimurium DT 104 gastroenteritis at a holiday banquet — Virginia, 2003. Presented at the 53rd Annual Epidemic Intelligence Service Conference; 2004 Apr 19-23; Atlanta.

41. Centers for Disease Control and Prevention. Outbreak of histoplasmosis among industrial plant workers — Nebraska, 2004. MMWR 2004;53:1020–2.

42. Becker KM, Moe CL, Southwick KL, MacCormack JN. Transmission of Norwalk virus during a football game. N Engl J Med 2000;343;1223–7.

43. Taylor DN, Wachsmuth IK, Shangkuan YH, Schmidt EV, Barrett TJ, Schrader JS, et al. Salmonellosis associated with marijuana: a multistate outbreak traced by plasmid fingerprinting. New Engl J Med 1982;306:1249–53.

44. MacDonald KL, Spengler RF, Hatheway CL, Hargrett NT, Cohen ML. Type A botulism from sauteed onions. JAMA 1985;253:1275–8.

45. Nash D, Mostashari F, Fine A, Miller J, O'Leary D, Murray K, et al. The outbreak of West Nile virus infection in the New York City area in 1999. N Engl J Med 2001;344:1807–14.

46. Roehrig JT, Nash D, Maldin B, Labowitz A, Martin DA, Lanciotti RS, et al. Persistence of virus-reactive serum immunoglobulin M antibody in confirmed West Nile virus encephalitis cases. Emerg Infect Dis 2003;9:376–9.

47. Klee AL, Maldin B, Edwin B, IPoshni I, Mostashari F, Fine A, et al. Long-term prognosis for clinical West Nile Virus infection. Emerg Infect Dis 2004;10:1405–11.

48. Fraser DW, Tsai TF, Orenstein W, Parkin WE, Beecham HJ, Sharrar RG, et al. Legionnaires' disease: description of an epidemic of pneumonia. N Engl J Med 1977;297:1189–97.

49. Bopp DJ, Saunders BD, Waring AL, Waring AL, Ackelsberg J, Dumas N, et al. Detection, isolation, and molecular subtyping of *Escherichia coli* O157:H7 and *Campylobacter jejuni* associated with a large waterborne outbreak. J Clin Microbiol 2003;41:174–80.

50. Division of Tuberculosis Elimination [Internet]. Atlanta: CDC; [updated 1999 Oct; cited 2006 Sep 19]. Self study modules on Tuberculosis, Module 7: Confidentiality in Tuberculosis Control: Background. Available from: http://www.cdc.gov/nchstp/tb/pubs/ssmodules/module7/ss7background.htm.

Websites

For more information on:	Visit the following websites:
Average and minimum incubation periods	http://www.cdc.gov/az.do

GLOSSARY

A

active immunity see immunity, active.

active surveillance see surveillance, active.

age-adjusted mortality rate see mortality rate, age-adjusted.

agent a factor (e.g., a microorganism or chemical substance) or form of energy whose presence, excessive presence, or in the case of deficiency diseases, relative absence is essential for the occurrence of a disease or other adverse health outcome.

age-specific mortality rate see mortality rate, age-specific.

alternative hypothesis see hypothesis, alternative.

analytic epidemiology see epidemiology, analytic.

analytic study see study, analytic.

antibody any of a variety of proteins in the blood that are produced in response to an antigen as an immune response.

antigen any substance (e.g., a toxin or the surface of a microorganism or transplanted organ) recognized as foreign by the human body and that stimulates the production of antibodies.

applied epidemiology see epidemiology, applied.

arbovirus any of a group of viruses that are transmitted between hosts by mosquitoes, ticks, and other arthropods.

arithmetic mean see mean, arithmetic.

arithmetic-scale line graph see line graph, arithmetic-scale.

arthropod an organism that has jointed appendages and segmented external skeleton (e.g., flies, mosquitoes, ticks, or mites).

association the statistical relation between two or more events, characteristics, or other variables.

asymmetrical a type of distribution where the shape to the right and left of the central location is not the same. Often referred to as a skewed distribution; the mean, median, and mode of an asymmetrical distribution are not the same.

asymptomatic without symptoms.

attack rate a form of incidence that measures the proportion of persons in a population who experience an acute health event during a limited period (e.g., during an outbreak), calculated as the number of new cases of a health problem during an outbreak divided by the size of the population at the beginning of the period, usually expressed as a percentage or per 1,000 or 100,000 population (see also **incidence proportion**).

attack rate, secondary a measure of the frequency of new cases of a disease among the contacts of known patients.

attributable proportion see **proportion, attributable**.

attributable risk percent see **proportion, attributable**.

attribute a risk factor that is an intrinsic characteristic of the individual person, animal, plant, or other type of organism under study (e.g., genetic susceptibility, age, sex, breed, weight).

axis one of the dimensions of a graph in a rectangular graph, the x-axis is the horizontal axis, and the y-axis is the vertical axis.

B

bar chart a visual display in which each category of a variable is represented by a bar or column bar charts are used to illustrate variations in size among categories.

bar chart, 100% component a stacked bar chart in which all bars or columns are the same length, and the measured axis represents 0%–100%.

bar chart, deviation a bar chart displaying either positive or negative differences from a baseline.

bar chart, grouped a bar chart displaying quantities of two variables, represented by adjoining bars or columns (i.e., a group) of categories of one variable, separated by space between groups.

bar chart, stacked a bar chart displaying quantities of two variables, represented by subdivided bars or columns (the subdivisions representing the categories of one variable) separated by space between bars or columns.

bias a systematic deviation of results or inferences from the truth or processes leading to such systematic deviation; any systematic tendency in the collection, analysis, interpretation, publication, or review of data that can lead to conclusions that are systematically different from the truth. In epidemiology, does not imply intentional deviation.

bias, information systematic difference in the collection of data regarding the participants in a study (e.g., about exposures in a case-control study, or about health outcomes in a cohort study) that leads to an incorrect result (e.g., risk ratio or odds ratio) or inference.

bias, selection systematic difference in the enrollment of participants in a study that leads to an incorrect result (e.g., risk ratio or odds ratio) or inference.

bimodal having two data peaks.

biologic transmission see **transmission, biologic**.

birth cohort see **cohort, birth**.

birth rate, crude the number of live births during a specified period divided by the mid-period population, usually expressed per 1,000 population.

box plot a visual display that summarizes data by using a "box and whiskers" format to indicate the minimum and maximum values (ends of the whiskers), interquartile range (length of the box), and median (line through the box).

C

carrier a person or animal that harbors the infectious agent for a disease and can transmit it to others, but does not demonstrate signs of the disease. A carrier can be asymptomatic (never indicate signs of the disease) or can display signs of the disease only during the incubation period, convalescence, or postconvalescence. The period of being a carrier can be short (a transient carrier) or long (a chronic carrier).

case an instance of a particular disease, injury, or other health conditions that meets selected criteria (see also **case definition**). Using the term to describe the person rather than the health condition is discouraged (see also **case-patient**).

case-control study see **study, case-control**.

case definition a set of uniformly applied criteria for determining whether a person should be identified as having a particular disease, injury, or other health condition. In epidemiology, particularly for an outbreak investigation, a case definition specifies clinical criteria and details of time, place, and person.

case-fatality rate (also called **case-fatality ratio**) the proportion of persons with a particular condition (e.g., patients) who die from that condition. The denominator is the number of persons with the condition; the numerator is the number of cause-specific deaths among those persons.

case, index the first case or instance of a patient coming to the attention of health authorities.

case-patient in a case-control study, a person who has the disease, injury, or other health condition that meets the case definition (see also **case**).

case, source the case or instance of a patient responsible for transmitting infection to others; the instance of a patient who gives rise to an outbreak or epidemic.

cause, component a factor that contributes to a sufficient cause (see also **cause, sufficient**).

cause of disease a factor (e.g., characteristic, behavior, or event) that directly influences the occurrence of a disease. Reducing such a factor among a population should reduce occurrence of the disease.

cause, necessary a factor that must be present for a disease or other health problem to occur.

cause-specific mortality rate see **mortality rate, cause-specific**.

cause, sufficient a factor or collection of factors whose presence is always followed by the occurrence of a particular health problem.

census the enumeration of an entire population, usually including details on residence, age, sex, occupation, racial/ethnic group, marital status, birth history, and relationship to the head of household.

central location (also called **central tendency**) a statistical measurement to quantify the middle or the center of a distribution. Of the multiple ways to define central tendency, the most common are the mean, median, and mode.

chain of infection the progression of an infectious agent that leaves its reservoir or host through a portal of exit, is conveyed by a mode of transmission, and then enters through an appropriate portal of entry to infect a susceptible host.

"chartjunk" unnecessary or confusing visual elements in charts, illustrations, or graphs. The term was first used by Edward Tufte in his book, *The Visual Display of Quantitative Information* (1983).

class interval the span of values of a continuous variable that are grouped into a single category (see also **class**), usually to create a frequency distribution for that variable.

class limits the values at the upper and lower ends of a class interval.

clinical criteria the medical features (e.g., symptoms, medical examination findings, and laboratory results) that are used in a case definition.

clinical disease a disease that has been manifested by its symptoms and features.

clinical trial see **trial, clinical**.

cluster an aggregation of cases of a disease, injury, or other health condition (particularly cancer and birth defects) in a circumscribed area during a particular period without regard to whether the number of cases is more than expected (often the expected number is not known).

cohort a well-defined group of persons who have had a common experience or exposure and are then followed up, as in a cohort study or prospective study, to determine the incidence of new diseases or health events.

cohort, birth a group of persons born during a particular period or year.

cohort study see **study, cohort**.

common-source outbreak see **outbreak, common-source**.

community immunity see **immunity, herd**.

community trial see **trial, community**.

comparison group a group in an analytic study (e.g., a cohort or case-control study) with whom the primary group of interest (exposed group in a cohort study or case-patients in a case-control study) is compared. The comparison group provides an estimate of the background or expected incidence of disease (in a cohort study) or exposure (in a case-control study).

confidence interval a range of values for a measure (e.g., rate or odds ratio) constructed so that the range has a specified probability (often, but not necessarily, 95%) of including the true value of the measure.

confidence limits the end points (i.e., the minimum and maximum values) of a confidence.

confounding the distortion of the association between an exposure and a health outcome by a third variable that is related to both.

contact exposure to a source of an infection; a person who has been exposed.

contact, direct exposure or transmission of an agent from a source to a susceptible host through touching (e.g., from a human host by kissing, sexual intercourse, or skin-to-skin contact) or from touching an infected animal or contaminated soil or vegetation.

contagious capable of being transmitted from one person to another by contact or close proximity.

contingency table a two-variable table of cross-tabulated data.

continuous variable see **variable, continuous**.

control in a case-control study, a member of the group of persons without the health problem under study (see also **comparison group** and **study, case-control**).

crude when referring to a rate, an overall or summary rate for a population, without adjustment.

crude birth rate see **birth rate, crude**.

crude death rate see **mortality rate, crude**.

crude mortality rate see **mortality rate, crude**.

cumulative frequency in a frequency distribution, the number or proportion of observations with a particular value and any smaller value.

cumulative frequency curve a plot of the cumulative frequency rather than the actual frequency for each class interval of a variable. This type of graph is useful for identifying medians and quartiles and other percentiles.

D

death-to-case ratio the number of deaths attributed to a particular disease, injury, or other health condition during a specified period, divided by the number of new cases of that disease, injury, or condition identified during the same period.

decision analysis application of quantitative methods to decision-making.

decision tree a branching chart that represents the logical sequence or pathway of a clinical or public health decision.

demographic information personal characteristics of a person or group (e.g., age, sex, race/ethnicity, residence, and occupation) demographic information is used in descriptive epidemiology to characterize patients or populations.

dendrogram see **phylogenetic tree**.

denominator the lower portion of a fraction; used in calculating a ratio, proportion, or rate. For a rate, the denominator is usually the midinterval population.

dependent variable see **variable, dependent**.

descriptive epidemiology see **epidemiology, descriptive**.

determinant any factor that brings about change in a health condition or in other defined characteristics (see also **cause** and **risk factor**).

direct transmission see **transmission, direct**.

discrete variable (or **data**) see **variable** (or **data**), **discrete**.

distribution in epidemiology, the frequency and pattern of health-related characteristics and events in a population. In statistics, the frequency and pattern of the values or categories of a variable.

dose-response association between an exposure and health outcome that varies in a consistently increasing or decreasing fashion as the amount of exposure (dose) increases.

dot plot a visual display of the specific data points of a variable.

droplet nuclei the residue of dried droplets of infectious agents that is easily inhaled and exhaled and can remain suspended in air for relatively long periods or be blown over great distances.

droplet spread the direct transmission of an infectious agent by means of the aerosols produced in sneezing, coughing, or talking that travel only a short distance before falling to the ground.

E

effect the result of a cause.

effectiveness the ability of an intervention or program to produce the intended or expected results in the field.

efficacy the ability of an intervention or program to produce the intended or expected results under ideal conditions.

efficiency the ability of an intervention or program to produce the intended or expected results with a minimum expenditure of time and resources.

EIS Epidemic Intelligence Service; CDC's 2-year training program in applied epidemiology for public health professionals (http://www.cdc.gov/eis).

endemic the constant presence of an agent or health condition within a given geographic area or population; can also refer to the usual prevalence of an agent or condition.

environmental factor an extrinsic factor (e.g., geology, climate, insects, sanitation, or health services) that affects an agent and the opportunity for exposure.

epidemic the occurrence of more cases of disease, injury, or other health condition than expected in a given area or among a specific group of persons during a particular period. Usually, the cases are presumed to have a common cause or to be related to one another in some way (see also **outbreak**).

epidemic curve a histogram that displays the course of an outbreak or epidemic by plotting the number of cases according to time of onset.

epidemic period the time span of an outbreak or epidemic.

epidemiologic triad the traditional model of infectious disease causation having three components: an external agent, a susceptible host, and an environment that brings the host and agent together so that disease occurs.

epidemiology the study of the distribution and determinants of health conditions or events among populations and the application of that study to control health problems.

epidemiology, analytic the aspect of epidemiology concerned with why and how a health problem occurs. Analytic epidemiology uses comparison groups to provide baseline or expected values so that associations between exposures and outcomes can be quantified and hypotheses about the cause of the problem can be tested (see also **study, analytic**).

epidemiology, applied the application or practice of epidemiology to control and prevent health problems.

epidemiology, descriptive the aspect of epidemiology concerned with organizing and summarizing data regarding the persons affected (e.g., the characteristics of those who became ill), time (e.g., when they become ill), and place (e.g., where they might have been exposed to the cause of illness).

epidemiology, field applied epidemiology (i.e., the application or practice of epidemiology to control and prevent health problems), particularly when the epidemiologist(s) must travel to and work in the community in which the health problem is occurring or has occurred.

evaluation systematic and objective examination of activities to determine their relevance, effectiveness, and impact.

excess risk risk difference, calculated as the risk among the exposed group minus the risk among the unexposed group.

experimental study see **study, experimental**.

exposed group a group whose members have had contact with a suspected cause of, or possess a characteristic that is a suspected determinant of, a particular health problem.

exposure having come into contact with a cause of, or possessing a characteristic that is a determinant of, a particular health problem.

F

false-negative a negative test result for a person who actually has the condition similarly, a person who has the disease (perhaps mild or variant) but who does not fit the case definition, or a patient or outbreak not detected by a surveillance system.

false-positive a positive test result for a person who actually does not have the condition. Similarly, a person who does not have the disease but who nonetheless fits the case definition, or a patient or outbreak erroneously identified by a surveillance system.

field epidemiology see **epidemiology, field**.

follow-up study see **study, cohort**.

fomite an inanimate object that can be the vehicle for transmission of an infectious agent (e.g., bedding, towels, or surgical instruments).

forest plot a graph that displays the point estimates and confidence intervals of individual studies included in a meta-analysis or systematic review as a series of parallel lines.

frequency the amount or number of occurrences of an attribute or health outcome among a population.

frequency distribution a complete summary of the frequencies of the values or categories of a variable, often displayed in a two-column table with the individual values or categories in the left column and the number of observations in each category in the right column.

frequency polygon a graph of a frequency distribution in which values of the variable are plotted on the horizontal axis, and the number of observations are plotted on the vertical axis. Data points are plotted at the midpoints of the intervals and are connected with straight lines.

G

geometric mean see **mean, geometric**.

graph a visual display of quantitative data arranged on a system of coordinates.

H

health a state of complete physical, mental, and social well-being and not merely the absence of disease or other infirmity.

health indicator any of a variety of measures (e.g., mortality rate) that indicate the state of health of a given population.

health information system a combination of health statistics from different sources. Data from these systems are used to learn about health status, health care, provision and use of services, and the impact of services and programs on health.

healthy worker effect the observation that employed persons generally have lower mortality rates than the general population, because persons with severe, disabling disease (who have higher mortality rates) tend to be excluded from the workforce.

herd immunity see **immunity, herd**.

high-risk group a group of persons whose risk for a particular disease, injury, or other health condition is greater than that of the rest of their community or population.

HIPAA the Health Insurance Portability and Accountability Act, enacted in 1996, which addresses the privacy of a person's medical information as well as postemployment insurance and other health-related concerns.

histogram a visual representation of the frequency distribution of a continuous variable. The class intervals of the variable are grouped on a linear scale on the horizontal axis, and the class frequencies are grouped on the vertical axis. Columns are drawn so that their bases equal the class intervals (i.e., so that columns of adjacent intervals touch), and their heights correspond to the class frequencies.

host a person or other living organism that is susceptible to or harbors an infectious agent under natural conditions.

host factor an intrinsic factor (e.g., age, race/ethnicity, sex, or behaviors) that influences a person's exposure, susceptibility, or response to an agent.

hyperendemic the constant presence at high incidence and prevalence of an agent or health condition within a given geographic area or population.

hypothesis a supposition, arrived at from observation or reflection, that leads to refutable predictions; any conjecture cast in a form that will allow it to be tested and refuted.

hypothesis, alternative the supposition that an exposure is associated with the health condition under study. The alternative is adopted if the null hypothesis (see also **hypothesis, null**) proves implausible.

hypothesis, null the supposition that two (or more) groups do not differ in the measure of interest (e.g., incidence or proportion exposed); the supposition that an exposure is not associated with the health condition under study, so that the risk ratio or odds ratio equals 1. The null hypothesis is used in conjunction with statistical testing.

I

immunity, active resistance developed in response to an antigen (i.e., an infecting agent or vaccine), usually characterized by the presence of antibody produced by the host.

immunity, herd the resistance to an infectious agent of an entire group or community (and, in particular, protection of susceptible persons) as a result of a substantial proportion of the population being immune to the agent. Herd immunity is based on having a substantial number of immune persons, thereby reducing the likelihood that an infected person will come in contact with a susceptible one among human populations, also called **community immunity**.

immunity, passive immunity conferred by an antibody produced in another host This type of immunity can be acquired naturally by an infant from its mother or artificially by administration of an antibody-containing preparation (e.g., antiserum or immune globulin).

incidence a measure of the frequency with which new cases of illness, injury, or other health condition occurs among a population during a specified period.

incidence proportion the fraction of persons with new cases of illness, injury, or other health condition during a specified period, calculated as the number of new cases divided by the size of the population at the start of the study period (see also **attack rate**).

incidence rate a measure of the frequency with which new cases of illness, injury, or other health condition occur, expressed explicitly per a time frame. Incidence rate is calculated as the number of new cases over a specified period divided either by the average population (usually mid-period) or by the cumulative person-time the population was at risk.

incubation period the time interval from exposure to an infectious agent to the onset of symptoms of an infectious disease.

independent variable see **variable, independent**.

index case see **case, index**.

indirect transmission see **transmission, indirect**.

individual data values or observations from each record (also called raw data).

infant mortality rate see **mortality rate, infant**.

infection invasion of the body tissues of a host by an infectious agent, whether or not it causes disease.

infectivity the ability of an infectious agent to cause infection, measured as the proportion of persons exposed to an infectious agent who become infected.

information bias see bias, information.

interquartile range a measure of spread representing the middle 50% of the observations, calculated as the difference between the third quartile (75th percentile) and the first quartile (25th percentile).

isolation the separation of infected persons to prevent transmission to susceptible ones. Isolation refers to separation of ill persons; **quarantine** refers to separation of potentially exposed but well persons.

L

latency period the time from exposure to a causal agent to onset of symptoms of a (usually noninfectious) disease (see also **incubation period**).

life expectancy a statistical projection of the average number of years a person of a given age is expected to live, if current mortality rates continue to apply.

line graph, arithmetic-scale a graph that displays patterns or trends by plotting the frequency (e.g., number, proportion, or rate) of a characteristic or event during some variable, usually time. The y-axis, measuring frequency, uses an arithmetic scale.

line graph, semilogarithmic-scale a graph that displays patterns or trends by plotting the frequency (e.g., number, proportion, or rate) of a characteristic or event during some variable, usually time. The y-axis, measuring frequency, uses a logarithmic scale.

line listing a type of epidemiologic database, organized similar to a spreadsheet with rows and columns in which information from cases or patients are listed each column represents a variable, and each row represents an individual case or patient.

logarithmic transformation conversion of nominal or ordinal data to logarithmic data. The purpose is to examine rate of change instead of amount of change only.

M

map, area (shaded, choropleth) a visual display of the geographic pattern of a health problem, in which a marker is placed on a map to indicate where each affected person lives, works, or might have been exposed.

mean (or average) commonly called the average; it is the most common measure of central tendency.

mean, arithmetic the measure of central location, commonly called the average, calculated by adding all the values in a group of measurements and dividing by the number of values in the group.

mean, geometric the mean, or average, of a set of data measured on a logarithmic scale.

measure of association a quantified relationship between exposure and a particular health problem (e.g., risk ratio, rate ratio, and odds ratio).

measure of central location a central value that best represents a distribution of data. Common measures of central location are the mean, median, and mode also called the measure of central tendency.

measure of dispersion see **measure of spread**.

measure of spread a measure of the distribution of observations out from its central value. Measures of spread used in epidemiology include the interquartile range, variance, and the standard deviation.

measurement scale the complete range of possible values for a measurement.

mechanical transmission see **transmission, mechanical**.

median the measure of central location that divides a set of data into two equal parts, above and below which lie an equal number of values (see also **measure of central location**).

medical surveillance see **surveillance, medical**.

midrange the halfway point, or midpoint, in a set of observations. For the majority of data, the midrange is calculated by adding the smallest observation and the largest observation and dividing by two. The midrange is usually calculated as an intermediate step in determining other measures.

mode the most frequently occurring value in a set of observations (see also **measure of central location**).

mode of transmission the manner in which an agent is transmitted from its reservoir to a susceptible host (see also **transmission**).

morbidity disease; any departure, subjective or objective, from a state of physiological or psychological health and well-being.

mortality death.

mortality rate a measure of the frequency of occurrence of death among a defined population during a specified time interval.

mortality rate, age-adjusted a mortality rate that has been statistically modified to eliminate the effect of different age distributions among different populations.

mortality rate, age-specific a mortality rate limited to a particular age group, calculated as the number of deaths among the age group divided by the number of persons in that age group, usually expressed per 100,000.

mortality rate, cause-specific the mortality rate from a specified cause, calculated as the number of deaths attributed to a specific cause during a specified time interval among a population divided by the size of the midinterval population.

mortality rate, crude a mortality rate from all causes of death for an entire population, without adjustment.

mortality rate, infant the mortality rate for children aged <1 year, calculated as the number of deaths reported among this age group during a given period divided by the number of live births reported during the same period, and expressed per 1,000 live births. Infant mortality rate is a universally accepted indicator of the health of a nation's population and the adequacy of its health-care system.

mortality rate, neonatal the mortality rate for children from age birth up to, but not including, 28 days. In calculating neonatal mortality rates, the numerator is the number of deaths among this age group during a given period, and the denominator is the number of live births reported during the same period. The neonatal mortality rate is usually expressed per 1,000 live births.

mortality rate, postneonatal the mortality rate for children from age 28 days up to, but not including, 1 year. In calculating postneonatal mortality rates, the numerator is the number of deaths among this age group during a given period, and the denominator is the number of live births during the same period.. The postneonatal mortality rate is usually expressed per 1,000 live births.

mortality rate, race/ethnic-specific a mortality rate limited to a specified racial or ethnic group both numerator and denominator are limited to that group.

mortality rate, sex-specific a mortality rate among either males or females.

N

natural history of disease the progression of a disease process in a person from the time it begins to the time it resolves, in the absence of treatment.

NCHS The National Center for Health Statistics, the US governmental organization responsible for national vital statistics and multiple national health surveys. Organizationally, NCHS is a component of the Centers for Disease Control and Prevention, one of the agencies of the US Department of Health and Human Services.

NHANES The National Health and Nutrition Examination Survey, a representative survey of the civilian, noninstitutionalized US population conducted by the National Center for Health Statistics, designed to (1) estimate the proportion of the US population and designated groups with selected disease and risk factors; (2) monitor trends in selected behaviors, exposures, and diseases; and (3) study the associations among diet, nutrition, and health.

necessary cause see **cause, necessary**.

neonatal mortality rate see **mortality rate, neonatal**.

nominal scale see **scale, nominal**.

normal curve the bell-shaped curve that results when a normal distribution is graphed.

normal distribution a distribution represented as a bell shape, symmetrical on both sides of the peak, which is simultaneously the mean, median, and mode, and with both tails extending to infinity.

notifiable disease a disease that, by law, must be reported to public health authorities upon diagnosis.

null hypothesis see **hypothesis, null**.

numerator the upper portion of a fraction (see also **denominator**).

O

observational study see **study, observational**.

odds ratio a measure of association used in comparative studies, particularly case-control studies, that quantifies the association between an exposure and a health outcome; also called the cross-product ratio.

ordinal scale see **scale, ordinal**.

outbreak the occurrence of more cases of disease, injury, or other health condition than expected in a given area or among a specific group of persons during a specific period. Usually, the cases are presumed to have a common cause or to be related to one another in some way. Sometimes distinguished from an epidemic as more localized, or the term less likely to evoke public panic (see also **epidemic**).

outbreak, common-source an outbreak that results from persons being exposed to the same harmful influence (e.g., an infectious agent or toxin). The exposure period can be brief or can extend over days, weeks, or longer, with the exposure being either intermittent or continuous.

outbreak, point-source a common source outbreak in which the exposure period is relatively brief so that all cases occur within one incubation period.

outbreak, propagated an outbreak that spreads from person to person rather than from a common source.

outcome(s) any or all of the possible results that can stem from exposure to a causal factor or from preventive or therapeutic interventions; all identified changes in health status that result from the handling of a health problem.

outlier a value substantively or statistically different from all (or approximately all) of the other values in a distribution.

P

***P* value** the probability of observing an association between two variables or a difference between two or more groups as large or larger than that observed, if the null hypothesis were true. Used in statistical testing to evaluate the plausibility of the null hypothesis (i.e., whether the observed association or difference plausibly might have occurred by chance).

pandemic an epidemic occurring over a widespread area (multiple countries or continents) and usually affecting a substantial proportion of the population.

passive immunity see **immunity, passive**.

passive surveillance see **surveillance, passive**.

pathogenicity the ability of an agent to cause disease after infection, measured as the proportion of persons infected by an agent who then experience clinical disease.

percentile a set of cut points used to divide a distribution or a set of ranked data into 100 parts of equal area with each interval between the points containing 1/100 or 1% of the observations. For example, the 5th percentile is a cut point with 5% of the observations below it and the remaining 95% above it.

period prevalence see **prevalence, period**.

person-time rate the incidence rate calculated as the number of new cases among a population divided by the cumulative person-time of that population, usually expressed as the number of events per persons per unit of time.

person-time the amount of time each participant in a cohort study is observed and disease-free, often summed to provide the denominator for a person-time rate.

phylogenetic tree a branching chart that indicates the evolutionary lineage or genetic relatedness of organisms.

pie chart a circular graph of a frequency distribution in which each segment of the pie is proportional in size to the frequency of corresponding category.

point prevalence see **prevalence, point**.

point-source outbreak see **outbreak, point-source**.

population the total number of inhabitants of a geographic area or the total number of persons in a particular group (e.g., the number of persons engaged in a certain occupation).

population pyramid a graphical display of the age-sex distribution of a population, constructed with a horizontal histogram of the age distribution of males pointing to the left, and the corresponding horizontal histogram of age distribution of females pointing to the right.

portal of entry a pathway into the host that gives an agent access to tissue that will allow it to multiply or act.

portal of exit a pathway by which an agent can leave its host.

postneonatal mortality rate see **mortality rate, postneonatal**.

predictive value positive the proportion of cases identified by a test, reported by a surveillance system, or classified by a case definition that are true cases, calculated as the number of true-positives divided by the number of true-positives plus false-positives.

prevalence the number or proportion of cases or events or attributes among a given population.

prevalence rate the proportion of a population that has a particular disease, injury, other health condition, or attribute at a specified point in time (point prevalence) or during a specified period (period prevalence).

prevalence, period the amount of a particular disease, chronic condition, or type of injury present among a population at any time during a particular period.

prevalence, point the amount of a particular disease, chronic condition, or type of injury present among a population at a single point in time.

privacy rule a set of regulations based on the Health Insurance Portability and Accountability Act to protect the privacy of individually identifiable health information.

propagated outbreak see **outbreak, propagated**.

proportion a ratio in which the numerator is included in the denominator; the ratio of a part to the whole, expressed as a "decimal fraction" (e.g., 0 2), a fraction (1/5), or a percentage (20%).

proportion, attributable a measure of the impact of a causative factor on the public health; the proportion of a health state or event among exposed persons that can be attributed to the exposure also called attributable risk percent.

proportionate mortality the proportion of deaths among a population attributable to a particular cause during a selected period. Each cause of death is expressed as a percentage of all deaths, and the sum of the proportionate mortality for all causes must equal 100%. These proportions are not mortality rates because, in proportionate mortality, the denominator is all deaths instead of the population among whom the deaths occurred.

prospective study see **study, prospective**.

Q

quarantine the separation of well persons who have been exposed or are suspected to have been exposed to a communicable disease, to monitor for illness and to prevent potential transmission of infection to susceptible persons during the incubation period. Quarantine refers to separation of potentially exposed but well persons; **isolation** refers to separation of ill persons.

R

race/ethnic-specific mortality rate see **mortality rate, race/ethnic-specific**.

random sample see **sample, random**.

range in statistics, the difference between the largest and smallest values in a distribution; in common use, the span of values from smallest to largest.

rate an expression of the relative frequency with which an event occurs among a defined population per unit of time, calculated as the number of new cases or deaths during a specified period divided by either person-time or the average (midinterval) population. In epidemiology, it is often used more casually to refer to proportions that are not truly rates (e.g., attack rate or case-fatality rate).

rate ratio a measure of association that quantifies the relation between an exposure and a health outcome from an epidemiologic study, calculated as the ratio of incidence rates or mortality rates of two groups.

ratio the relative size of two quantities, calculated by dividing one quantity by the other.

record in a line listing, each row is a record or observation. A record represents data related to a single case.

relative risk a general term for measures of association calculated from the data in a two-by-two table, including risk ratio, rate ratio, and odds ratio (see also **risk ratio**).

representative sample see **sample, representative**.

reservoir the habitat in which an infectious agent normally lives, grows, and multiplies, which can include humans, animals, or the environment.

retrospective study see **study, retrospective**.

risk the probability that an event will occur (e.g., that a person will be affected by, or die from, an illness, injury, or other health condition within a specified time or age span).

risk factor an aspect of personal behavior or lifestyle, an environmental exposure, or a hereditary characteristic that is associated with an increase in the occurrence of a particular disease, injury, or other health condition.

risk ratio a measure of association that quantifies the association between an exposure and a health outcome from an epidemiologic study, calculated as the ratio of incidence proportions of two groups.

S

sample a selected subset of a population a sample can be random or nonrandom and representative or nonrepresentative.

sample, random a sample of persons chosen in such a way that each one has the same (and known) probability of being selected.

sample, representative a sample whose characteristics correspond to those of the original or reference population.

scale, interval a measurement scale consisting of quantitative categories whose values are measured on a scale of equally spaced units, but without a true zero point (e.g., date of birth).

scale, nominal a measurement scale consisting of qualitative categories whose values have no inherent statistical order or rank (e.g., categories of race/ethnicity, religion, or country of birth).

scale, ordinal a measurement scale consisting of qualitative categories whose values have a distinct order but no numerical distance between their possible values (e.g., stage of cancer, I, II, III, or IV).

scale, ratio a measurement scale consisting of quantitative categories whose values are intervals with a true zero point (e.g., height in centimeters or duration of illness).

scatter diagram (or **scattergram**) a graphical display of the association between two variables in which a dot is plotted on the graph for each set of paired values for two continuous variables, with one variable plotted on the horizontal axis, and the other plotted on the vertical axis.

seasonality change in physiologic status or in the occurrence of a disease, chronic condition, or type of injury that conforms to a regular seasonal pattern.

secondary attack rate see **attack rate, secondary**.

secular trend see **trend, secular**.

selection bias see **bias, selection**.

semilogarithmic-scale line graph see **line graph, semilogarithmic-scale**

sensitivity the ability of a test, case definition, or surveillance system to identify true cases; the proportion of people with a health condition (or the proportion of outbreaks) that are identified by a screening test or case definition (or surveillance system).

sentinel surveillance see **surveillance, sentinel**.

sex-specific mortality rate see **mortality rate, sex-specific**.

skewed a distribution that is not symmetrical.

source (of infection) the person, animal, object, or substance from which an infectious agent is transmitted to a host.

source case see **case, source**.

specificity the ability or a test, case definition, or surveillance system to exclude persons without the health condition of interest; the proportion of persons without a health condition that are correctly identified as such by a screening test, case definition, or surveillance system.

spectrum of illness the range of manifestations a disease process can take (e.g., from asymptomatic to mild clinical illness to severe illness and death).

sporadic an event that occurs infrequently and irregularly.

spot map a visual display of the geographic pattern of a health problem, in which a marker is placed on a map to indicate where each affected person lives, works, or might have been exposed.

standard deviation a statistical summary of how dispersed the values of a variable are around its mean, calculated as the square root of the variance.

standard error (of the mean) the standard deviation of a theoretical distribution of sample means of a variable around the true population mean of that variable. Standard error is computed as the standard deviation of the variable divided by the square root of the sample size.

statistical inference generalizations developed from sample data, usually with calculated degrees of uncertainty.

statistical significance the measure of how likely it is that a set of study results could have occurred by chance alone. Statistical significance is based on an estimate of the probability of the observed or a greater degree of association between independent and dependent variables occurring under the null hypothesis (see also *P* **value**).

study, analytic a study, usually observational, in which groups are compared to identify and quantify associations, test hypotheses, and identify causes. Two common types are cohort studies and case-control studies.

study, case-control an observational analytic study that enrolls one group of persons with a certain disease, chronic condition, or type of injury (case-patients) and a group of persons without the health problem (control subjects) and compares differences in exposures, behaviors, and other characteristics to identify and quantify associations, test hypotheses, and identify causes.

study, cohort an observational analytic study in which enrollment is based on status of exposure to a certain factor or membership in a certain group. Populations are followed, and disease, death, or other health-related outcomes are documented and compared. Cohort studies can be either prospective or retrospective.

study, cross-sectional a study in which a sample of persons from a population are enrolled and their exposures and health outcomes are measured simultaneously; a survey.

study, experimental a study in which the investigator specifies the type of exposure for each person (clinical trial) or community (community trial) then follows the persons' or communities' health status to determine the effects of the exposure.

study, observational a study in which the investigator observes rather than influences exposure and disease among participants. Case-control and cohort studies are observational studies (see also **study, experimental**).

study, prospective an analytic study in which participants are enrolled before the health outcome of interest has occurred.

study, retrospective an analytic study in which participants are enrolled after the health outcome of interest has occurred. Case-control studies are inherently retrospective.

subclinical without apparent symptoms.

surveillance, active public health surveillance in which the health agency solicits reports.

surveillance, medical monitoring of a person who might have been exposed to an infectious, chemical, radiologic, or other potentially causal agent, for the purpose of detecting early symptoms.

surveillance, passive public health surveillance in which data are sent to the health agency without prompting.

surveillance, sentinel a surveillance system that uses a prearranged sample of sources (e.g., physicians, hospitals, or clinics) who have agreed to report all cases of one or more notifiable diseases.

surveillance, syndromic (1) the monitoring of the frequency of illnesses with a specified set of clinical features among a given population without regard to the specific diagnoses, if any, that are assigned to them by clinicians. (2) A system for early detection of outbreaks whereby health department staff, assisted by automated acquisition of data routinely collected for other purposes and computer generation of statistical signals, monitor disease indicators, particularly those associated with possible terrorism-related biologic and chemical agents, continually or at least daily to detect outbreaks earlier than would otherwise be possible with traditional public health methods.

survey a systematic canvassing of persons to collect information, often from a representative sample of the population.

survival curve a line graph that begins with 100% of the study population and displays the percentage of the population still surviving at successive points in time. A survival curve can also be used to depict freedom from a health problem, complication, or another endpoint.

symmetrical a type of distribution where the shapes to the right and left of the central location are the same. Normal, bell-shaped distributions are symmetrical; the mean, median, and mode are the same.

symptom any indication of disease noticed or felt by a patient.

syndrome a combination of symptoms characteristic of a disease or health condition; sometimes refers to a health condition without a clear cause (e.g., chronic fatigue syndrome).

syndromic surveillance see **surveillance, syndromic**.

T

table an arrangement of data in rows and columns. In epidemiology, the data are usually summaries of the frequency of occurrence of an event or characteristic occurring among different groups.

table shell a table that is completely drawn and labeled but contains no data.

table, two-by-two a two-variable table with cross-tabulated data, in which each variable has only two categories. Usually, one variable represents a health outcome, and one represents an exposure or personal characteristic.

transmission (of infection) any mode or mechanism by which an infectious agent is spread to a susceptible host.

transmission, airborne transfer of an agent suspended in the air, considered a type of indirect transmission.

transmission, biologic indirect transmission by a vector in which the infectious agent undergoes biologic changes inside the vector as part of its life cycle before it is transmitted to the host (see also **transmission, mechanical**).

transmission, direct immediate transfer of an agent from a reservoir to a host by direct contact or droplet spread.

transmission, indirect transfer of an agent from a reservoir to a host either by being suspended in air particles (airborne), carried by an inanimate objects (vehicleborne), or carried by an animate intermediary (vectorborne).

transmission, mechanical indirect transmission by a vector in which the infectious agent does not undergo physiologic changes inside the vector (see also **transmission, biologic**).

transmission, vectorborne transmission of an agent by a living intermediary (e.g., tick, mosquito, or flea); considered a type of indirect transmission.

transmission, vehicleborne transmission of an agent by an inanimate object; considered a type of indirect transmission; includes foodborne and waterborne transmission.

trend movement or change in frequency over time, usually upwards or downwards.

trend, secular changes occurring over a substantial period, generally years or decades.

trial, clinical an experimental study that uses data from individual persons. The investigator specifies the type of exposure for each study participant and then follows each person's health status to determine the effects of the exposure.

trial, community an experimental study that uses data from communities. The investigator specifies the type of exposure for each community and then follows the communities' health status to determine the effects of the exposure.

trial, randomized clinical a clinical trial in which persons are randomly assigned to exposure or treatment groups.

two-by-two table see **table, two-by-two.**

V

validity the degree to which a measurement, questionnaire, test, or study or any other data-collection tool measures what it is intended to measure.

variable any characteristic or attribute that can be measured and can have different values.

variable (or **data**), **discrete** a variable that is limited to a finite number of values; data for such a variable.

variable, continuous a variable that has the potential for having an infinite number of values along a continuum (e.g., height and weight).

variable, dependent in a statistical analysis, a variable whose values are a function of one or more other variables.

variable, independent an exposure, risk factor, or other characteristic being observed or measured that is hypothesized to influence an event or manifestation (the dependent variable).

variance a measure of the spread in a set of observations, calculated as the sum of the squares of deviations from the mean, divided by the number of observations minus 1 (see also **standard deviation**).

vector a living intermediary that carries an agent from a reservoir to a susceptible host (see also **transmission, biologic** and **transmission, mechanical**) (e.g., mosquitoes, fleas, or ticks).

vehicle an inanimate object that can carry an agent from a reservoir to a susceptible host (e.g., food, water, blood products, and bedding) (see also **transmission, indirect**).

virulence the ability of an infectious agent to cause severe disease, measured as the proportion of persons with the disease who become severely ill or die.

vital statistics systematically tabulated data about recorded births, marriages, divorces, and deaths.

X

x-axis the horizontal axis of a rectangular graph, usually displaying the independent variable (e.g., time).

Y

y-axis the vertical axis of a rectangular graph, usually displaying the dependent variable (e.g., frequency — number, proportion, or rate).

years of potential life lost (YPLL) a measure of the impact of premature death on a population, calculated as the sum of the differences between a predetermined minimally acceptable age (e.g., 65 years or current life expectancy) and the age at death for everyone who died earlier than that age.

Z

zoonosis an infectious disease that is transmissible from animals to humans.